To: Dr Ross : a good
friend + colleague

From: Winita.

9/20/91

CONTEMPORARY ISSUES IN CHRONIC PAIN MANAGEMENT

CURRENT MANAGEMENT OF PAIN

P. PRITHVI RAJ, SERIES EDITOR

The series, *Current Management of Pain*, is intended by the series editor and the publishers to provide up-to-date information on advances in the clinical management of acute and chronic pain and related research as quickly as possible. Both the series editor and the publishers felt that, although comprehensive texts are now available, they do not always cover the rapid advances in this field. Another format was needed to publish advances in basic sciences and clinical modalities, and to bring them rapidly to the practitioners in the community. A questionnaire was sent to selected clinicians and, based on their responses, topics were chosen by the series editor. Editors of each volume were chosen for their expertise in the field and their ability to encourage other active pain specialists to contribute their knowledge.

Ghia J.N. ed. The Multidisciplinary Pain Center: Organization and Personnel Functions for Pain Management, 1988. ISBN 0-89838-359-5.

Lynch N.T., Vasudevan S.V., eds. Persistent Pain: Psychosocial Assessment and Intervention, 1988. ISBN 0-89838-363-3.

Abram S.E. ed. Cancer Pain, 1988. ISBN 0-89838-389-7.

Racz G.B. ed. Techniques of Neurolysis, 1989. ISBN 0-89838-397-8.

Stanton-Hicks M. ed. Pain and the Sympathetic Nervous System, 1989. ISBN 0-7923-0304-0.

Rawal N., Coombs D.W. eds. Spinal Narcotics, 1989. ISBN 0-7923-0374-1.

Stanton-Hicks M., Janig W. eds. Reflex Sympathetic Dystrophy, 1989. ISBN 0-7923-0527-2.

Janisse T. ed. Pain Management of AIDS Patients, 1991. ISBN 0-7923-1056-X.

Parris W. ed. Contemporary Issues in Chronic Pain Management, 1991. ISBN 0-7923-1182-5.

CONTEMPORARY ISSUES IN CHRONIC PAIN MANAGEMENT

Edited by
WINSTON C.V. PARRIS
Vanderbilt University
Nashville, TN 37232

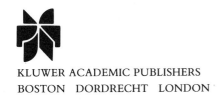

KLUWER ACADEMIC PUBLISHERS
BOSTON DORDRECHT LONDON

Distributors for North America:
Kluwer Academic Publishers
101 Philip Drive
Assinippi Park
Norwell, Massachusetts 02061 USA

Distributors for all other countries:
Kluwer Academic Publishers Group
Distribution Centre
Post Office Box 322
3300 AH Dordrecht, THE NETHERLANDS

Library of Congress Cataloging-in-Publication Data

Contemporary issues in chronic pain management/edited by Winston
  C.V. Parris.
      p.   cm.—(Current management of pain; 9)
    Includes bibliographical references.
    Includes index.
    ISBN 0-7923-1182-5
    1. Intractable pain.   I. Parris, Winston C.V.   II. Series.
    [DNLM: 1. Chronic Disease.   2. Pain—therapy. W1 CU788LW v. 9/
WL 704 C761]
  RB127.C67 1991
  616'.0472—dc20
  DNLM/DLC
  for Library of Congress   91-4653
                                                                  CIP

CONTENTS

CONTRIBUTING AUTHORS

Bennett Blumenkopf, M.D.
Assistant Professor of Neurosurgery
Department of Neurosurgery
Vanderbilt University Medical Center
Nashville, Tennessee 37232

Steven F. Brena, M.D.
Clinical Professor of Rehabilitation Medicine
Emory University School of Medicine
Atlanta, Georgia 30322

Thomas G. Burish, Ph.D.
Associate Provost for Academic Affairs
Professor of Psychology
Vanderbilt University
Nashville, Tennessee 37232

Stanley L. Chapman, Ph.D.
Clinical Associate Professor of Rehabilitation Medicine
Emory University
Atlanta, Georgia

Joachim Chrubasik, M.D.
Professor of Anesthesiology
Department of Anesthesiology
University Hospital of Zurich
Zurich, Switzerland

Hans Christian Colov, M.D.
Medical Director, Pain Clinic
Skodsborg Sanatorium
Skodsborg, Denmark

Martha W. Davis, Ph.D.
Fred Hutchinson Cancer Research Center
University of Washington Medical Center
Seattle, Washington 98195

Ris Dirksen, M.D.
Consultant Anesthesiologist
Institute for Anesthesiology
Raboud University Hospital
Nijmegen, Holland

Neal Goldberger, M.D.
Chief of Anesthesiology
Blanchfield Army Community Hospital
Fort Campbell, Kentucky 42223

Joseph Harrison, J.D., Ph.D.
P.O.Box 6397
Delray Beach, Florida
33484-6397

William B. Hobbins, M.D.
5510 Medical Circle
Madison, Wisconsin

Joel Katz, Ph.D.
Department of Psychology
McGill University
Montreal, Quebec
Canada

Howard S. Kirshner, M.D.
Professor & Vice-Chairman of Neurology
Department of Neurology
Vanderbilt University Medical Center
Nashville, Tennessee 37232

Jonathan Lipman, Ph.D.
Research Assistant Professor
Departments of Medicine and Surgery
Vanderbilt University School of Medicine
Nashville, Tennessee 37232

David Longmire, M.D.
Neurologist/Algologist
The Pain Institute of Northwest Alabama
Russellville, Alabama 35653

Professor Marco Maresca
Servizio di Algologia
Clinical Medical
1 Viale Morgagni
50139 Florence, Italy

Ronald Melzack, Ph.D.
Professor of Psychology
Department of Psychology
McGill University
Stewart Biological Sciences Bldg.
Montreal, PQ, Canada

Winston C.V. Parris, M.D.
Professor of Anesthesiology
Director, Pain Control Center
Department of Anesthesiology
Vanderbilt University Medical Center
Nashville, Tennessee 37232

Professor Paolo Procacci
Pain Center
University of Florence
Florence, Italy

B.V. Rama Sastry, Ph.D.
Professor of Pharmacology
Department of Pharmacology
Vanderbilt University Medical Center
Nashville, Tennessee 37232-6600

David P. Schwartz, Ph.D.
Clinical Psychologist
Cincinnati, Ohio

Janos Szolcsanyi, M.D.
Professor of Pharmacology
University Medical School of PECS
Pecs, Hungary

Leanne Wilson, Ph.D.
Fred Hutchinson Cancer Research Center
University of Washington Medical Center
Seattle, Washington

FOREWORD

PROFESSOR SIR KENNETH L. STUART

Pain control has become one of medicine's most rapidly growing disciplines, and I welcome the opportunity to write this foreword to a book that I am sure will make its own unique contribution to advancing this discipline.

My pleasure in writing it is heightened by my pride in the fact that its editor was at one time an undergraduate student of mine at the University of the West Indies in Jamaica. One of the uncertainties teachers always face is that they can never predict how their charges will turn out. This uncertainty has been happily resolved. Dr. Parris' professional career has been marked by the same dedication and commitment that characterized his undergraduate days and that clearly has been brought to the preparation of this scholarly and practical work.

Pain relief has been until recently a comparatively neglected field. Its neglect was determined not so much by lack of professional awareness of its importance but mainly because so little could be done about it in the past.

The advances in its management and control that are described in this text, and to which Dr. Parris and his coauthors have made such outstanding contributions, meet an important need. It is a need that has been long-standing and has been becoming progressively critical; a need that has been heightened by more than the additional demands that could be anticipated as the ages of populations increased. It is heightened also by the very humanism and compassion in medicine that the capacity itself to relieve pain has fostered.

The diversity of pain-controlling approaches now open to medicine are well reflected in the chapters of this book. They range from drug therapy, electronic, and mechanical devices to psychotherapy. There are also useful chapters on diverse approaches to pain management and evaluation, and also on its biochemical, cultural, and psychosocial implications.

Dr. Parris has been able to call upon an impressive range of contributors, which has ensured not only that all aspects of pain control are covered, but that they are covered by experts. There is hardly an aspect of the subject for which the reader will not find authoritative comment and instruction.

The value and significance of its contributions are further enhanced by the fact that many of the techniques it deals with were comparatively unknown two decades ago. Many of these, therefore, are more than mere refinements of existing approaches. They are new contributions to medical scientific advancement. Measurement of substance P, for instance, promises to provide a new and reliable tool as a reproducible biological marker for chronic pain.

Dr. Parris and his colleagues are to be congratulated on this admirable textbook. It will be a valuable compendium of information on its subject for many years for students and practitioners of medicine alike, and it will fill important gaps in our knowledge about pain and its control. But it will achieve more than this. The success with which it links scholarship and research to the practical and utilitarian should ensure for it a lasting place as a resource for those who are called upon to provide service to the millions of people whose daily suffering has been until now so inadequately confronted.

FOREWORD

BRADLEY E. SMITH, M.D.

... the world ... hath really neither joy, nor love, nor light, nor certitude, nor peace, nor help for pain; and we are here, as on a darkling plain, swept with confused alarms of struggle and flight, where ignorant armies clash by night.

Dover Beach
Matthew Arnold c.1847–1851

"Help for pain" has been one of humanity's unanswered prayers since first we could pray. For the first time in the thousand centuries of the existence of modern man, these prayers were partially answered at about the same time *Dover Beach* was written, when the effectiveness of surgical anesthesia by inhalation of ether was demonstrated. Yet in the following century, further progress was relatively slow, despite the appearance of cocaine, procaine, aspirin, meperidine, and a host of cults and charlatans, along with a number of misdirected, but well-intended and ethical physicians.

In the past few short years, however, amazing progress toward escape from this darkling plain is at last being offered by a new and exciting group of scientists and practitioners who specialize in pain control. They are characterized by an ability to synthesize and apply a wealth of new information, science, and clinical experience from many disciplines in an effective new format to provide "help for pain."

Many have attributed the birth of this new specialty to Dr. John J. Bonica, who in 1953 published a prodigious encyclopedia of pain syndromes and treatments, many of which are still unmodified standards today [1]. In his book, and in his famous clinic, he demonstrated that pain is many faceted, that physical pain may lead to psychic overlay, that psychogenic sources may manifest as physical pain, and that "help for pain" may best be found in the combined resources of physicians of many specialties, psychologists, and others.

A major factor in the exponential expansion of this knowledge base has been the increasing sophistication of the art of investigation. Pain, being subjective, has been notorious for the unreliability of enthusiastic reports concerning new modalities of therapy. Thus, a real antipathy arose in much of the medical community as a reaction to disappointment when many of these modalities failed to pass the test of time. This antipathy, unforunately, has on occasion blanketed the whole field of pain research and pain therapists as well.

However, a revolution in the science of pain investigations, exemplified by the insightful works of Henry K. Beecher [2], has now provided us with increasingly effective methods for defining the results of alternative therapies and recognizing valuable tools, and has made us more agile in the rejection of useless ones. As a result, there is a growing awareness in both the medical community and the public that this impressive new armamentarium is at last genuine. As evidence of this new awareness, nearly every major medical center now boasts a busy "Pain Control Center," and scholarly journals and books are devoted to this new body of experience and research with increasing frequency.

Of course, the battle against pain is not yet won, but for the first time in the history of modern human kind, significant advances are appearing with increasing frequency. Many of the world's foremost contributors to this marvelous progress are represented among the authors gathered here by the editor. Their discussions amount to a declaration of "the state of the art" in "help for pain." They are clearly no longer soldiers of ignorant armies that clash with pain by night on a darkling plain, but our enlightened champions for whose victories we all owe great thanks.

Final thanks should be extended to the editor, by whose stature these eminent authorities were convinced to participate, and by whose labors the manuscripts were molded into an integrated whole.

REFERENCES

1. Bonica J. 1953. The Management of Pain. Philadelphia, Lea & Febiger.
2. Beecher HK. 1959. Measurement of Subjective Responses: Quantitative Effects of Drugs. New York, Oxford University Press,

PREFACE

Ten years ago and before, it would have been fairly accurate to state that chronic pain represented a failure of modern medical science. Although the pain puzzle, its mechanisms, and its effective treatment have not yet been solved, there has been great progress in this area. Testimony of this progress is borne out by the several textbooks and publications dealing with the issues of pain management that have been published recently. The idea of producing *Contemporary Issues in Chronic Pain Management* originated after a planned symposium on pain management had been postponed inevitably as a result of the devastation by Hurricane Gilbert of the planned venue of that symposium. Since a great deal of effort had gone into the preparation for that proposed symposium, I speculated that the material prepared by the speakers of that symposium should form the nucleus of a proposed book: *Contemporary Issues in Chronic Pain Management.* With that concept in the mind, I decided to expand the existing material by supplementation with reviews of some old issues, as well as discussions of some new issues in chronic pain management. I hope that these issues may be stimulating and provocative for the reader and for health-care providers involved in chronic pain management.

The contributing authors come from different specialties, different countries, have different opinions on identical issues, but have one common and unifying goal, and that is the advancement of the discipline of chronic pain management and the courage to expand their views in an open forum. The diversity in background of the different authors is obvious and deliberate;

my aim has been the production of a book that would be diverse, informative, and useful to various personnel in the arena of chronic pain management. I feel very proud to have the world-renowned pain scientist, Dr. Ronald Melzack, as a contributor to this work. His chapter, Recent Physiological Studies on Pain, is excellent and of customary high quality. I am equally proud to have my mentor, colleague, and friend, Dr. Steven Brena, discuss pain, ethnicity, and culture. I believe that this work may mark the beginning of a series of research projects that might help bridge the gap and narrow the differences in attitudes to pain and approaches to its management at a world level. I believe that there are several chapters in which authors present new or relatively new information, relating directly to chronic pain management and that I hope the reader will find useful. Some of those chapters are provocative and some of them present new aspects of old issues in pain management. I am delighted to have Dr. Janos Szolcsanyi, of University of Pecs in Hungary, present his work, Perspectives of Capsaicin-Type Agents in Pain Therapy and Research. Dr. Szolcsanyi is, without question, one of the world authorities on capsaicin and pain research, and his expertise is unquestioned. I am also proud to have him as part of this work, particularly in this new political age of *glasnost* and *perestroika.*

A work of this nature cannot be accomplished without the unselfish and competent assistance of many people. In that regard, I owe my debt and gratitude to several people. First of all, I would like to thank Dr. Prithvi Raj for his support and encouragement in helping me initiate, develop, and produce this book. I would also like to thank Ms. Lorie Savel, the editorial consultant at Kluwer Publications, for her untiring assistance and talented competence in working out all the less glamorous activities that are absolutely necessary to attempt and to complete a project of this kind. If any one person is due immeasurable gratitude, it is my chairman, colleague, and more importantly my friend, Dr. Bradley E. Smith. I am truly indebted to Dr. Smith for his encouragement and assistance in developing my interest in pain management over the past 12 years. His unparalleled support of my activities and his total confidence in me was without question one of the single most important factors in my undertaking this project. As recently as last year, he graciously arranged for me to take my sabbatical so that I could devote some time to this work. To him I am eternally grateful.

When I first started medical school I was, as a neophyte, truly impressed with one giant of a man who had the gentility of a lamb, as far as his empathy and devotion to his patients were concerned. This was Professor Sir Kenneth Stuart. I was also truly touched by his compassion for and competence towards his patients, and I am delighted that Her Majesty Queen Elizabeth II has recently recognized his talents and honored him with a knighthood for his contributions to medicine in the Caribbean. It is an honor and a pleasure to have my former teacher, Professor Stuart, write the Foreword to this book. I would also like to thank Dr. Irving Glick of the United States Tennis Association for his support, encouragement, and friendship during the preparation of this book and for his collaboration with me in several sports-related pain projects. My secretary, Sherry Duke, has had to put up with me through it all and has had to spend long and tiring hours on the computer and on the telephone co-ordinating this effort from my office with the many contributing authors. Her competence is unquestioned and her efforts are greatly appreciated by me. I would like to thank all the contributing authors for their contribution, support, and the efforts that they put into meeting our deadlines. I would also like to thank you, the reader, for taking the time to read this work, and I sincerely hope that you enjoy it.

Finally, but without doubt most importantly, I would like to thank very very sincerely, my tolerant and patient wife, Shirley, for the many hours that I was away from her during the pursuit of this work and other tasks, and even the many hours when I was with her but preoccupied with this project. I can truly say that without her constant support and caring, and also the patience of my children — Wayne, Wendell, and Sharon — this book would still be in its embryonic stages.

Winston C.V. Parris

CONTEMPORARY ISSUES IN CHRONIC PAIN MANAGEMENT

1. HISTORICAL PERSPECTIVES ON PAIN MANAGEMENT

DAVID P. SCHWARTZ AND WINSTON C.V. PARRIS

For all the happiness mankind can gain, it is not in pleasure but in rest from pain.

John Dryden.

Pain is as old as humankind. Therefore the history of pain may well represent a review of part of the history of the world. Humankind has been suffering from the days of Adam and Eve through the ravages of war and pestilence right into Christianity through the "scourging at the pillar," and including all the great historic periods of this world into the modern era. Humans have always sought ways to alleviate the pain of disease, inflammation, and trauma. The causes, mechanisms, and treatment of pain have been elusive, however, from earliest times until now. The conceptual models for the causes in origin of pain, as well as its treatment, have run parallel to physical models of the universe in each period of history. Great strides have been made in dealing with acute pain mechanisms, but this is definitely not the case for chronic pain. Modest strides in unraveling the puzzle of chronic pain have been made in the past decade, but much more work needs to be done in an attempt to solve not only those complex mechanisms of chronic pain, but to devise effective and safe methods of providing sustained, reliable, and reproducible pain relief for patients with chronic pain.

The purpose of this chapter is to review some of the major historical events that have influenced pain and its management, and to trace the major phases of conceptualizing pain and its treatment. Four major phases will be arbitrarily considered in this theoretical development. These include:

1. Ancient history through the Scientific Revolution
2. The Scientific Revolution through the mid-20th century
3. Mid-20th century through the end of World War II
4. End of World War II through the present time

In each historical period, significant events will be highlighted, and in the contemporary era the development of pain management as an independent discipline will be examined. The contemporary trends, associated problems, and the conventional position on major medical issues relating to pain will be discussed.

ANCIENT HISTORY THROUGH THE SCIENTIFIC REVOLUTION
It is clear that pain has been recognized as a part of human existence since the time of the earliest archeological data available [1]. Prehistoric humans attempted to treat pain resulting from both illness and injury with many techniques we would still recognize today, such as heat, cold, and pressure [1,2]. Pain was felt to be caused by forces outside the individual, such as evil spirits, and treatment therefore included deliberate wounding or opening of the body, such as trephining, to allow the negative forces to escape. Spells and magic were employed by medicine men or shamans to cast out the evil. The use of natural pain-relieving herbs, such as opium, came to be employed as well [3]. Of central importance throughout prehistoric conceptualizations of pain and its treatment was the belief that pain was the result of evil forces located outside the individual. This belief was also held in ancient Egypt [4], India [5], and China [6]. The Egyptians and Indians believed pain was experienced in the heart, whereas the Chinese identified multiple points in the body where pain might dwell. Attempts to drain the pain from the body by means of needle insertion may have been the origin of acupuncture therapy.

The ancient Greeks were the first to consider pain as a sensory function, which could arise from peripheral stimulation. Aristotle, in particular, believed that pain was a central sensation arising from some type of stimulation of the flesh. Although Plato suggested the brain as the destination of these messages, Aristotle preferred the concept that the heart was the originating source or processing center for pain. His belief was that an excess of vital heat was conducted by the blood to the heart, there to be felt as pain. Greek philosophers following Aristotle, such as Straton, saw the brain as the site of pain perception. The Egyptians, Heraphilus and Eistratus, also supported this view, bolstered by actual anatomical studies showing the connections of the peripheral and central nervous system. Some 400 years later, the Roman philosopher Galen rediscovered the Egyptian work, and greatly expanded the model of the nervous system. His work, however, was little recognized until the 20th century.

Thus, through the period of the Roman empire, a progression occurred in terms of better understanding pain as a sensation, similar to other sensations of the body. A parallel growth in the development of therapeutic modalities can be seen. The Egyptians used opium as early as 1550 BC [2], as well as trephining, heat, cold, massage, and exercise, to treat painful illnesses. The Romans, Greeks, and Chinese described the use of drugs for pain, as well as surgery. Electricity was first used by the Greeks of that era as they exploited the use of the electrogenic torpedo fish (*Scribonius longus*) to treat the pain of headache and arthritis. Electrostatic generators were used in the late Middle Ages, along with the Leyden jar, and these strategies resulted in the reemergence of electrotherapy as a modality for managing medical problems, including pain. Effectively, no other advances utilizing electrotherapy were made following this practice of using electrostatic generators until the discovery of the electric battery in the 19th century. At that time, attempts to revive the use of electrotherapy in medicines were not very successful, and the practice was mainly relegated to application by charlatans and obscure scientists.

From a historical perspective, then, it would appear that as we emerge from ancient history, a trend has developed whereby the treatment of the external causes of pain, conceptualized by removing evil humors or spirits, was no longer popular. Pain, instead, seemed to evolve into being seen as an experience in its own right, and its treatment began to focus on reducing the experience of pain per se for the patient.

In the Middle Ages and Renaissance, the debate continued as to the seat of sensation of pain. William Harvey, known for his discovery of the circulation, supported the heart as the focus of pain sensation, while Descartes emphasized the brain. Descartes' description of pain conduction from peripheral damage through nerves to the brain preceded the specificity theory [7] by some two centuries. Despite these theoretical explorations, however, there were no real advances in pain therapy until the 18th century.

THE SCIENTIFIC REVOLUTION
Advances in pain theory and treatment in the 18th and 19th centuries proceeded along two related lines: the discovery of the analgesic properties of nitrous oxide, followed by local anesthetic agents such as cocaine, and the discovery of the anatomic division of the spinal cord into sensory (dorsal) and motor (ventral) divisions. Together, these two new areas of knowledge initiated the beginnings of the modern understanding and management of pain.

In terms of the latter, Muller [8] was the first to propose (based on anatomical studies) a straight-through system of specific nerve energies, in which specific energy from a sensation was transmitted along the sensory nerves to the brain. From this point, two physiological theories of pain sensation emerged: the specificity theory and the intensive theory.

The specificity theory, originally proposed by Descartes, was formalized by Schiff [7] based upon animal research. The cornerstone of this theory was that each sensory modality, including pain, was transmitted along independent pathways. By examining the effect of incisions in the spinal cord, Schiff demonstrated that touch and pain were independent, and that sectioning the cord differentially resulted in the loss of one modality without affecting the other. Continued research by Blix [9], Goldscheider [10], and von Frey [11] contributed to the concept of separate receptors for the four modalities of touch, warmth, cold, and pain.

The intensive theory, on the other hand, maintained that the sensation of pain was not a separate modality, but instead resulted from a sensory overload of sufficient intensity for any modality. First proposed by Darwin [12], and formalized by Erb [13], the theory was expanded by Goldscheider [10] to include the roles of stimulus, intensity, and central summation of stimuli. The controversy between the specificity and intensive theories gradually swung towards specificity theory, with this becoming universally accepted by the mid-20th century.

For a variety of reasons (some valid, others not), the specificity theory became predominant and pain therapies began to focus on identifying and interrupting pain pathways. Letievant [14], in the late 19th century, first described specific neurectomy techniques for neuralgic pain. In the following 50 or so years, a variety of surgical interventions for chronic pain were developed and reported [15]. One major liability of the approach is still present in modern times; this is the notion that pain can be "fixed" by a surgical procedure, drug, or other procedure. At the same time, the discovery of both general and local anesthetic agents led to an ever-emerging technology of nerve blockade approaches for pain control. In 1888, Corning wrote the first book on the use of a local anesthetic (cocaine) for nerve pain, followed by a more comprehensive treatise in 1894. A rapid proliferation of local and regional anesthetic techniques for both surgery and pain disorders followed. By 1907, Scholosser reported relief of neuralgic pain for long periods via alcohol injection to the affected nerves. Reports of similar treatment of pain from cancer and tuberculosis were also made [2]. Swetlow in 1926 and White in 1928 reported on the use of alcohol injection into the thoracic sympathetic ganglia for chronic angina, and Dogliotti [16] used alcohol in the subarachnoid space for cancer pain. The increasing prevalence of causalgic injuries prompted work by Leriche [17] to develop the use of sympathetic block with procaine. Bonica [3] also points out that the period before 1940 marked a proliferation in the practice of nerve blocks and regional anesthesia by anesthesiologists for surgery. This produced a body of physicians skilled in the knowledge, art, and practice of interrupting nerve conduction.

Thus, the period of time between 1900 and 1950 saw pain come to be treated as a discrete sensory phenomenon, with attempts to determine an anatomical basis for its transmission and thereby its treatment. Both the understanding and the management of pain came to be based on scientific medical principles, grounded in basic sciences such as anatomy and physiology. Most important was the increasing recognition that pain could be a disorder over and above that caused by illness and injury, and that the pain required treatment in its own right. The stage was thus set for the emergence of pain management as a discipline in its own right.

THE DEVELOPMENT OF PAIN MANAGEMENT AS A DISCIPLINE

The period between the two great world wars saw an unusually large number of young men and women who had sustained many traumatic lesions as a result of military or civilian casualties of the war. The frustrating attempts to deal with those problems created a major problem in chronic pain management. The many reports of frostbite and associated vascular injuries, particularly to the German and Russian troops fighting on the eastern front in the winning days of the Second World War, presented a major problem in pain management. The practice of nerve blocks, notably Bier blocks or intravenous regional sympathetic blocks and sympathetic ganglionic blocks, increased in an attempt to control the various sympathetically mediated pain problems that occurred in that era. It was in that background that significant development was made. In that era, regional anesthesia techniques, as developed by Corning, Quincke, Bier, and others, were already well-established practice. The subsequent contributions of Pitkin and Etherington-Wilson, Barker, and Adriani, all produced tremendous gain as far as the management of pain was concerned.

In 1946, Dr. John Bonica began the first multidisciplinary pain center in Tacoma, Washington, based out of a private practice. It arose from his recognition that chronic pain was optimally treated by a team of specialists. For the first time, patients suffering pain were routinely evaluated by different medical specialties, physical therapists, and psychiatrists. Treatment involved input from all the specialties, and they met to discuss their patients on a regular basis. This experience led to the publication of the historic book, *The Management of Pain* in 1953 by Dr. John Bonica. The treatment of pain by a team of specialists became an acceptable idea, although not widely known to either the general medical audience or the lay public. Other multidisciplinary pain programs began to emerge around the country, carrying forward the original Bonica model. However, the lack of an adequate theory to explain the phenomena of pain still proved a stumbling block. Although it was becoming accepted that both pain sensation and resulting dysfunction were affected by more than observable tissue pathology, this remained a "phenomenon in search of a theory" until 1965. With the publication of the gate control theory by Melzack and Wall, a unifying theory was available. In particular, the theory's emphasis on both ascending and descending modulating systems laid down a framework into which multiple disciplines, such as medicine, psychology, and physical therapy, could fit their contributions. Interest began to grow in both the theory and practice of pain management. Training programs in medical pain management began, the first at the University of Washington. At the same time, Fordyce [18] and Sternbach [19] were demonstrating the crucial role of psychological and behavioral factors in understanding and managing chronic pain.

Fordyce demonstrated that pain-related disability could be modulated by environmental factors, as well as tissue pathology, and set forth the beginnings of the behavioral pain management programs seen today. Sternbach showed that many of the psychological factors earlier thought to be causative of intractable pain from a psychosomatic model were, in fact, a *result* of the pain. Their work evolved into the more comprehensive biopsychosocial or multi-axial models of conceptualizing pain (i.e., Turk et al. [20]), which are accepted practice today.

ORGANIZATIONAL DEVELOPMENT

In 1974, the International Association for the Study of Pain (IASP) was formed and began publication of its journal, *Pain*, in 1975. The American chapter of the IASP, the American Pain Society, was established in 1977 and held its first annual meeting in 1979. This organization, comprising both clinicians and researchers from many disciplines, including medicine, psychology, physical therapy, and nursing, further promoted the study and treatment of pain. Both the IASP and the APS chose not to become involved in accreditation of either pain clinicians or pain treatment programs, although the organization did attempt to survey and classify existing facilities offering pain treatment. Instead, both organizations attempted to function primarily as a forum for research, education, and exchanging of ideas among both clinicians and basic researchers, while avoiding politically charged issues such as training and accreditation. This created a void, as the growth of pain management as a clinical entity began to necessitate that standards be set. Some criteria were needed for consumers, insurers, and peer reviewers of pain management therapy, as many began to ask, What is acceptable pain treatment? Who should provide it? and Who should be paid for it?

The Commission on Accreditation of Rehabilitation Facilities (CARF) was the first to offer a system of accreditation for pain treatment centers in 1983. Given CARF's background in rehabilitation models, it was evident that the CARF model would be oriented towards physical and psychosocial rehabilitation of patients suffering pain, as opposed to modality treatment to reduce pain sensation. Indeed, CARF standards mandate that only multidisciplinary pain management programs, representing at a minimum medicine, psychology or psychiatry, and physical therapy, are eligible for accreditation. However, CARF specifically does not accredit clinicians in pain management, aiming instead at the programs and facilities as entities. For example, the CARF model requires that medical directors of pain management programs have at least 2 years experience in pain management, participate in ongoing education and training, and be board certified in their specialty. The actual accreditation of pain physicians, however, is not codified by CARF.

The CARF model is gaining acceptance among insurers, primarily because of its emphasis on accountability and program evaluation, and because objective goals, such as increased physical function, reduced medication intake, and return to work, are emphasized. Several states now require CARF accreditation reimbursement of any chronic pain therapy for reimbursement under Worker's Compensation, and in some cases private insurers are also adopting the CARF standard as well.

During this time period, a growing number of physicians in the United States came to believe that neither CARF nor the American Pain Society completely met their practice or professional needs. In particular, there was a vacuum in respect to evaluating the competence of pain-oriented physicians, since there were no agreed-upon standards for the training and credentialing of these physicians. To deal with these growing needs, although recognizing the important roles of the American Pain Society and CARF, a group of physicians proposed the idea of the formation of the American Academy of Algology. This academy was formed by and for physicians interested in pain management, and the inaugural meeting was held in 1983 in Washington, D.C. The birth of the American Academy of Algology provided physician-algologists a forum in which to discuss their specific concerns and to deal exclusively with pain from a medical standpoint. Naturally, the creation of the American Academy of Algologists created some political friction between both physician and nonphysician members of the American Pain Society. Advocates of the creation of the American Academy of Algologists argued that the reimbursement issues, the fee scheduling issues, and the medical management issues were completed different when the interest of a pain physician was compared with other health-care providers. The opponents of the creation of the American Academy of Algology argued that this academy was divisive in nature and would polarize opinion and result in controversy in the ranks of pain-oriented health-care providers. Nothwithstanding, the organization grew and developed. Because of a semantic dislike for the term *American Academy of Algology*, this term was changed in 1986 and is currently known as the *American Academy of Pain Medicine*. Today the American Academy of Pain Medicine still flourishes and its membership is growing slowly but surely. This organization is now recognized by the American Medical Association and has a seat in its House of Delegates. This organization has grown to have its own clinical journal, i.e., *The Clinical Journal of Pain*, and attempts are currently underway to address the issues of training, credentialing, and certification of competently trained pain physicians.

It is hoped that this process will be successful and that pain management will develop and grow into a fully accredited, appropriately credentialed, and highly respected discipline in modern medicine.

The history of medicine, and in particular the history of many specialities in medicine, is characterized by special interest polarization, which has never served the interest of the profession or the specialty. In fact, this polarization, when carried to extremes, has actually impeded progress in medicine. It is hoped that the discipline of pain medicine may recognize those potential, politically undesirable situations and avoid the unnecessary and unpleasant consequences of such polarization. While differences of opinion are acceptable and healthy, a heated debate of those differences of opinion is counterproductive to the growth of a specialty, and destructive polemics and selfish behavior are to be avoided at all costs. If these potential pitfalls are bypassed and if the growth of pain medicine continues as predicted, then the future of pain medicine looks very promising. Testimony of that future is reflected by the quality and quantity of papers that are usually produced at the triannual World Congress of Pain and at the annual American Academy of Pain Medicine and the American Pain Society Meetings. This situation is not only present in the United States, but is reflected by the various national pain organizations that are developing and being productive throughout the world. As the accreditation, credentialing and socioeconomic issues are solved, one could predict that the building blocks for the solution of the pain puzzle would be in place. When this is the case, not only the history but also the future of pain medicine will be very bright indeed.

REFERENCES

1. Bonica JJ. 1953. The Management of Pain. Philadelphia, Lea — Febiger.
2. Keele KD. 1957. Anatomies of Pain. Oxford, Blackwell.
3. Bonica JJ. 1985. Evolution of pain concepts and pain clinics. In SF Brena, SL Chapman (eds), Clinics in Anesthesiology: Chronic Pain: Management Principles, Vol. 3. pp. 1–16
4. Castiglioni A. 1947. A History of Medicine. New York, AA Knopf.
5. Lin Y. 1949. The Wisdom of India. London, Joseph.
6. Veith I. 1949. Huang Ti Ne Ching Su Wen. Baltimore, William — Wilkens.
7. Schiff M. 1848. Lerbuch der Physiologie, Muskel, und Nervenphysiologie. Schavenburg, Lahr.
8. Muller J. 1840. In Baly W (trans) Handbuch der Physiologie des Menschen. London, Taylor and Walton.
9. Blix M. 1884. Experimentelle bietrag zur losung der frage uber die specifische energie der hautnerven. Z Biol 20:141–156.
10. Goldscheider A. 1884. Die spezifische energie der gefuhlsnerven de haut. Monatsschrift Prakt Germatol 3:282.
11. von Frey M. 1894. Ber. Verhandl. Konig. Sachs. Ges. Wiss. Leipzig. Beitrage Zur Physiologie des Schmerzsinnes 46:185–196.
12. Darwin E. 1794. Zoonomia, or the Laws of Organic Life. London, J. Johnson.
13. Erb WH. 1874. Krankhetender peipherischen cerebrospinalen nerven in Luckey G, Some recent studies of pain. Am J Psychol 7:109.
14. Letievant E. 1873. Traites des Sections Nerveuses. Paris, JB Bailliere.
15. White JC, Sweet WH. 1969. Pain and the Neurosurgeon. A forty-year experience. Springfield, IL, Charles C. Thomas.
16. Dogliotti AM. 1931. Traitement des syndromes douloureux de la périphérie par alcoholisation sub-arachnoïdienne. Presse Médicale 39:1249–1252.
17. Leriche R. 1939. Surgery of Pain. Baltimore, William — Wilkins.
18. Fordyce WE. 1976. Behavioral Methods for Chronic Pain and Illness. St. Louis, CV Mosby.
19. Sternbach RA. 1974. Pain Patients: Traits and Treatment. New York, Academic Press.
20. Turk DC, Meichenbaum D, Genest M. 1983. Pain and Behavioral Medicine: A Cognitive-Behavioral Perspective. New York, Guilford.

2. PAIN, ETHNICITY, AND CULTURE

STEVEN F. BRENA, AND STANLEY L. CHAPMAN

In his classical book, *A Study of History*, historian Arnold Toynbee defined society as the "total network of relationships among individuals"; he also defined culture as "identifiable patterns of behaviors, overt and covert, of members of a society"; in turn, *civilization* is defined as a culture primarily developed in urban communities (from the Latin, *civis* = city). Obviously, these definitions stress the role of behaviors in determining social-cultural characteristics. On the other hand, *ethnicity* (Greek, *ethnos* = race or group) is a much broader term, including not only social and cultural factors but also racial, ethical, and moral variables.

A state of wellness is based on the three cornerstones of sound mind, fit body, and supportive environment. Breakdown in any of all of these cornerstones can lead to the experience of pain and suffering. While the physical and mental factors involved in the painful experience have been widely studied, relatively few studies have empirically documented the role of the environment, as reflected in ethnic and sociocultural factors. In this chapter, a brief review of existing literature on such factors is presented.

PAIN AND RELIGION

The term *religion* is derived from the Latin word *religare*, meaning "to bind together." Religion indeed can be said to bind together groups of people by ethical and moral codes reinforced through the performance of special rituals.

Before the rise of modern science and technology, pain was seen largely in a religious context. Indeed, the very word *pain* is derived from the Latin word *poena* meaning punishment; the Latin word, in turn, has a Sanskrit root *pu*, meaning sacrifice or purification. Obviously, these terms indicate a symbolic religious component in the evolution of human views of pain as an existential phenomenon. Christians, for example, historically have spiritualized pain in the name of Christ, and have seen in the cross the perfect model for suffering and triumph over suffering. Followers of Christianity have frequently taught the concept that pain and suffering are necessary for atonement for personal sins and for the sins of others. For example, the pain of childbirth was seen as a necessary atonement for the sins of Eve, and it is reported that Queen Victoria was criticized widely in the 19th century for her decision to receive chloroform during childbirth. Suffering was seen by many as a part of human life and as an instrument of purification, not as something to be cured or alleviated on a physical or mental level.

Other religions have developed their own concepts of pain. For example, Islamic religion teaches that pain and suffering are a manifestation of Allah's will to be accepted without question. Islamic teachings emphasize forbearance, silence, and steadfastness in counseling sufferers to refrain from complaints and to "welcome illness as if it were health." Both Hindu and Buddhist philosophies stress the role of meditation as a way to relieve pain and suffering by bringing the body and the mind into a state of balance.

In more primitive societies, control of pain often has been viewed as a test of manhood. The "hook swinging ceremony," which was characteristic of some American Indian tribes and apparently still is practiced in some Latin American groups, is a good illustration of the influence of religious beliefs on pain perceptions. In this ceremony, an individual is chosen to represent the divine power. Two hooks are inserted into the victim's back and he is hoisted into the air by a crane connected to the hooks. He then is made to swing in the air so that the appears to fly. The victim must not display any sign of suffering. In this example, through the support of the community and a strong desire to be part of a specific group, the individual appears able to detach himself from visible signs of pain and suffering [1].

Actually, some philosophies of management of chronic pain patients at pain rehabilitation centers have some parallels to the teachings of the world's great religions. For example, the appeal to self-control through devotional practice is a keystone of religious teachings and is rooted in the Bible, Koran, and the *Bhahavad Gita* of the Hindus [2]. In the religious context, self-control is deemed to be essential to "purify" the individual and to prepare him or her for a personal spiritual experience; in pain rehabilitation, development of control over one's own bodily functions, emotions, and thoughts through various psychophysiological interventions is an accepted and well-researched prerequisite for healthy living and control of suffering, even in the presence of bodily damage. The commandment to live morally is common to all religions, expressed as "the will of God" in the Ten Commandments of the Jewish and Christian religions, in the Hindu *Yoga Sutras of Patanjali*, and in the rules of the Koran. But to live according to moral and ethical codes means also to grow more integrated in physical, emotional, and intellectual functioning. This integration demands the capability to maintain a state of wellness without "breaking down" into existential suffering, even in the face of pain and stress [3].

The call for sensual moderation is another cornerstone of all religions. Examples include various Christian rules of sexual containment, rules of fasting during Lent for Catholics, the ban of alcohol in many Christian-Protestant and Muslim churches, the dawn-to-dusk fast during the Muslim Ramadan, and the rules for food preparations and avoidance of the Jews and the Hindus. On a similar note, modern health science has well documented the threat to health generated by excessive or improper drinking and eating. Obesity is a common complicating factor in chronic low back pain, and there is some evidence that excessive smoking may aggravate headache pain [4]. Stress management, now a well-recognized modality in pain control, teaches moderation and balance in work, rest, and recreational activities.

PAIN AND ETHNICITY

In a classic paper published in 1952, Zborowski compared "old Americans" (families who had lived in the United States for many generations and who were of Anglo-Saxon ancestry), with Italian-Americans and American Jews. All were patients in a Veterans Administration Hospital in New York [5,6]. The author found that "old Americans" tended to be distraught and to withdraw more from social contacts when in pain than those in the other two groups. Italians tended loudly to demand pain relief and could demonstrate satisfaction when such relief was obtained through medications. In contrast, Jews would also request relief but would continue to remain skeptical that relief achieved through medication would last. Zborowski concluded that the Italians were "present-oriented," while Jews and "old Americans" were "future-oriented." The "old Americans" were more optimistic about eventual outcome than Jews.

In 1965, Sternbach and Tursky [7] studied changes in skin potentials and pain responses following electrical stimulation in 60 housewives divided into four ethnic groups: Yankees (third-generation Americans of British Protestant descent) and three groups of first-generation Americans, including Irish Roman Catholics, Italian Roman Catholics, and Jews. All subjects were socially "middle class," and there were no significant differences among the groups for various physical factors. The authors found significant differences among the groups for pain tolerance, with the Yankees having the highest mean tolerance levels, followed by the Jews and the Irish, with Italians yielding the lowest tolerance mean level. Yankees also produced a more rapid and greater decrease in skin potentials than the other groups. The authors concluded that attitudinal factors accounted for these psycho-physical and autonomic differences. Borrowing from Zborowski's hypothesis about present and future orientations, they argued that Yankees had a matter-of-fact attitude toward pain; Jews, because they were future-oriented, were not upset by the short-term experimental pain; Irish were undemonstrative with respect to pain; and Italians, being present-oriented, were the most upset by the experimental pain setting.

In a series of studies, Lambert et al. [8] tried to determine the relationship of religious affiliation, ethnic group membership, and self-perception in respect to pain tolerance and "pain sensitivity range," i.e., the difference between pain tolerance and pain threshold. These investigators used 80 Jews and 80 Christian women, applying pressure pain experimentally. Each group was further subdivided into three subgroups of 30, 30, and 20 members, respectively, with the latter serving as a control group. They observed no significant differences in mean baseline pain tolerance among all subgroups. Then subjects in one experimental subgroup were informed that subjects of the other religious groups could tolerate less pain than they could, while subjects in other subgroup were told that subjects of the other religious subgroup could tolerate more pain. The control subgroups received no change in instruction from baseline. The authors found that the Jewish subgroup that has been told that Jews could tolerate less pain than Christians significantly increased their pain tolerance scores over baseline, while the other Jewish subgroup that had been informed that Jews could tolerate more pain showed no significant changes. In contrast, both Christian subgroups increased their main pain tolerance significantly. Lambert et al. suggested that religious affiliation interacts with group perception in creating a differential pain response pattern.

In a more clinical setting, Zola [9] interviewed 196 patients and their families to determine responses and attitudes toward pain. He found that lower socioeconomic status Irish patients tended to deny pain and emphasized the physical effects of illness. The lower socioeconomic status Italian patients emphasized the importance of their pain. They had diffuse complaints and were vocal and dramatic in describing the effects of pain on their daily lives. The Anglo-Saxon patients fell between the Irish and the Italians in their responses, but were more similar to the Irish.

Koopman et al. [10] studied the same subjects and found age to be a significant moderating variable. Specifically, Italian-Americans over 60 years of age were highly distinct from the Irish and Anglo-Saxon groups, while the younger Italian-Americans, who likely had fewer cultural ties to the "old country," did not differ significantly from the Irish and Anglo-Saxons.

Studying blacks, Irish, Italian, Jewish, and Puerto Rican patients with facial pain, Lipton and Marbach [11] also found that the degree of assimilation to American norms was a significant predictor of attitudinal and behavioral responses to pain. Social class also made a difference; higher socioeconomic classes tended to show higher pain tolerance, even within the same ethnic group.

SOCIAL MODELING

A number of investigators have pointed to the importance of observational learning in the development of chronic pain responses. Studying 11,000 English school children with chronic abdominal pain, Apley [12] demonstrated that those children without clear medical evidence to account for their pain came from families who visited physicians with medical complaints far more often than did those children with clear medical evidence for abdominal pain. He inferred that children complaining of pain in the absence of physical evidence had learned to focus on pain through observation of behavior in their families. Violon and Giurgen [13] found a family history of chronic pain in 78% of a mixed group of chronic pain sufferers in comparison with 44% of controls with chronic illness in the absence of pain. While genetic predisposition for pain could be analyzed in this latter study, Apley's results do not support the hypothesis that genetic factors would be primary; they fit much better with a social learning hypothesis.

Two reports have suggested that sexual or physical abuse can be significant factors in the development of pain, particularly pelvic pain problems in women. Murphy [14] reported that 65 of 100 women with chronic pelvic pain gave a history of incest, rape, or sexual molestation, with 40% reporting an incestuous relationship. In the same vein, Haber and Roos [15] found that 56% of 53 women with chronic pain had been sexually or physically abused prior to the onset of their pain problem. Women with abdominal or vaginal pain of unknown etiology were found to have the highest percentage of previous abuse. Unfortunately, control groups of nonmedical patients or medical nonpain patients were not included in these studies.

More direct evidence for the role of social modeling in pain responses has come from studies in which groups of subjects observed models who had been exposed to experimental painful stimuli. Observation of models who successfully tolerated or controlled painful stimulation resulted in reduced subsequent pain behavior in the observer [16,17]. The dependent measure in many of the social modeling studies and virtually all of the studies on pain and religion or ethnicity has been a verbal pain report. While verbal responses are important because they can critically affect the reactions of others to the person in distress, they do not necessarily describe the subject's subjective experience, which can diverge from verbal behavior. Signal detection methods, in which the ratings of pain responses to repeated trials of stimuli of varying intensity are analyzed, have been suggested as a way to separate sensory responses from responses related to subjective bias or attitude, social desirability, response sets, willingness to report distress or pain, etc. Unfortunately, the validity and meaning of these methods remain controversial [18,19].

CROSS-CULTURAL ASSESSMENT OF PAIN AND FUNCTION

Most of the early research on pain responses among ethnic groups has been focused on experimentally induced pain. Instruments that permit direct evaluation of clinical pain have been lacking until the last two decades, which have seen a proliferation of reliable and valid measures for chronic pain assessment. Some of them appear to be promising for cross-cultural studies [20].

Two important instruments that permit direct evaluation of subjective pain intensity have been introduced into the pain field. These are the visual analog scale (VAS) [21] and the McGill Pain Questionnaire (MPQ) [22]. The former allows a nonverbal graphic representation of pain along a line by having the patient mark the degree of pain intensity, while the latter uses adjectives as verbal descriptors of the quality of pain experienced by the patient. Both methods have been widely used, but the VAS has the advantage of not requiring a good vocabulary or knowledge of English. It thus is easy to adapt to a patient's native language. The MPQ has been translated into Italian, German, and Finnish languages with demonstration of its usefulness in measuring the semantics of pain in populations speaking these languages [23–26]; however, it has been shown that the same word, for example, *pain*, can have different meanings across cultural groups and even among individuals [27]. Languages differ greatly in their use of descriptive terms for pain. For example, it was found that English had four basic terms to describe a painful experience — *pain, hurt, sore*, and *ache* — while the Japanese had three and the Thais had only two [28]. Such findings suggest the potential linguistic difficulties involved in cross-cultural research.

The Sickness Impact Profile (SIP) is an example of a test that has demonstrated reliability and validity in cross-cultural study [29]. The SIP is a behaviorally based self-report test that measures the effects of health problems on functioning along a variety of dimensions [30,31]. It contains 136 statements about health-related dysfunction across 12 categories. The 12 category scores are combined into three major subscales (physical, psychosocial, and other), which in turn are combined to form an overall score. The lower the scores, the less impairment is present across scales. So far, the SIP has been translated into Japanese and Spanish languages.

The Multidimensional Pain Inventory (MPI) is another test with good psychometric properties that is likely to be useful for cross-cultural study [32]. The MPI is comprised of three parts: Part I is a global assessment of the impact of pain upon a patient's lifestyle. Part II measures patient perceptions of the range and frequency of responses of significant others to their display of pain and suffering. Part III is comprised of a daily activity checklist.

One problem in cross-cultural studies of pain is the assessment of medical findings in pain patients across cultures. Compared with the relative abundance of instruments designed to measure various other variables that are significant in the overall pain experience, few have been developed to assess physical signs [20]. In 1988 Rudy et al. [33] developed a Medical Examination and Diagnostic Information Coding System (MEDICS) and demonstrated its reliability and validity. With some minor modifications, this instrument also has been found useful for assessment of physical signs in cross-cultural studies

[30]. Scored by the physician, it contains 20 items, each of which represents a particular medical finding and is scored "normal-absent" or "abnormal-present" in a binary fashion. The lower the scores, the less pathology is likely to be present. The 20 items are summated in a linear fashion, with all combined to yield an overall scale score.

CROSS-CULTURAL STUDIES ON PAIN

Few authors have tried to determine responses to the experience of pain across different cultures. In one study, differences in health control attitudes between chronic low back patients in the United States and New Zealand were researched through the use of the Health Locus of Control Questionnaire (HLC) [34]. The HLC is an 11-item instrument that assesses general beliefs regarding cotrol over health. Factor analysis indicated three distinct subscales, measuring degree of belief that health is controlled by one's own self, by powerful others such as physicians, or by luck, fate, or chance [35]. New Zealanders rated their health as less dependent on physicians than did Americans, and New Zealand women saw themselves as having less personal control over their health than did New Zealand men.

In a second study, the same authors tested 198 patients suffering from chronic low back pain in New Zealand and in the United States, all of whom completed comparable outpatient treatment programs [36]. Approximately 55% of the sample from each country returned a follow-up questionnaire 1 year later. Results indicated that despite nearly similar reports of subjective pain intensity in the two different cultures, the U.S. patients reported significantly greater emotional and behavioral disruptions associated with their pain. Specifically, American patients consistently reported using more medications, experiencing more dysphoric mood states, and being more hampered in social, sexual, recreatioal, and vocational functioning.

The authors also examined the role of financial compensation among patients from both cultures. At the onset of treatment, 49% of the American sample and only 17% of the New Zealand sample were receiving pain-related compensation. Within both cultures, patients receiving compensation were less likely to report a return to full activity at follow-up than those who were not, with the relationship being particularly pronounced in the U.S. sample. The authors hypothesized that the key to understand the differences found among patients in the two countries is contained in the respective disability and rehabilitation systems. In New Zealand, full health benefits are available to any wage earner, with no need to prove injury at work; with the absence of an adversarial relationship among employer, insurer, and claimant, there tends to be an early rehabilitation intervention.

In 1985, a large-scale study of migraine epidemiology was carried out in 22 rural ethnic minority communities of 21 provinces of the Peoples' Republic of China [37]. The data were compared with epidemiological findings in the United States. The authors documented a lower prevalance and incidence of migraines among Chinese than among Americans, while other variables, such as age and sex distribution, were found to be similar in China and in the United States.

Using the MEDICS and SIP instruments, Brena et al. [38] studied responses to low back pain in comparable groups of American, Japanese, and Mexican patients [40]. Results revealed no significant differences between American and Japanese groups in overall score and all four subscale scores of MEDICS. By contrast, the Mexicans rated significantly lower on all five MEDICS scores. Similarly, the Mexican group scored significantly lower that the Japanese and American samples on the physical subscale of the SIP. In comparison with both the Japanese and Mexican groups, the American group showed significantly higher scores on the overall SIP score and on the psychosocial and other scales of the SIP. In the discussion, the authors pointed out differences among the cultures that could have influenced the results. These include a more coherent and cohesive family structure in the Japanese and Mexican cultures. The work structure also is very different among the three cultures. In Japan, productivity and loyalty to the employer is emphasized, while in Mexico, unemployment is high and employment thus is considered a treasured privilege. The health-care delivery systems in Japan and in Mexico are less aggressive, less technologically oriented, and by far less defensive against possible litigation than the American system.

PAIN AND WORK

Cultural values regarding work are likely to influence responses to the painful experience considerably. Seres and Newman [39] correlated changes in the value placed on work in the United States with data suggesting declines in job tenure, increases in the healing periods from injuries, increases in pain-related claims for early retirement, and the skyrocketing increase in compensation costs. In a recent review of the literature on pain and litigation, Chapman and Brena [40] reviewed evidence that factors such as cultural values and family structure, in addition to educational level, income, regional unemployment rates, and the ability of the worker to control the pace of work, often are more important than medical findings in predicting return to work, particularly in the lower and middle ranges of injury or disease severity. The wisdom of the New Zealand Workers' Compensation legislation and the usefulness of the cooperative relationship between employers and employees in Japan are well supported by Dworkin's et al. [41] results, which show that prolonged unemployment lowers the likelihood of return to work.

CONCLUSIONS

In summary, pain cannot be separated from its ethnic, social, and cultural context. The manner in which pain is defined, expressed, and treated always has depended on the basic values of the culture in which it has occurred. In an age when the world is rapidly becoming a giant village with instant communication across the globe, it is amazing that so little attention has been pain in the pain literature to ethnic and cross-cultural responses to clinical pain. Our understanding of factors involved in chronic pain could be enhanced by studies comparing its incidence and expression in different cultures around the world. There is a particular need for large-scale epidemiological studies in different cultures on chronic back pain patients similar to the headache study in the Peoples' Republic of China. With added and greater cross-cultural information available, it may be possible to identify empirically those factors that exert positive influences in containing pain behaviors and to apply them to curb the current epidemic of chronic pain and disability in the industrialized Western nations, while at the same time relieving patients in all nations from unnecessary suffering.

REFERENCES

1. Beltrutti D. 1984. Cultural factors in chronic pain. Pan Minerva Med 26:87–92.
2. Yogananda P. 1987. The Science of Religion, 8th ed. Los Angeles, Self-Realization Fellowship.
3. Brena S. 1972. Pain and religion. Springfield, IL, Charles C. Thomas.
4. Saper J. 1986. Personal communication.
5. Zborowski M. 1952. Cultural components in response to pain. J Soc Issues 8:16–30.
6. Zborowski M. 1969. People in Pain. San Franscisco, Jossey-Bass.
7. Sternbach RA, Tursky B. 1965. Ethnic differences among housewives in psychophysical and skin potential responses to electric shock. Psychophysiology 1:241–246.
8. Lambert WE, Libman E, Poser G. 1960. The effect of increased salience of a membership group on pain tolerance. J Pers 38:350–357.
9. Zola J. 1966. Culture and symptoms. An analogy of patients presenting complaints. Am Sociol Rev 31:615–620.
10. Koopman C, Eisenthal S, Stoeckle JD. 1984. Ethnicity in the report of pain, emotional distress and requests of medical outpatients. Soc Sci Med 18:487–490.
11. Lipton JA, Marbach JJ. 1984. Ethnicity and the pain experience. Soc Sci Med 19:1279–1298.
12. Apley J. 1975. The Child with Abdominal Pain. Oxford, Blackwell Press.
13. Violon A, Giurgen D. 1984. Familial models for chronic pain. Pain 18:199–203.
14. Murphy TM. 1981. Profiles of pain patients, including chronic pelvic pain. In LKY Ng (ed), New Approaches to Treatment of Chronic Pain: A Review of Multidisciplinary Pain Clinics and Pain Centers. Washington DC, NIDA Research Monograph 36, pp. 122–129.
15. Haber J, Roos C. 1984. Effects of spouse abuse and/or sexual abuse in the development and maintenance of chronic pain in women. Presentation at the Fourth World Congress on Pain. Seattle, Washington.
16. Craig KD, Weiss SM. 1971. Vicarious influences on pain-threshold determination. J Psychol 19:53–59.
17. Vernon, DTA. 1974. Modeling and birth order in responses to painful stimuli. J Pers Soc Psychol 29:794–799.
18. Wolff BB. 1978. Behavioral measurement of human pain. In RA sternbach (ed), The Psychology of Pain. New York, Raven Press, pp. 129–168.
19. Wolff BB. 1980. Measurement of human pain. In JJ Bonica (ed), Pain. New York, Raven Press, pp. 173–184.
20. Williams RC. 1988. Toward a set of reliable and valid measures for chronic pain assessment in outcome research. Pain 35:239–251.
21. Huskisson EC. 1974. Measurement of pain. Lancet 2:1127–1131.
22. Melzack R. 1975. The McGill Pain Questionnaire: Major properties and scoring methods. Pain 1:277–299.
23. Ketovuori H, Pontinen PG. 1981. Pain vocabulary in Finnish: The Finnish pain questionnaire. Pain 11:247–253.
24. Kiss I, Muller H, Abel M. 1987. The McGill Pain Questionnaire — German version. A study

on cancer pain. Pain 29:195–207.

25. Radvila A, Adler RH, Galeassi RL, Vorkanf H. 1987. The development of a German language pain questionnaire and its application in a situation causing acute pain. Pain 28:185–195.
26. Maiani G, Sanavio E. 1985. Semantics of pain in Italy: The Italian version of the McGill Pain Questionnaire. Pain 22:399–405.
27. Diller A. 1980. Cross-cultural pain semantics. Pain 9:9–26.
28. Gaston-Johansson F. 1984. Pain assessment: Differences in quality and intensity of the words pain, ache and hurt. Pain 20:69–76.
29. Fabrega H, Tyma S. 1976. Culture, language and the shaping of illness: An illustration based on pain. J Psychosom Res 20:323–327.
30. Sanders SH, Brena SF. 1989. The pain center patient: Cross-cultural similarities and differences. Presentation at the Eighth Annual Meeting of the American Pain Society. Phoenix, Arizona.
31. Follick MJ, Smith TW, Hern DK. 1985. The Sickness Impact Profile: A global measure of disability in chronic low back pain. Pain 21:67–76.
32. Kerns RD, Turk DC, Rudy TE. 1985. The West Haven-Yale Multidimensional Pain Inventory (WHYMPI). Pain 23:345–356.
33. Rudy DE, Turk DC, Brena SF. 1988. The differential utility of medical procedures in the assessment of chronic pain patients. Pain 34:53–60.
34. Tait R, DeGood D, Carron H. 1982. A comparison of health locus of control beliefs in low back patients from the U.S. and New Zealand. Pain 14:53–61.
35. Wallston KA, Wallston BS, DeVellis B. 1978. Development of the Multidimensional Health Locus of Control (MHLC) scales. Health Educ Monogr 6:160–170.
36. Carron H, DeGood D, Tait R. 1985. A comparison of low back patients from the U.S. and New Zealand; psychosocial and economic factors affecting severity of disability. Pain 21:77–89.
37. Zhao F, Tsay J, Chang X, Wong W, Li S, Yao S, Chang S, Schoenberg B. 1988. Epidemiology of migraines: A survey in 21 provinces of the Peoples' Republic of China. Headache 28:558–565.
38. Brena SF, Motoyama H, Spier CG. 1990. Cross-cultural assessment of pain and function: East and West. Presentation to the Sixth World Congress on Pain. Adelaide, Australia.
39. Seres JL, Newman RI. 1983. Negative influences of the disability compensation system: Perspectives for the clinician. Semin Neurol 3:360–369.
40. Chapman SL, Brena SF. 1989. Pain and litigation. In PD Wall, R Melzack (eds), Textbook of Pain, 2nd ed. Edinburgh, Churchill-Livingstone, pp. 1032–1041.
41. Dworkin RH, Handlin DS, Richlin DM, Brand L, Vannucci C. 1985. Unraveling the effects of compensation, litigation and employment on treatment response in chronic pain. Pain 23:49–59.

3. RECENT PHYSIOLOGICAL STUDIES OF PAIN

RONALD MELZACK AND JOEL KATZ

Pain is a subjective experience that is influenced by cultural learning, the meaning of the situation, attention, and other cognitive activities [1]. Stimulation of receptors, then, does not mark the beginning of the pain process. Rather, stimulation produces neural signals that enter an active nervous system that is already the substrate of past experience, culture, anxiety, and so forth. These brain processes actively participate in the selection, abstraction, and synthesis of information from the total sensory input. Pain, therefore, is not the end product of a simple, linear sensory transmission system, but is a dynamic process that involves continuous interactions among complex ascending and descending systems.

THE GATE-CONTROL THEORY OF PAIN

The traditional specificity theory of pain, which is still taught in many medical schools, proposes that pain is a specific sensation and that the intensity of pain is proportional to the extent of tissue damage. This theory implies a fixed, straight-through transmission system from somatic pain receptors to a pain center in the brain. Recent evidence, however, shows that pain is not simply a function of the amount of bodily damage alone. Consequently, Melzack and Wall [2] proposed the gate control theory of pain, which suggests that neural mechanisms in the dorsal horns of the spinal cord act as a gate that can increase or decrease the flow of nerve impulses from peripheral fibers to the spinal cord cells that project to the brain. Somatic input is therefore subjected to the modulating influence of the gate *before* it evokes pain perception and response.

The gate-control theory suggests that large-fiber inputs (such as gentle rubbing or vibration) tend to close the gate, while small-fiber inputs (evoked by intense stimulation) generally open it, and that the gate is also profoundly influenced by descending controls from the brain. It further proposes that the sensory input is modulated at successive synapses throughout its projection from the spinal cord to the brain areas responsible for pain experience and response. Pain occurs when the number of nerve impulses that arrive at these areas exceeds a critical level. Melzack and Wall [1] have recently assessed the present-day status of the gate-control theory in the light of new physiological research. It is clear that the theory has continued to thrive and evolve despite considerable controversy. The concept of gating (or input modulation) is stronger than ever.

SPINAL CORD MECHANISMS

The dorsal horns, which receive fibers from the body and project impulses towards the brain, provide valuable clues about information processing at the spinal cord level. The dorsal horns comprise several layers or laminae, each or which is now known to have specialized functions. The inputs and outputs of each lamina are not entirely understood. But the picture that emerges reveals that the input is modulated in the dorsal horns before it is transmitted to the brain.

The substantia gelatinosa (laminae 1 and 2) is of particular interest because it represents a unique system on each side of the spinal cord that appears to have a modulating effect on the input. Many afferent fibers from the skin terminate in the substantia gelatinosa, and the dendrites of many cells in lower laminae, the axons of which project to the brain, lie within the substantia gelatinosa. This region, then, is situated between a major portion of the peripheral nerve fiber terminals and the spinal cord cells that project to the brain. There is convincing physiological evidence [1] that the substantia gelatinosa has a modulating effect on transmission from peripheral fibers to spinal cells.

Although cells in all laminae undoubtedly play a role in pain processes, lamina 5 cells are particularly responsive when noxious stimuli are applied within their receptive fields. Their fields have a remarkably complex organization, and they respond with characteristic firing patterns to stimulation over a wide range of intensities. Moreover, lamina 5 cells receive multiple inputs. There is reason to believe that they receive inputs from the lamina 4 cells, which respond readily to light touch. In addition, they receive inputs from the small myelinated and unmyelinated fibers from the skin, from deeper tissues such as blood vessels and muscles, and from the viscera [3].

It is now known that virtually all dorsal horn cells are under the control of fibers that descend from the brain. These cells, moreover, with the exception of the substantia gelatinosa, have extensive projections to the brain. In primates, the majority project through the spinothalamic tract, while some appear to project through the dorsolateral and dorsal column systems.

The small (A–delta and C–) fibers, in this conceptual framework, play a highly specialized and important role in pain processes. The activity of high-threshold small fibers, during intense stimulation, may be especially important in raising the T-cell output above the critical level necessary for pain. But the small fibers are believed [1] to do much more than this. They facilitate transmission ("open the gate") and thereby provide the basis for summation, prolonged activity, and spread of pain to other body areas. This facilitatory influence at the dorsal horns provides the small fibers with greater power than any envisaged in the concept of "pain fibers." It is also well known that endorphins and enkephalins are dorsal-horn neurotransmitters, thereby providing the neural basis for epidural morphine infusion as a way to treat severe chronic pain [4].

The C-fibers, in particular, have recently been shown [5] to play an especially important role in pain produced by injury of deep tissues. Stimulation of C-fibers emanating from subcutaneous structures, such as joints and muscles, produce changes in spinal excitability that may persist for hours and may produce a spread of excitability to adjacent cells so that the receptive fields that trigger abnormal firing may expand to include areas far beyond the injured tissue. The fact that these striking effects of stimulation of C-fibers in deep tissues does not occur when the nerves from the injured tissue are sectioned provides a rationale for the observation that regional anesthetic blocks may prevent a subsequent occurrence of pathological pain [6,7]. Kehlet [8] has recently reviewed convincing clinical evidence to support his contention that regional or epidural blocks prior to a surgical incision diminish morbidity and mortality in patients who undergo a variety of surgical procedures.

THE DIMENSIONS OF PAIN EXPERIENCE

The problem of pain, since the beginning of this century, has been dominated by the concept that pain is purely a sensory experience. Yet pain also has a distinctly unpleasant, affective quality. It becomes overwhelming, demands immediate attention, and disrupts ongoing behavior and thought. It motivates or drives the organism into activity aimed at stopping the pain as quickly as possible. To consider only the sensory features of pain and ignore its motivational-affective properties is to look at only part of the problem. Even the concept of pain as a perception, with full recognition of past experience, attention, and other cognitive influences, still neglects the crucial motivational dimension.

These considerations suggest that there are three major psychological dimensions of pain: sensory-discriminative, motivational-affective, and cognitive-evaluative. Melzack and Casey [9] have proposed that these dimensions are subserved by physiologically specialized systems in the brain (Figure 3-1).

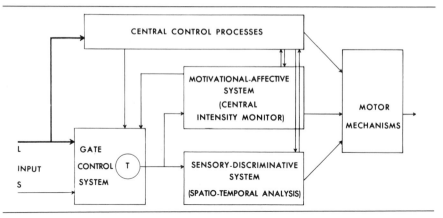

Figure 3-1. Conceptual model of the sensory, motivational, and central control determinants of pain. The output of the T (transmission) cells of the gate-control system projects to the sensory-discriminative system and the motivational-affective system. The central control trigger is represented by a line running from the large fiber system to central control processes; these, in turn, project back to the gate control system and to the sensory-discriminative and motivational-affective systems. All three systems interact with one another and project to the motor system.

The sensory-discriminative dimension

Physiological and behavioral studies suggest that several rapidly conducting systems — the neospinothalamic tract, the spinocervical tract, and the post-synaptic neurons in the dorsal column system — contribute to the sensory-discriminative dimension of pain. Neurons in the ventrobasal thalamus, which receive a large portion of their afferent input from these systems, show discrete somatotropic organization. Studies in human patients and in animals [1], taken together, suggest that the rapidly conducting projection systems have the capacity to transmit precise information about the spatial, temporal, and magnitude properties of the input that characterize the sensory-discriminative dimension of pain.

The motivational-affective dimension

There is convincing evidence [9] that the brainstem reticular formation and the limbic system, which receive projections from the spinoreticular and paleo-spinothalamic components of the anterolateral somatosensory pathway, play a particularly important role in the motivational-affective dimension of pain. These medially coursing fibers, which comprise a "paramedial ascending system" [9], tend to be short and to connect diffusely with one another during their ascent from the spinal cord to the brain. They are not organized to carry discrete spatial and temporal information. Their target cells in the brain usually have wide receptive fields, sometimes covering half or more of the body surface. In addition to the convergence of somatosensory fibers, inputs from other sensory systems, such as vision and audition, also arrive at many of these cells.

Reticular formation

It is now well established that the reticular formation is involved in aversive drive and similar pain-related behavior. Stimulation of nucleus gigantocellularis in the medulla [10] and the central grey and adjacent areas in the midbrain [11] produces strong aversive drive and behavior typical of responses to naturally occurring painful stimuli. In contrast, lesions of the central grey or spinothalamic tract produce marked decreases in responsiveness to noxious stimuli [12]. Similarly, at the thalamic level, "fearlike" responses associated with escape behavior have been elicited by stimulation in the medial and adjacent intralaminar nuclei of the thalamus [13]. In the human, lesions in the medial thalamus (parafascicular and centromedian complex) and intralaminar nuclei have provided relief from intractable pain [14].

Limbic system

The reciprocal interconnections between the reticular formation and the limbic system is of particular importance in pain processes [9]. The midbrain central grey, which is traditionally part of the reticular formation, is also a major gateway to the limbic system. It is part of the "limbic midbrain" area [15] that projects to the medial thalamus and hypothalamus, which in turn project to limbic forebrain structures. Many of these areas also interact with portions of the frontal cortex that are sometimes functionally designated as part of the limbic system.

It is now firmly established [9] that the limbic system plays an important role in pain processes. Electrical stimulation of the hippocampus, amygdala, or other limbic structures may evoke escape or other attempts to stop stimulation [16]. After ablation of the amygdala and overlying cortex, cats show marked changes in affective behavior, including decreased responsiveness to noxious stimuli [17]. Surgical section of the cingulum bundle, which connects the frontal cortex to the hippocampus, also produces a loss of "negative affect" associated with intractable pain in human subjects [18]. This evidence indicates that limbic structures, although they play a role in many other functions, provide a neural basis for the aversive drive and affect that comprise the motivational dimension of pain.

The cognitive-evaluative dimension

We have already noted that cognitive activities, such as cultural values, anxiety, attention, and suggestion, all have a profound effect on pain experience. These activities, which are subserved in part at least by cortical processes, may affect the sensory-discriminative dimension or the motivational-affective dimension. Thus, excitement in games or war appears to block both of these dimensions of pain, while suggestion and placebos may modulate the motivational-affective dimension and leave the sensory-discriminative dimension relatively undisturbed.

Cognitive functions, then, are able to act selectively on sensory processing or motivational mechanisms. In addition, there is evidence that the sensory input is localized, identified in terms of its physical properties, evaluated in terms of past experience, and modified *before* it activates the discriminative or motivational systems. Soldiers wounded in battle may feel little or no pain from the wound but may complain bitterly about an inept vein puncture [19]. Dogs that repeatedly receive food immediately after the skin is shocked, burned, or cut soon respond to these stimuli as signals for food and salivate, without showing any signs of pain, yet howl as normal dogs would when the stimuli are applied to other sites on the body [20].

The neural system that performs these complex functions of identification, evaluation, and selective input modulation must conduct rapidly to the cortex so that somatosensory information has the opportunity to undergo further analysis, interact with other sensory inputs, and activate memory stores and preset response strategies. It must then be able to act selectively on the sensory and motivational systems in order to influence their response to the information being transmitted over more slowly conducting pathways. Melzack and Wall [2] have proposed that the dorsal-column and dorsolateral projection pathways act as the "feed-forward" limb of this loop. Moreover, the powerful descending inhibitory influences exerted on dorsal-horn cells in the spinal cord [21] can modulate the input before it is transmitted to the discriminative and motivational systems (Figure 3-1). These rapidly conducting ascending and descending systems can thus account for the fact that psychological processes play a powerful role in determining the quality and intensity of pain.

The conceptual model

The physiological and behavioral evidence described above led Melzack and Casey [9] to extend the gate-control theory to include the motivational dimension of pain (Figure 3-1). They proposed that

1. The sensory-discriminative dimension of pain is influenced primarily by the rapidly conducting spinal systems.
2. The powerful motivational drive and unpleasant affect characteristic of pain are subserved by activities in reticular and limbic structures that are influenced primarily by the slowly conducting spinal systems.
3. Neocortical or higher central nervous system processes, such as evaluation of the input in terms of past experience, exert control over activity in both the discriminative and motivational systems.

It is assumed that these three categories of activity interact with one another to provide *perceptual information* regarding the location, magnitude, and spatio-temporal properties of the noxious stimulus, *motivational tendency* toward escape or attack, and *cognitive information* based on analysis of multimodal information, past experience, and probability of outcome of different response strategies. All three forms of activity could then influence motor mechanisms responsible for the complex pattern of overt responses that characterize pain.

CHRONIC AND ACUTE PAIN

The time course of pain is profoundly important in determining its psychological effects on an organism. Acute pain, which is usually associated with a well-defined cause (such as a burned finger or a ruptured appendix), normally has a characteristic time course and vanishes after healing has occurred. The pain usually has a rapid onset — the *phasic* component — and the subsequent *tonic* component that persists for variable periods of time. Chronic pain states, such as low back pain, the neuralgias, or phantom limb pain, may begin as acute pain and pass through both the phasic and tonic phases. The tonic pain, however, may persist long after the injury has healed. It is then labelled as *chronic pain* and appears to involve neural mechanisms that are far more complex than those of acute pain. The pain not only persists but may spread to adjacent or more distant body areas. It is resistant to surgical control and its prolonged time course is characteristically associated with high levels of anxiety and depression. We will first deal with the neural mechanisms of acute pain and then briefly examine some of the properties of chronic pain.

Dennis and Melzack [22] reviewed the properties of the spinal cord pain-signalling pathways and speculated on some of their possible functions. One set of pathways, the "lateral" pathways, is rapidly conducting and seems to be particularly well suited to convey phasic information. The value of rapidly conducting, direct pain-signalling systems is obvious: Unless an organism reacts quickly, a stimulus that only threatens tissue damage may become overtly damaging.

A second set of pathways is slowly conducting. These pathways are unlikely to signal the need for immediate action. Instead, they are more likely to play a role in chronic, deeply unpleasant, diffuse pain, as well as to contribute to the longer lasting motivational-affective dimension of pain. These "medial pathways" seem best adapted to carry *tonic* information on the state of the organism. Thus, they continue to send messages as long as the wound is susceptible to reinjury. These messages may prevent further damage, and foster rest, protection, and care of the injured areas, thereby promoting healing and recuperative processes.

MEMORY MECHANISM IN PAIN

A memorylike mechanism may account for pain in the absence of a detectable lesion or any other peripheral input that can account for the pain. A patient in whom a memorylike mechanism such as this is active may be diagnosed as a malingerer or a conversion hysteric when, in fact, a central neural mechanism, such as self-sustaining neural activity, may be the major underlying cause of the pain.

There is now a growing literature on the neural mechanisms of prolonged, memorylike activity related to referred pain. An injury of a hindpaw in the rat produces a heightened sensitivity to pain (hyperalgesia) in the same paw *and* in the opposite paw [23,24]. Surprisingly, the hyperalgesia in the contralateral paw persists even after all the nerves from the injured area are completely sectioned. These results show clearly that the hyperalgesia is dependent on abnormal activity in the central nervous system, probably the spinal cord. There is excellent evidence, moreover, that the changes in central neural activity continue for many weeks or longer after injury [25]. Thus, there is a growing body of data to show that surgical patients who receive an epidural block, in addition to a general anesthetic, have significantly less pain and fewer pain-related complications during and after recovery than patients who have surgery with only a general anesthetic.

HYPERSTIMULATION ANALGESIA

It is an assumption that memorylike circuits plays a role in pain. However, it is a fact that chronic pain can be controlled by relatively brief decreases or increases of the sensory input. This clinical fact can be explained in terms of a disruption of memorylike mechanisms.

It is well known that short-acting, local anesthetic blocks of trigger points often produce prolonged, sometimes permanent relief of some forms of myofascial or visceral pain [26,27]. Astonishingly, brief, intense stimulation of trigger points by dry needling [27], intense cold [27], or injection of normal saline [28] often produces prolonged relief of some forms of myofascial or visceral pain. This type of pain relief, which may be generally labelled as *hyperstimulation analgesia* [29], is one of the oldest methods used for the control of pain. It is sometimes known as *counterirritation*, and includes such methods of folk medicine as application of mustard plasters, ice packs, hot cups, or blistering agents to parts of the body.

This interest in folk medicine gained enormous impetus in recent years by the rediscovery of the ancient Chinese practice of acupuncture — inserting needles into specific body sites and twirling them manually. More recently, the Chinese have practiced electroacupuncture, in which electrical pulses are passed through the needles. We now know that the original claims that acupuncture produces surgical analgesia (or anesthesia) have not been borne out by later investigation. However, acupuncture stimulation has been shown in several well-controlled clinical and experimental investigations [30] to provide substantial relief of pain. This is not surprising because it is now evident that there is nothing mysterious or magical about acupuncture; it is a form of *hyperstimulation analgesia* comparable to cupping or blistering the skin.

Transcutaneous electrical nerve stimulation has recently been found to provide a powerful technique for the control of pain. When it is administered the same way as acupuncture — for brief periods of time at moderate-to-high stimulation intensities (just below painful levels) — it frequently produces pain relief that outlasts the 20-minute period of stimulation by several hours, occasionally for days or weeks [29,31]. Daily stimulation carried out at home by the patient sometimes provides gradually increasing relief over periods of weeks or months. A further study [32] examined the correlation between trigger points and acupuncture points for pain. The results of the analysis showed that every trigger point reported in the Western medical literature has a corresponding acupuncture point. Furthermore, there is a close correspondence, 71%, between the pain syndromes associated with the two kinds of points. This close correlation suggests that trigger points and acupuncture points for pain, though discovered independently and labelled differently, represent the same phenomenon and can be explained in terms of the same underlying neural mechanisms.

There are three major properties of hyperstimulation analgesia: 1) a moderate-to-intense sensory input is applied to the body to alleviate pain, 2) the sensory input is sometimes applied to a site distant from the site of pain, and 3) the sensory input, which is usually of brief duration (ranging from a few

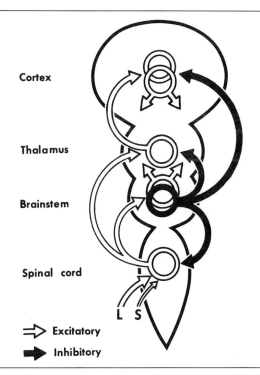

Figure 3-2. Schematic diagram of the central biasing mechanism. Large and small fibers from a limb activate a neuron pool in the spinal cord, which excites neuron pools at successively higher levels. The central biasing mechanism, represented by the inhibitory projection system that originates in the brainstem reticular formation, modulates activity at all levels. When sensory fibers are destroyed after amputation or peripheral nerve lesion, the inhibitory influence decreases. This results in sustained activity at all levels that can be triggered repeatedly by the remaining fibers. Stimulation of the central biasing mechanism increases descending inhibition and tends to "close the gate" to pain-signaling inputs. L = large fibers; S = small fibers.

seconds to 20 or 30 minutes) may relieve chronic pain for days, weeks, or sometimes permanently.

The relief of pain by brief, intense stimulation of distant trigger points (or acupuncture points) can be explained physiologically in terms of the gate control theory. The most plausible explanation [1] seems to be that the brainstem areas that are known to exert a powerful inhibitory control over transmission in the pain signalling system may be involved (Figure 3-2). The descending controls, which have been labelled as a "central biasing mechanism" [29] or as "diffuse noxious inhibitory controls" [21], receive inputs from widespread parts of the body and, in turn, project to widespread parts of the spinal cord. The stimulation of particular nerves or tissues by transcutaneous electrical stimulation or any other form of stimulation that activates small fibers could bring about an increased input to the central biasing mechanism, which would close the gates to pain signals from selected body areas.

There has been recent support for this hypothesis. Direct electrical stimulation of the brainstem areas that produce behavioral analgesia inhibits the transmission of nerve impulses in dorsal horn cells that have been implicated in gate-control mechanisms. Bilateral lesions of the dorsolateral spinal cord abolish these inhibitory effects and also abolish or reduce the analgesia produced by brainstem stimulation and morphine [33]. Furthermore, the analgesia-producing brainstem areas are known to be highly sensitive to morphine, and the effect of stimulation is partially reduced by the administration of naloxone, an opiate antagonist [33]. The demonstration that naloxone also reduces the analgesic effects of transcutaneous electrical stimulation and acupuncture is consistent with the hypothesis that intense stimulation activates a neural feedback loop through the brainstem analgesia-producing areas.

CENTRAL PATTERN-GENERATING MECHANISMS

The complexity of the interacting sensory and psychological factors in pain and its management is highlighted by studies of chronic phantom body pain in paraplegics with total spinal cord lesions. Melzack and Loeser [34] reviewed cases of patients who had sustained total spinal cord sections at thoracic or lumbar levels, yet continued to suffer severe pain in the abdomen, groin, or legs. The completeness of the lesion was verified visually during surgical removal of injured tissue or as a result of segmental cordectomy (the removal of an entire section of the spinal cord) to prevent nerve impulses produced by injured tissues from reaching the brain. Nevertheless, pain returned immediately or as long as 11 years later. The pain was usually felt in definite parts of the body phantom and was often described as burning, crushing, or cramping. The sympathetic ganglia, the only other possible route for nerve impulses from the legs, were also blocked in several patients without effect on the pain. Since there is no known anatomical substrate for sensory input from the lower abdomen or legs to enter the spinal cord above midthoracic levels, it is evident that peripheral input from levels below the total transection is not the cause of pain in these patients. Although many of the patients were severely depressed by their physical status as paraplegics, there was no evidence that the pain was caused by depression or neurosis. On the basis of the clinical data, Melzack and Loeser proposed that the loss of input to central structures after deafferentation may play an important role in producing pain.

The effects of deafferentation on the activity of central neurons have been investigated in several contexts. Loeser and Ward [35] showed that cutting several dorsal roots in the cat produces abnormal bursts of firing in dorsal horn cells that persist for as long as 180 days after the root section. Furthermore, single shock pulses to adjacent intact roots produce prolonged firing that persists for hundreds of milliseconds. These abnormal patterns are commonly seen after deafferentation. Non-noxious input also has the ability to trigger the high-frequency firing patterns. It is of particular interest that this abnormal activity has been recorded from lamina 5 cells, which are known to be involved in sensory transmission processes related to pain. Similar abnormal activity in trigeminal cells in the cat is also seen after extraction of all the teeth on one side [34].

The abnormal firing patterns observed in the deafferented spinal cord in cats have also been observed in humans [34]. In one case, just prior to cordectomy, the deafferented cord was examined physiologically with microelectrodes. The cells showed abnormal bursting activity that resembled that seen after chronic deafferentation in the cat spinal cord.

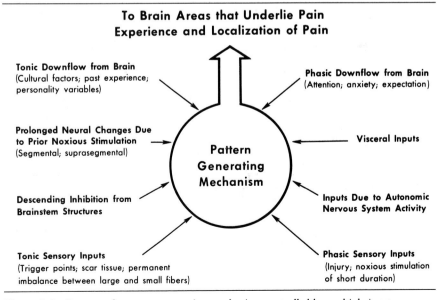

Figure 3-3. Concept of a pattern-generating mechanism controlled by multiple inputs.

These observations led Melzack and Loeser to suggest a concept (Figure 3-3) of pain to explain the clinical data. They proposed that neuron pools at many levels of the spinal cord and brain can act as *pattern-generating mechanisms*. These neuron pools are assumed to comprise the dorsal horns (i.e., the entire gate system) in the spinal cord and the homologous interacting systems associated with the cranial nerves. They proposed that other nuclei along the course of the major somatosensory projection systems can act as pattern-generating mechanisms. These cells are normally under sensory and downstream control. When deafferentation occurs, however, the cells fire spontaneously in abnormal bursts for prolonged periods of time. They proposed that the pattern-generating mechanisms, in paraplegics, must lie above the level of spinal transection or cordectomy. Furthermore, those regions responsible for pattern generation are assumed to project to the regions of the brain involved in precise localization of sensory inputs, that is, those neural areas that subserve the body schema, as well as to the areas that subserve pain experience.

The concept of central pattern-generating mechanisms provides an explanation for those pain states that are characterized by degeneration of sensory nerve fibers, dorsal root pathology, or spinal injury. Many of the neuralgias occur after partial nerve injury, and causalgia occurs more frequently after partial than after total peripheral nerve lesions [1]. Even phantom limb pain is associated with partial nerve damage, since a portion of the fibers in a nerve bundle degenerates after total section, while the remainder regenerates into the stump tissue [1]. Partial deafferentation, therefore, may alter the activity of cells in the spinal cord and brain, and produce the nerve impulse patterns that subserve pain.

There is now convincing evidence [36] of "pain memories" in phantom limbs, that is, phantom limb sensations that resemble somatosensory events experienced in the limb before amputation. These somatosensory memories are predominantly replicas of distressing preamputation lesions and pains that were experienced at, or near, the time of amputation, and are described as having the same qualities of sensation as the preamputation pain. The patients who experience these pains emphasize that they are suffering real pain that they can describe in vivid detail, and insist that the experience is not merely a cognitive recollection of an earlier pain. Among the somatosensory memories reported are cutaneous lesions, deep tissue injuries, bone and joint pain, and painful preamputation postures. These findings suggest that somatosensory inputs of sufficient intensity and duration can produce long-term changes in central neural structures.

These data have recently received support from studies with animals [37]. Peripheral neurectomy in rats is followed by self-mutilation (autotomy) in which the animal chews and scratches the distal portions of the insensitive paw to the point of amputation. It is well established that autotomy is a response to painful or dysesthetic sensations referred to the denervated limb. Several studies have found that the onset of autotomy is earlier if the paw is injured prior to nerve section. Katz et al. [37] have shown that electrical stimulation of the sciatic nerve prior to neurectomy results in a significantly greater incidence of autotomy and even changes the pattern of autotomy. These results suggest that the central excitability produced by sciatic nerve stimulation prior to nerve section is retained in CNS structures as a somatosensory pain memory. They complement reports of amputees with phantom limb pain characterized by the persistence of a painful preamputation lesion.

REFERENCES

1. Melzack R, Wall PD. 1988. The Challenge of Pain. New York, Penguin Books.
2. Melzack R, Wall PD. 1965. Pain mechanisms: A new theory. Science 150:971–979.
3. Pomeranz B, Wall PD, Weber WV. 1968. Cord cells responding to fine myelinated afferents from viscera, muscle and skin. J Physiol 199:511–532.
4. Yaksh TL, Stevens CW. 1988. Properties of the modulation of spinal nociceptive transmission by receptor-selective agents. In R Dubner, GF Gebhart, MR Bond (eds), Proceedings of the Vth World Congress on Pain. Amsterdam, Elsevier Press, pp. 417–435.
5. Wall PD. 1988. Stability and instability of central pain mechanisms. In R Dubner, GF Gebhart, MR Bond (eds), Proceedings of the Vth World Congress on Pain. Amsterdam, Elsevier Press, pp. 13–24.
6. McQuay HJ, Carroll D, Moore RA. 1988. Postoperative orthopaedic pain — the effect of opiate premedication and local anaesthetic blocks. Pain 33:291–295.
7. Bach S, Noreng MF, Tjellden NU. 1988. Phantom limb pain in amputees during the first 12 months following amputation, after preoperative lumbar epidural blockade. Pain 33:297–301.
8. Kehlet H. 1988. Modification of responses to surgery by neural blockade: Clinical implications. In MJ Cousins, PO Bridenbaugh (eds), Neural Blockade. C Philadelphia, pp. 145–188.
9. Melzack R, Casey KL. 1968. Sensory, motivational, and central control determinants of pain: A new conceptual model. In D Kenshalo (ed), The Skin Senses. Springfield, IL, Charles C. Thomas, pp. 423–443.
10. Casey KL. 1970. Somatosensory responses of bulboreticular units in awake cat: Relation to escape-producing stimuli. Science 173:77–80.
11. Delgado JMR. 1955. Cerebral structures involved in transmission and elaboration of noxious stimulation. J Neurophysiol 18:261–275.
12. Melzack R, Stotler WA, Livingston WK. 1958. Effects of discrete brainstem lesions in cats on perception of noxious stimulation. J Neurophysiol 21:353–357.
13. Roberts WW. 1962. Fear-like behavior elicited from dorsomedial thalamies of cat. J Comp Physiol Psychol 55:191–197.
14. White JC, Sweet WH. 1969. Pain and the Neurosurgeon. Springfield, IL Charles C. Thomas.
15. Nauta WJH. 1958. Hippocampal projections and related neural pathways to the midbrain in the cat. Brain 81:319–340.
16. Delgado JMR, Rosvold HE, Looney E. 1956. Evoking conditioned fear by electrical stimulation of subcortical structures in the monkey brain. J Comp Physiol Psychol 49:373–380.
17. Schreiner L, Kling A. 1953. Behavioral changes following rhinencephalic injury in cat. J Neurophysiol 15:643–659.
18. Foltz EL, White LE. 1962. Pain "relief" by frontal cingulumotomy. J Neurosurg 19:89–100.
19. Beecher HK. 1959. Measurement of Subjective Responses. New York, Oxford University Press.
20. Pavlor IP. 1928. Lectures on Conditional Reflexes. New York, International Publishers.
21. Le Bars D, Dickenson AH, Besson JM. 1983. Opiate analgesia and descending control systems. In JJ Bonica, U Lindblom, A Iggo (eds), Advances in Pain Research and Therapy, Vol. 5. New York, Raven Press, pp. 341–372.
22. Dennis SG, Melzack R. 1977. Pain-signalling systems in the dorsal and ventral spinal cord. Pain 4:97–132.
23. Coderre TJ, Melzack R. 1985. Increased pain sensitivity following heat injury involves a central mechanism. Behav Brain Res 15:259–262.
24. Coderre TJ, Melzack R. 1986. Procedures which increase acute pain sensitivity also increase

autotomy. Exp Neurol 92:713–722.

25. Dennis SG, Melzack R. 1979. Self-mutilation after dorsal rhizotomy in rats: Effects of prior pain and pattern of root lesions. Exp Neurol 65:412–421.
26. Livingston WK. 1943. Pain Mechanisms. New York, Macmillan.
27. Travell JG, Simons DG. 1983. Myofascial Pain and Dysfunction: The Trigger Point Manual. Baltimore, Williams & Wilkins.
28. Frost FA, Jessen B, Siggaard-Andersen J. 1980. A control, double-blind comparison of mepivacaine injections versus saline injection for myofascial pain. Lancet 8:499–501.
29. Melzack R. 1975. Prolonged relief of pain by brief, intense transcutaneous somatic stimulation. Pain 1:357–373.
30. Chapman CR, Colpitts YM, Benedetti C, Kitaeff R, Gehrig JD. 1980. Evoked potential assessment of acupunctural analgesia: Attempted reversal with naloxone. Pain 9:183–197.
31. Fox EJ, Melzack R. 1976. Transcutaneous electrical stimulation and acupuncture: Comparison of treatment for low back pain. Pain 2:141–148.
32. Melzack R, Stillwell DM, Fox EJ. 1977. Trigger points and acupuncture points for pain: Correlations and implications. Pain 3:3–23.
33. Basbaum AI, Marley NJE, O'Keefe J, Clanton CH. 1977. Reversal of morphine and stimulus produced analgesia by subtotal spinal cord lesions. Pain 3:43–56.
34. Melzack R, Loeser JD. 1978. Phantom body pain in paraplegics: Evidence for a central "pattern generating mechanism" for pain. Pain 4:195–210.
35. Loeser JD, Ward AA. 1967. Some effects of deafferentation on neurons of the cat spinal cord. Arch Neurol 17:629–636.
36. Katz J, Melzack R. 1990. Pain "memories" in phantom limbs: Review and clinical observations. Pain 43:319–336.
37. Katz J, Vaccarino AL, Coderre TC, Melzack R. 1991. Injury prior to neurectomy alters the pattern of autonomy in rats. In preparation.

4. ANALGESIOLOGY: A NEW APPROACH TO PAIN

RIS DIRKSEN

Pain has been defined as an unpleasant sensory and emotional experience associated with actual or potential tissue damage, or described in terms of such damage [1]. Conditions of insensitivity to pain are usually discovered before the age of 20 [2], because the absence of any reaction to avoid noxious stimulation results in injuries. In this context, pain and the perception of pain are not isolated phenomena, but parts of regulatory systems that protect the individual against violations of homeostasis. The second aspect of pain is that it disturbs the normal sensory state of a living being. The normal state can be regarded as the normosensoperceptive condition to be maintained in the physiological range by means of various cooperative and coordinated mechanisms (sensory homeostasis).

These two aspects of pain involve two distinct parts of the central nervous system. As Figure 4-1 illustrates, the pain system is hierarchically organized in serial and parallel tracts, and relay nuclei. It also shows that the two parts of the sensory system, referred to as the nociperception and loop system, do not function separately. Functional balance and neuronal connections exist between both parts.

THE ROLE OF NOCICEPTION IN GENERAL HOMEOSTASIS
Nociperception is the awareness of pain. This means that a signal generated in the peripheral nerve endings has acted as an input to the integrative circuits of the sensory cortex (see Figure 4-1). The connections that serve this purpose

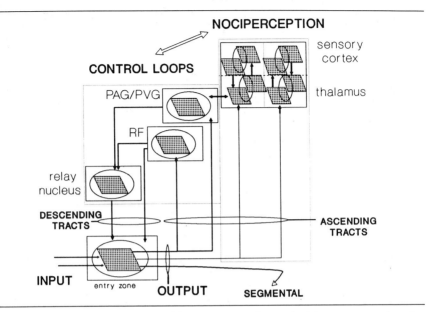

Figure 4-1. Schematic presentation of the "pain system" organized in two parts subserving control loops and nociperception. PAG/PVG = periaqueaductal/periventricular gray; RF = reticular formation; segmental = segmental output (e.g., to a flexor muscle); dotted areas = neuronal mazes; arrows = (functional) connections.

include the sensory tracts that synapse in the spinal cord, the nuclei of the brain stem, the sensory nuclei of the thalamus, and the cortex [3]. Noticably, only part of the projections of these systems maintains somatotopic organization.

The medial lemniscus systems synapse in the spinal cord and the sensory information ascend in the somatotopically organized gracile and cuneate fascicles. The fascicles terminate in synapses of the corresponding nuclei in the most caudal part of the medulla oblongata and ascend further in the medial lemniscus [3]. These fascicles and spinothalamic projections have terminal fields organized in clusters in the principal ventroposterolateral nucleus of the thalamus. Similarly, somatotopic organization is maintained in the cortical projections to and within the columns of the primary somatosensory cortex. The protopathic system subserves pain and temperature, and yields ungraded, diffuse impressions of an all-or-none character. The protopathic system is distinguished from the epicritic system, which subserves a discriminative function. The signal transfer of the protopathic system occurs along the spino-thalamic tract of the anterolateral system. The terminal fields of this tract are located in the medial division of the posterior group of the thalamus and are not somatopically organized [3,4]. The spatially separate areas of the thalamus with their different patterns of nerve endings give origin to complementary thalamic outputs to the cortex that maintain the different patterns [5].

The different hierarchic levels of the nociperceptive part of the pain system participate in the transfer and recognition of noxious signals. This process is essential to maintaining general homeostasis. The intrinsic control systems of homeostasis have basic components: the controlled variable, a sensor, a comparator, and an effector [6]. The purpose of a control system is to maintain the controlled variable within narrow limits.

A noxious stimulus is the controlled variable for the nociperceptive part of the central nervous system, and its presence activates, even in the absence of nociperception, nocifensive mechanisms leading to an effort of the organism to avoid the noxious cause by means of an effector. For example, the flexor muscles are the effector(s) in a noxious induced withdrawal reaction (Figure 4–2). When the period that the signal has served as a warning signal has elapsed, the persisting sensation of pain causes suffering. This indicates that there are limits to the effectiveness of the control mechanisms of sensory homeostasis.

REGULATION OF THE SENSORY HOMEOSTASIS

Analgesic or antinociceptive effects of stress or electrical stimulation indicate that intrinsic mechanisms can be activated to minimize a deviation from the normosensoperceptive condition [7–10]. The presence of interindividual differences in the state of activity of such endogenous control mechanisms is illustrated by the uncommon inherited syndrome of insensitivity to pain [11]. A high level of tonic activity of endorphinergic controls has been proposed to cause the shift of the set point of the threshold to pain, as naloxone has resulted

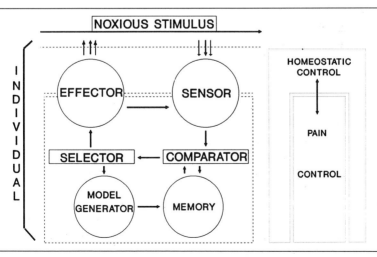

Figure 4-2. Scheme of the control system of an individual. The controlled variable of nociperception is the noxious stimulus and that of the loop systems is the (resulting) activity of the neurones in the entry zone. The presence of the two parts of the "pain system" is indicated with dotted lines.

in a return of that set point to normal [12]. Although endorphinergic and other endogenous pain control mechanisms (see sections on loop systems and endorphin systems) are responsive in normal humans as well, the persistence of pain in states of ongoing activation of the primary afferents indicates that there are limits to the extent that the regulatory mechanisms can effect a return of sensory perception to its setpoint. If limits of regulation are violated too long or too heavily, an uncontrolled state will develop. In chronic pain the uncontrolled state results in dysfunction, disuse, and trophic and sudomotor changes in and outside the affected area. In the acute state of pain, the uncontrolled state can result in life-threatening pain shock. These hazards of the uncontrolled state make it obvious that one should always provide adequate pain relief, and that one should not rely on the presence of endogenous pain control mechanisms. However, adequate pain treatment acknowledges the organization and directions of efforts of endogenous control mechanisms, because it is important to decide whether therapeutic efforts should supplement, augment, or rather reduce activities of intrinsic mechanisms.

Various endogenous mechanisms that act to change the processing of the afferent inputs have been recognized. Some of these will be described below as contingents of recognized functional and neuroanatomical entities: 1) the type of information carried in the primary afferent fibers (primary afferent channels, 2) secondary activation of the loop systems (loop systems), and 3) the endorphinergic mechanisms (endorphin systems). These entities are generally thought to act in a single direction of effect, i.e., the primary afferents are thought to excite and transfer the evoked stimulus; the descending tracts are proposed to exert an inhibitory influence in case of a noxious stimulus (negative feedback); and, as the opiates are powerful analgesics, the endorphins of the endorphin systems have been popularly designated as causing a pain-inhibitory effect.

Primary afferent channels

The primary afferent input in the central nervous system evoked by the noxious stimuli is a result of activation of the peripheral sensors. Owing to differences in the type of primary afferent nerves of these peripheral sensors [13] and consequently the differences in speed of signal transmission and type of neurotransmitter substances, the release of the neurotransmitters in the terminal fields of the primary afferents has a time-dependent pattern. The marginal zone and the substantia gelatinosa of the dorsal horn are regarded as the sites where C- and A-delta primary afferent fibers have terminal fields [14–16]. However, the area surrounding the central canal (lamina X) is similar in many ways to the dorsal horn and functions as an additional site where the primary afferents have terminal fields [17]. The terminal fields of primary afferents constitute their functional entry zone (see Figure 4-1).

The numerous neurotransmitter substances released from the various primary afferent fibers in the entry zone of the spinal cord are diverse and include excitatory amino acids, such as glutamic acid, peptides [18], and even combinations of excitatory substances [19]. Some types of noxious stimuli (electrical stimuli, noxious heat, mechanical or visceral stimuli) cause the release of the "modality-specific substances," e.g., somatostatin, calcitonin gene-related peptide (CGRP), substance P, or vasoactive intestinal peptide (VIP) [20–24]. The administration of the primary afferent excitatory transmitter in the vicinity of the entry zone can be expected to mimic the function of the natural substance, and to cause an increase in the response to and perception of a noxious stimulus ("hyperalgesia"). This was illustrated by numerous data on spinal effects of various substances. For example, VIP depolarizes dorsal root terminals and decreases the reaction time of nociceptive responses in the rat [24]. Similarly, substance P and substance-P agonists cause a decrease in reaction time in the tail-flick reflex and vocalization in rats [25]. Somatostatin has caused scratching, and an increase in the hamstring reflex and conditioned C-fiber activation [26,27]. Also, a diminished availability of endogenous primary afferent excitatory transmitter substances will enhance the nociceptive threshold. Antiserum to CGRP produced this effect and was found to reduce hyperalgesia in rats with an induced arthritis [23].

The administration of modality-specific excitatory primary afferent transmitter substances, however, does not necessarily result in a mimicry of the physiological function of pain mediation. Antinociception or a biphasic effect of antinociception and hyperalgesia may actually be obtained. An antinociceptive effect was found after the selective administration of somatostatin and substance P [28–30]. The biphasic effect was reported after intrathecal injections of substance P [31] and CCK-8 [32]. In humans, the controversial treatment with perispinal somatostatin has resulted in pain relief [33].

These paradoxical effects can be explained by appreciating the fact that a signal of pain is necessary to the maintenance of general homeostasis. This function, tied to the part of the sensory system engaged in nociperception (see Figure 4-1), ensures that the signal of pain acquires priority for its transfer and processing. A warning signal will be more evident when other types of information that comprise a continuous input at the entry zone are silenced, i.e., attention focusing. It can be assumed that inhibitory mechanisms of primary afferent excitatory transmitters are accomplished by activation of inhibitory interneurons, such as the enkephalinergic or GABA-ergic (gamma amino butyric acid). Another explanation is that, although a substance identical to the primary afferent excitatory transmitter addresses the postsynaptic receptor after its injection, the access to these sites and signal transfer across the synaptic cleft will not be synchronized [34]. The paradoxical effect may therefore evolve from a remaining modulatory (protracted) or inhibitory action, as the signal of pain is not generated. Also, the transfer of the noxious signal may involve multiple transmitters rather than a single modality specific substance [35,36].

Loop systems

Each entry zone of the central nervous system is part of loop systems that include the neurogenic tracts ascending to supraspinally located neuronal populations and the descending tracts (see Figure 4-1). Examples of the supraspinal relay nuclei are the nucleus reticularis gigantocellularis, the mesencephalic reticular formation, the periaqueductal and periventricular grey matter, and the locus coeruleus [37,38]. These neuronal groups give origin to descending tracts to the spinal cord, with the nucleus raphe magnocellularis as an intermediate relay for an essential part of them [39] (see Figure 4-1). Further, the spinothalamic and spinocortical projections are known to be elements of loops that connect the spinal cord to higher hierarchic levels and then allow the processed signal to be fed back onto the spinal cord [40.41]. It is worth noting that: 1) there are different numbers and types of synaptic connections, 2) signal transfer occurs along neuronal tracts of different lengths, and 3) different functions are assigned to the two parts of nociperception and loop system (see Figure 4-1). Therefore, the loop systems provide the spinal cord with a signal that is a multifunction of relay and time (multispatiotemporal feedback).

Electrical stimulation of several of the nuclei that are components of the loop systems selectively suppresses nociception and activity in ascending axons in the spinal cord evoked by afferent A-delta and C-fiber stimulation in animals [42] as well as pain in humans [9,10,43]. Selective injection of opioid agonists in these nuclei also produces analgesia, but not necessarily by an action that involves the site within the nuclei where electrical stimulation takes effect, or by the same mechanism or effect as that of electrical stimulation [42,44,45]. Numerous transmitter and modulatory substances participate in these inhibitory descending tracts, and especially noradrenalin, dopamine, and serotonin are considered to contribute significantly to inhibitory mechanisms [46]. Yet, the activation of the descending tracts also enhances noxious afferent signal transfer [47–50]. Although facilitation of noxious signal transfer and pain inhibition caused by the descending tracts are obviously opposite in effect, similar inhibitory mechanisms are involved. The major difference is the site at which the inhibition is effected. For instance, if the levels above and below a level of input are inhibited, attention focusing is effected (see Figure 4-3A). Conversely, if the input at a level of entrance is inhibited (see Figure 4-3B), then antinociception is effected. It is consistent with the function of attention focusing that activation of descending tracts also results in a diminished activity of non-noxious neurons and ascending projection neurons [51,52], as such a diminished activity emphasizes the contrast between noxious and other types of input.

Endorphin systems

At the present, distinct classes of endogenous opioid ligands with distinct patterns of distribution in the central nervous system are recognized and

ATTENTION FOCUSING

DESCENDING TRACTS

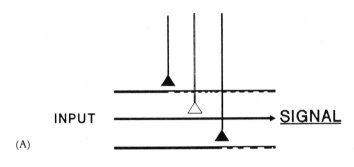

(A)

INHIBITORY CONTROL

DESCENDING TRACTS

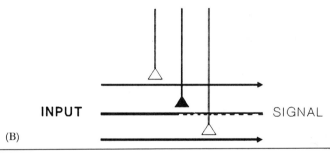

(B)

Figure 4-3. Scheme of descending tracts functional to (A) attention focusing (left) or (B) inhibitory control (right).

named after their precursor molecules, i.e., the proenkephalin–, the pro-dynorphin–, and the pro-opiomelanocortin-derived ligands. The accessory different types of receptor sites have been identified: μ_1-, μ_2-, σ-, δ-, K-, and ε- (sub)types. These sites act as the transducing factors in the actions of the active opioid ligands that derive from their precursor molecules [53]. At various sites of the above-described loop systems, μ_1-sites transduce powerful antinociceptive effects of locally injected specific agonistic ligands [54]. Drugs that bind selectively to receptor subtypes cause antinociception restricted to a specific type of afferent noxious stimulation [55] or cause antinociception by actions mainly at the supraspinal (e.g., pentazocine) or spinal level (e.g., morphine) [56]. Apart from these direct mechanisms resulting from an opioid receptor–agonist interaction, activation of descending noradrenergic and serotonergic inhibitory mechanisms (see Loop systems) results from specific μ-agonistic actions [57]. Indirect activation of descending tracts that involves the spinal release of met-enkephalin is caused by a supraspinal effect of β-endorphin only [58]. Also at the thalamic level, opioid mechanisms participate in nociception [59], although opiates administered in this site do not unequivocally cause an antinociceptive effect [60]. Finally, the neuronal proopiomelanocortin system that originates in the nucleus arcuatus is linked to the nociceptive system in the (PAG) periaqueductal grey area [61]. The neuronal part and the humoral part of the proopiomelanocortin system are activated in and contribute to the state of shock [62,63], and a similar activation can result from the excessive input of untreated pain (pain shock).

Even though the administration of a pharmacological dose of μ-agonistic drugs results in a reliable pain–inhibitory effect, the actions of these (and other types of) ligands for the receptors of the endorphin systems are complex, both in their mode of addressing the multiple receptor sites and in the resulting directions of effect. This latter effect also applies to the "simple" agonist morphine. Morphine has both excitatory and inhibitory effects on neurons of the spinal cord [64], causes a biphasic effect after intrathecal injection of a low dose [63], and causes analgesia or hyperalgesia [65]. Also, two directions of effect result from an interaction of the opioid antagonists within the endorphin systems. Along with hyperalgesic effects, the opioid antagonists have analgetic effects in humans and an antinociceptive effect in animals [66,67]. The antagonists augment or inhibit an antinociceptive effect of an agonistic drug [68,69]. The natural ligands may prove to be engaged in favoring the transfer of the noxious stimulus too, as indicated by recent data on dynorpin A$\{1-8\}$ [70].

Therefore, the direct effects of opioid ligands can be considered as functional according to two directions of effect. Similarly, the indirect effects of an opioid drug, i.e., those that involve the loop systems (see Loop systems), can be in two directions.

Attention focusing or inhibitory control

The simplified vision that the function of the primary afferents, loop, and endorphin systems is to accomplish a unidirectional change is not realistic. Although inhibitory mechanisms sometimes serve to indicate antinociception, neither inhibitory mechanisms nor excitatory mechanisms simply relate to (anti)nociception. Each part of the "pain" system participates in two directions to change the processing of noxious input signals. The inhibitory mechanisms may facilitate nociperception (attention focusing or pain permission) or be functional to antinociception (inhibitory control). Likewise, facilitatory mechanisms may prove to be functional to both (favoring signal transfer for the purpose of nociception or activation of analgesic mechanisms). Attention focusing and inhibitory control are dedicated to preserving general homeostasis and maintaining sensory homeostasis. As these two aspects of control are brought about by the activities of each of the above-outlined neuroanatomical and functional entities, one should be aware of the possibility of a "switch" between the two directions of effect. Such a switch of effect can cohere with a bidirectional effect of the transmitter concerned with the entity involved.

Several pitfalls are present in attributing such a complex function of bidirectional effectiveness to a substance that is injected. One should be aware of the functional presence of the various neurotransmitter or modulatory substances, not in a single, but in multiple parts of the central nervous system. Further, a single transmitter substance released or injected may cause changes in the breakdown or the release of one or more other substances [71–73]. Consequently, the effect can rely on the involvement of multiple systems, even when "selective" methods of drug administration, such as that of an intrathecal or intracerebroventricular injection, are used. Moreover, a pharmacological effect does not necessarily express the actual physiological function of a substance. Also, the effect of the natural agonists and the drugs injected may extend to more complex actions, which have been described as "system tuning" or modulation [74]. Such a system tuning may create a gradual transit between attention focusing and inhibitory control, and in the absence of pain carefully maintains a balance. Adequate therapeutic measures can reinstate this balance that is disturbed in condition of pain.

Many studies have shown that the suppression of a nocifensive reaction can be interpreted as relating to analgesia, but changes in the activation of motor responses should also be kept in mind as the cause for suppression of responses [75–77]. Various responses obviously depend on the integrity of the motor response, e.g., the tail-flick and withdrawal reflexes. Also, life-essential processes of flight, fight, and feeding can get priority and overrule the expression of a noxious impact.

CONTROL SYSTEMS THEORY AND PAIN

An integral part of a control system is the quantity being controlled, i.e., the controlled variable (Figure 4-2). When one is applying the control systems theory to pain, a main problem involves deciding on the number and the nature of the controlled variables. In order to determine the value of the controlled variable, a sensor has to be present. Based on the sensors recognized, we may distinguish two controlled variables: one for the nociperceptive system and one for the loop systems.

The nociperceptive system

Sensors capable of responding to an adequate stimulus are present in the distal endings of the peripheral nerves, e.g., the free nerve endings of the C-fibers, or morphological classified "receptors" such as the Pacinian corpuscles [78] (sensors: see Figure 4-2). The controlled variable recognized by a sensor is a noxious stimulus, for example, heat, pressure, electrical stimulation, or chemical irritation. The signal generated in the sensor is fed into the comparator. The value of the sensor signal is compared to the reference value (set point), which is kept in the memory of the control system. If a difference exists, an error signal (the difference between the detected value and the reference value) is generated. In the normal state, the error signal has to be zero, as the noxious stimulus is absent. If a noxious stimulus is present, the error signal activates an effector designated by the selector. The noxious stimulus then activates various effectors, such as the motor system and the cardiovascular system. Some of the responses mediated by the activation of effectors are used in pain research to assess an effect of a treatment. Examples are the motor responses elicited by the stimulus of the hot plate in behavioral studies, and the withdrawal reflexes elicited by heat or electricity. The function of the effectors is to enable the organism to remove the noxious stimulus, thus restoring the controlled variable within the physiological range.

The loop systems

A noxious input not only results in activation of the nociperceptive system (see section on), but also in the activation of loop systems (see Figure 4-1). The descending inhibitory tracts may act to restore the normosensoperceptive condition (negative feedback) (see Figure 4-3). The feedback is transmitted to the central neurons of the entry zone, such as those of the spinal cord. This means that the controlled variable of the loop systems is the activity of those neurons that can respond to a noxious stimulus. The nociceptive-driven neurons (Class III) and the wide dynamic range cells (Class II) of the entry zone have a basic state of activity and respond to the action potentials generated in the primary afferent channels [79–82]. The signal generated in the sensor is fed into the comparator. In the entry zone, complex neuronal connections, such as the internuncial cell pool of lamina VII of the spinal cord, are present. One can attempt to identify the functions of comparator, memory, or other components of the control system in such complex circuits. Specific functions of the involved second-order neurons are recognized. Examples of specific second-order neurons are the "inverse neurons" and "habituating cells" [83–85]. Examples of specific circuitry characteristics in which the neurons and the neuronal connections participate are "wind-up" [86,87], "reverberating circuits" (which may maintain an intrinsic signal), and "cascades" for sequential activation (which cannot maintain an intrinsic signal). We may conclude that knowledge of these interactions is increasing. However, the location and the mode of involvement in activities of some of the components of the control system is speculative for the time being.

The functions of the comparator, memory, and selector are nevertheless defined within the control systems. The value of the sensor signal is compared to the reference value (set point), which is kept in the memory of the control system. The comparison occurs both in the presence and absence of a noxious stimulus. The difference between the detected value and a reference value generates the error signal. As neuronal and circuitry activities fluctuate, even in the absence of the noxious stimulus, the primary setting of the control system should be regarded as a dynamic one. This means that an undulating error signal activates the selector. This is in accordance with a dynamic balance between attention focusing and inhibitory control (see Attention focusing or inhibitory control). The effectors are neurons that activate the descending tracts.

More control systems?

The present description limits itself to describing the "pain" system in two parts: nociperception and loop systems. However, one may consider applying the control systems theory to other aspects of the system, at different hierarchic levels. If these considerations are applied to the different subsystems, multiple sensors and effectors can be outlined as organized in a hierarchy of control systems, which in turn are organized in parallel and serial connections (see Figure 4-1). Each (sub)system will contain the components shown in Figure 4-2.

For example, reverberating circuits at the thalamic and the precortical level have proven to be engaged in a process of specific coding and subsequent decoding [88]. Decoders at the thalamic level can be regarded as the sensors, whereas the coders are the effectors that generate a complex signal to be decoded at the next level (sensors at the cortical level).

ANALGESIOLOGY

Until the present, pain has been described as a phenomenon caused by specific types of information arriving at a part of the nervous system (input). Motor responses, neuronal or tract activity, or evoked potentials have served to identify the impact of a noxious stimulus. Analgesia has been estimated, defined, and quantified by assessing the reduction of these responses effected with pharmacological or neurophysiological tools. The inhibitory controls and the presence of intrinsic pain-reducing mechanisms, as well as attention focusing, have been taken to indicate that when a noxious cause is present, then the regulatory systems are activated. Similarly, the control systems theory applied to pain acknowledges the input, the output, and efforts of regulatory mechanisms. However, the control systems theory also acknowledges the importance of the other components of the control system, e.g., memory and selectors (see Figure 4-2). The control systems are present at the different hierarchic levels of the central nervous system (see More control systems). Consequently, the components of the control system are not to be considered as resticted to a single level. For example, memory is a recognized function of the conscious mind. Yet it is present as a component of the control system of the loop system (see The loop systems) and may well prove to be present at the spinal level. Note that because of the cyclic nature of control systems, they are always in different states of activity [89].

The treatment of pain founded on the concept of the control systems theory

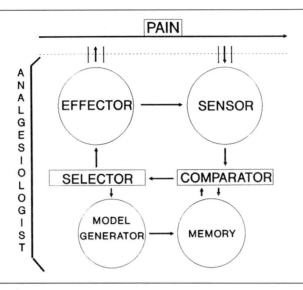

Figure 4-4. Scheme of an externalized control (the analgesiologist) which has the same components as the control system of an individual (see Figure 4-2). The controlled variable is the estimated quantity and quality of "pain."

is based on the establishment of an externalized control, which considers the intrinsic mechanisms (Figure 4-4). The externalized control (the analgesiologist) has components similar to those of the physiological control system. In humans, the controlled variable ("pain") has an estimated (scale) value and a characterized quality (e.g., the McGill questionnaire), as the actual measurement of pain is presently not feasible. The analgesiologist serves as the comparator by using information of the patient to compare the values obtained to an earlier reference value of the particular patient. If the analgesiologist decides that a shift beyond acceptable limits has occurred, he or she (the selector) selects adjusting measures to compensate for the detected perturbation. In order to be an adequate externalized control system and to prevent further perturbation, the analgesiologist bases his or her functioning on the knowledge of normal control and mode of involvement of the components of the control system in a condition of pain (system model). The task of adjusting and evaluating is cyclic, as is the intrinsic one, and acknowledges the dynamic character of the intrinsic systems. The effectiveness of the particular treatment (input/output relationship of pain therapy) adds to the understanding and models of the particular type of pain and the mode of system involvement (analgesiology: Figure 4-5). The evaluation of effect provides the feedback necessary for teaching, research, and renewing the models of pain. These are the tasks of the analgesiologist.

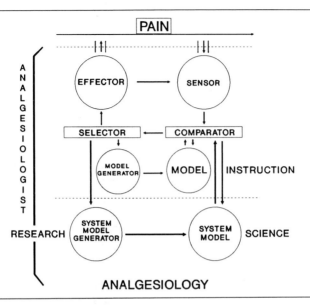

Figure 4-5. Scheme of analgesiology.

ACKNOWLEDGMENTS

The author gratefully acknowledges the discussions on the control systems theory with Dr. Jos Lerou and Gerard Nijhuis of the Institute for Anesthesiology of the University of Nijmegen.

REFERENCES

1. Merksey H. 1979. Pain terms; a list with definitions and notes on the usage. Recommended by the IASP Subcommittee on Taxonomy. Pain 6:249–252.
2. Thrush DC. 1973. Congenital insensitivity to pain. Brain Res 96:369–386.
3. Niewenhuys R, Voogd J, Van Huijzen C. 1978. The Human Central Nervous System. Berlin, Springer-Verlag.
4. Ralston HJ III. 1984. Synaptic organization of spinothalamic tract projections to the thalamus, with special reference to pain. In L Kruger, JC Liebeskind (eds), Advances in Pain Research and Therapy, Vol. 6. Neural mechanisms of Pain. New York, Raven Press, pp. 183–195.
5. Koralek K-A, Jensen KF, Killackey HP. 1988. Evidence for two complementary patterns of thalamic input to the rat somatosensory cortex. Brain Res 463:346–351.
6. Dirksen R, Lerou JGC, van Daele M, Nijhuis GMM, Crul JF. 1987. The clinical use of the Ohmeda Automated Anesthesia Record Keeper integrated in the Modulus II Anesthesia System. Int J Clin Mon Comp 4:135–139.
7. Spiaggi A, Bodnar RJ, Kelly DD, Glusman M. 1979. Opiate and non-opiate mechanisms of stress-induced analgesia: Cross tolerance between stressors. Pharm Biochem Behav 10:761–765.
8. Mayer DJ, Price DD. 1974. Pain reduction by focal electrical stimulation of the brain: An anatomical and behavioural analysis. Brain Res 68:73–93.
9. Hosobuchi Y, Adams JE, Linchitz R. 1977. Pain relief by electrical stimulation of the central gray matter in humans and its reversal by naloxone. Science 197:183–186.
10. Richardson DE, Akil H. 1977. Pain reduction by electrical brain stimulation in man. J

Neurosurg 47:178–183.

11. Dehen H, Willer JC, Prier S, Boureau F, Cambier J. 1978. Congenital insensitivity to pain and the "morphine-like" analgesic system. Pain 5:351–358.
12. Dehen H, Willer JC, Boureau F, Cambier J. 1977. Congenital insensitivity to pain, and endogenous morphine-like substances. Lancet ii:293–295.
13. Perl ER. 1984. Characterization of nociceptors and their activation of neurons in the superficial dorsal horn: First steps for the sensation of pain. In L Kruger, JC Liebeskind (eds), Advances in Pain Research and Therapy, Vol. 6. Neural mechanisms of Pain. New York, Raven Press, pp. 23–53.
14. LaMotte C. 1977. Distribution of the tract of Lissauer and the dorsal root fibres in the primate spinal cord. J Comp Neurol 172:529–562.
15. Kumazawa T, Perl ER. 1978. Excitation of marginal and substantia gelatinosa neurons in the primate spinal cord: Indications of their place in dorsal horn functional organization. J Comp Neurol 177:417–434.
16. Ralston HJ III, Ralston DD. 1979. The distribution of dorsal root axons in laminae I, II and III of the macaque spinal cord: A quantitative electron microscope study. J Comp Neurol 184:643–684.
17. LaMotte CC. 1988. Lamina X of primate spinal cord: Distribution of five neuropeptides and serotonin. Neuroscience 25:639–658.
18. Salt TE, Hill RG. 1983. Neurotransmitter candidates of somatosensory primary afferent fibres. Neuroscience 10:1083–1103.
19. Battaglia G, Rustioni A. 1988. Coexistence of glutamate and substance P in dorsal root ganglion neurons of the rat and monkey. J Comp Neurol 277:302–312.
20. Morton CR, Hutchison WD, Hendry IA. 1988. Release of immunoreactive somatostatin in the spinal dorsal horn of the cat. Neuropeptides 12:189–197.
21. Kuraishi Y, Hirato N, Sato Y, Hino Y, Satoh M, Takagi H. 1985. Evidence that substance P and somatostatin transmit separate information related to pain in the spinal dorsal horn. Brain Res 325:294–298.
22. Wiesenfeld-Hallin Z. 1986. Substance P and somatostatin modulate spinal cord excitability via physiological different sensory pathways. Brain Res 372:172–175.
23. Kuraishi Y, Nanayama H, Ohno H, Minami M, Satoh M. 1988. Antinociception induced in rats by intrathecal administration of antiserum against calcitonin gene-related peptide. Neurosci Lett 92:325–329.
24. Cridland RA, Henry JL. 1988. Effects of intrathecal administration of neuropeptides on a spinal nociceptive reflex in rat: VIP, galanin, CGRP, TRH, somatostatin and angiotensin II. Neuropeptides 11:22–32.
25. Cridland RA, Henry JL. 1986. Comparison of the effects of substance P, neurokinin A, physalaemin and eledoisin in facilitating a nociceptive reflex in the rat. Brain Res 381:93–99.
26. Seybold VS, Hylden JLK, Wilcox GL. 1982. Intrathecal substance P and somatostatin in rats: Behaviors indicative of sensation. Peptides 3:49–53.
27. Wiesenfeld-Hallin Z. 1985. Intrathecal somatostatin modulates spinal sensory and reflex mechanisms: Behavioural and electrophysiological studies in the rats. Neurosci Lett 62:69–74.
28. Dirksen R, Pol vd F, Nijhuis GMM. 1988. Control of the sensory input into the spinal cord. In (ed), Anesthesiology Feedback and Feedforeward. Nijmegen, pp. 97–110.
29. Starr MS, James TA, Gaytten D. 1978. Behavioural depressant and antinociceptive properties of substance P in the mouse: Possible implications of brain monoamines. Eur J Pharmacol 48:203–212.
30. Stewart JM, Getto CJ, Neldner K, Basil Reeve E, Krivoy WA, Zimmermann E. 1976. Substance P and analgesia. Nature 262:784–785.
31. Oehme P, Hecht K, Piesche L, Hilse H, Morgenstern E, Poppei M. 1980. Substance P as a modulator of physiological and pathological processes. In C Ajmone Marsan, WZ Traczyk (eds), Neuropeptides and Neuronal Transmission. New York, Raven Press, pp. 73–84.
32. Pittaway KM, Rodriquez RE, Hughes J, Hill RG. 1987. CCK 8 analgesia and hyperalgesia after intrathecal administration in the rat: Comparison with CCK-related peptides. Neuropeptides 10:87–108.
33. Chrubasik J. 1987. Clinical use of new peptides in pain relief. In The Pain Clinic II. Utrecht, VNU Science Press, pp. 123–134.
34. Dirksen R, Nijhuis GMM, Pinckaers JWM. 1985. Selective spinal analgesia: How close to physiological can we get? In Erdmann W (ed), The Pain Clinic I. Utrecht VNU Science Press, pp. 11–25.

35. Oku R, Satoh M, Fujii N, Otaka A, Yajima H, Takagi H. 1987. Calcitonin gene-related peptide promotes mechanical nociception by potentiating release of substance P from spinal dorsal horn in rats. Brain Res 403:350–354.
36. Wiesenfeld-Hallin Z, Hökfelt T, Lundberg JM, Forssmann WG, Reinecke M, Tschopp FA, Fischer JA. 1984. Immunoreactive calcitonin gene-related peptide and substance P coexist in sensory neurones to the spinal cord and interact in spinal behavioural responses of the rat. Neurosci Lett 52:199–204.
37. Reichling DB, Kwiat GC, Basbaum AI. 1988. Anatomy, physiology and pharmacology of the periaqueductal gray contribution to antinociceptive controls. In HL Fields, JM Besson (eds), Progress in Brain Research, Vol. 77. Amsterdam, Elsevier Science, pp. 31–46.
38. Iggo A, McMillan JA, Mokha SS. 1981. Spinal pathways for inhibition of multireceptive dorsal horn neurones by locus coeruleus and nucleus raphe magnus in the cat. J Physiol (London) 320:86P.
39. Bowker RM, Westlund KN, Sullivan MC, Wilber JF, Coulter JD. 1983. Descending serotonergic, peptidergic and cholinergic pathways from the raphe nuclei: A multiple transmitter complex. Brain Res 288:33–48.
40. Dickenson A. 1983. The inhibitory effects of thalamic stimulation on the spinal transmission of nociceptive information in the rat. Pain 17:213–224.
41. Casale EJ, Light AR, Rustioni A. 1988. Direct projection of the corticospinal tract to the superficial laminae of the spinal cord in the rat. J Comp Neurol 278:275–286.
42. Jurna I. 1980. Effect of stimulation in the periaqueductal grey matter on activity in ascending axons of the rat spinal cord: Selective inhibition of activity evoked by afferent A-delta and C fibre stimulation and failure of naloxone to reduce inhibition. Brain Res 196:33–42.
43. Hosobuchi Y, Adams JE, Rutkin B. 1973. Chronic thalamic stimulation for the control of facial anesthesia dolorosa. Arch Neurol 29:158–161.
44. Gebhart GF. 1982. Opiate and opioid peptide effects on brain stem neurons: Relevance to nociception and antinociceptive mechanisms. Pain 12:93–140.
45. Gebhart GF, Sandkuhler J, Thalhammer JG, Zimmermann M. 1984. Inhibition in the spinal cord of nociceptive information by electrical stimulation and morphine microinjection at identical sites in midbrain of the cat. J Neurophysiol 51:75–90.
46. Fitzgerald M. 1986. Monoamines and descending control of nociception. TINS 9:51–53.
47. LeBars D, Dickenson AH, Besson JM. 1979. Diffuse noxious inhibitory controls (DNIC). I. Effects on dorsal horn convergent neurons in the rat. Pain 6:283–304.
48. LeBars D, Dickenson AH, Besson JM. 1979. Diffuse noxious inhibitory controls (DNIC). II. Lack of effect on nonconvergent neurons, supraspinal involvement and theoretical implications. Pain 6:305–327.
49. Willis Jr WD. 1984. Modulation of primate spinothalamic tract discharges. In L Kruger, JC Liebeskind (eds), Advances in Pain Research and Therapy, Vol. 6. Neural Mechanisms of Pain. New York, Raven Press, pp. 217–241.
50. LeBars D, Villaneuva L. 1988. Electrophysiological evidence for the activation of descending inhibitory controls by nociceptive afferent pathways. In (eds), Progress in Brain Research, Vol. 77. Amsterdam, Elsevier, pp. 275–301.
51. Dostrovsky JO. 1980. Raphe and periaqueductal gray induced suppression of non-nociceptive neuronal responses in the dorsal column nuclei and trigeminal sub-nucleus caudalis. Brain Res 200:184–189.
52. Kajander KC, Ebner TJ, Bloedel JR. 1984. Effects of periaqueductal and raphe magnus stimulation on the responses of spinocervical and other projection neurons to non-noxious input. Brain Res 291:29–37.
53. Dirksen R. 1990. Opioid receptors and pain. Scientific Edition of the Farmaceutische Weekblad. Pharm Weekbl[su] 12:41–45.
54. Yaksh TL, Al-Rodhan NRF, Jensen TS. 1988. Sites of action of opiates in production of analgesia. In HL Fields, J-M Besson. (eds), Progress in Brain Research, Vol. 77. Amsterdam, Elsevier Science, pp. 371–395.
55. Schmauss C, Yaksh TL. 1984. In vivo studies on spinal opiate receptor systems mediating antinociception. II Pharmacological profiles suggesting a differential association of mu, delta and kappa receptors with visceral and cutaneous thermal stimuli in the rat. J Pharm Exp Ther 228:1–12.
56. Dirksen R, Lerou J, Nijhuis GMM, Booij LHDJ. 1990. Pentazocine: Not an agonist/antagonist analgesic. Eur J Anaesth S3:1–50.
57. Schmith DJ, Perrotti JM, Crisp T, Cabral MEY, Long JT, Scalzitti JM. 1988. The μ opiate

receptor is responsible for descending pain inhibition originating in the periaqueductal gray region of the rat brain. Eur J Pharmacol 156:47–54.
58. Tseng L-F, Towell JF, Fujimoto JM. 1986. Spinal release of immunoreactive Met-enkephalin by intraventricular betaendorphin and its analogues in anesthetized rats. J Pharm Exp Ther 237:65–75.
59. Jurna I. 1988. Dose dependent inhibition by naloxone of nociceptive activity evoked in the rat thalamus. Pain 35:349–354.
60. Walker GE, Yaksh TL. 1986. Studies on the effects of intrathalamically injected DADL and morphine on nociceptive threshold and electroencephalographic activity: A thalamic delta receptor syndrome. Brain Res 381:1–14.
61. Bloom F, Battenberg E, Rossier J, Ling N, Guillemin R. 1978. Neurons containing β-endorphin in rat brain exist separately from those containing enkephalin: Immunocytochemical studies. Proc Natl Acad Sci USA 75:1591–1595.
62. Dirksen R, Wood GJ, Nijhuis GMM. 1981. Mechanism of naloxone treatment in shock: A hypothesis. Lancet i:607–608.
63. Dirksen R. 1983. The clinical relevance of endorphin receptors — the antinociceptive effectiveness of epidurally or intrathecally injected endorphinomimetics. Thesis, Nijmegen.
64. Belcher G, Ryal RW. 1978. Differential excitatory and inhibitory effects of opiates on non-nociceptive and nociceptive neurones of the spinal cord of the cat. Brain Res 145:303–314.
65. Jacquet YF, Lajtha A. 1973. Morphine action at the central nervous system sites in rat: Analgesia or hyperalgesia depending on site and dose. Science 182:490–492.
66. Levine JD, Gordon NC, Fields HL. 1979. Naloxone dose-dependently produces analgesia and hyperalgesia in post-operative pain in man. Nature 278:740–741.
67. Taiwo YO, Basbaum AI, Perry F, Levine JD. 1989. Paradoxical analgesia produced by low doses of the opiate antagonist naloxone is mediated by interaction at a site with characteristics of the delta opioid receptor. J Pharm Exp Ther 249:97–101.
68. Vaccarino AL, Tasker RAR, Melzack R. 1989. Analgesia produced by normal doses of opioid antagonists alone and in combination with morphine. Pain 36:103–109.
69. Levine JD, Gordon NC, Taiwo YO, Coderra TJ. 1988. Potentiation of pentazocine analgesia by low-dose naloxone. J Clin Invest 82:1574–1577.
70. Iadarola MJ, Brady LS, Draisci G, Dubner R. 1988. Enhancement of dynorphin gene expression in spinal cord following experimental inflammation: Stimulus specificity, behavioural parameters, and opioid receptor binding. Pain 35:313–326.
71. Szreniawski S, Czlonowski A, Janicki P, Libich J, Gumulka SW. 1980. Substance P: Pain transmission and analgesia. In C Ajmone Marsan, WZ Traczyk (eds), Neuropeptides and Neuronal Transmission. New York, Raven Press, pp. 121–129.
72. Chrusciel TL. 1980. Metabolism of enkephalins and endorphins. In C Ajmone Marsan, WZ Traczyk (eds) Neuropeptides and Neuronal Transmission. New York, Raven Press, pp. 209–216.
73. Barclay RK, Phillips MA. 1980. Inhibition of enkephalin degrading aminopeptidases activity by certain peptides. Biochem Biophys Res Commun 96:1732–1738.
74. Barker JL, Neale JH, Smith TG Jr., MacDonald RL. 1978. Opiate peptide modulation of amino acid responses suggest novel form of neural communication. Science 199:1451–1454.
75. Holstege JC, Kuypers HGJM. 1987. Brainstem projections to spinal motoneurons: An update. Neuroscience 23:809–821.
76. Jurna I. 1988. Drug-induced dissociation of motor and sensory responses of the nociceptive system and its relevance to pain control in anesthesiology. In Anesthesiology-Feedback and Feedforeward. Nijmegen, pp. 65–77.
77. Duysens J, Dom R, Gybels J. 1989. Suppression of the hindlimb flexor reflex by stimulation of the medial hypothalamus and thalamus in the rat. Brain Res 499:131–140.
78. Chouchkov CN. 1978. Cutaneous receptors. Adv Anat Embryol Cell Biol 54:1–62.
79. Cervero F, Iggo A, Ogawa H. 1976. Nociceptive-driven dorsal horn neurons in the lumbar spinal cord of the cat. Pain 2:5–24.
80. Menétrey D, Giesler GJ, Besson J-M. 1977. An analysis of response properties of spinal cord dorsal horn neurons to non-noxious and noxious stimuli in the spinal rat. Exp Brain Res 27:15–33.
81. Pomeranz P, Wall PD, Weber WV. 1968. Cord cells responding to fine myelinated afferents from viscera, muscle and skin. J Physiol (London) 199:511–532.

82. Price DD, Dubner R. 1977. Neurons that subserve the sensory-discriminative aspects of pain. Pain 3:307–338.
83. Cervero F, Iggo A, Moloney V. 1979. An electrophysiological study of neurons in the substantia gelatinosa Rolandi of cat's spinal cord. Q J Exp Physiol 64:297–314.
84. Light AR, Trevino DL, Perl ER. 1979. Morphological features of functionally defined neurones in the marginal zone and substantia gelatinosa of the spinal dorsal horn. J Comp Neurol 186:151–172.
85. Wall PD, Merrill EG, Yaksh TL. 1979. Responses of single units in laminae 2 and 3 in the monkey. Brain Res 160:245–260
86. Chung JM, Kenshalo DR, Gerhart KD, Willis WT. 1979. Excitation of primate spinothalamic neurons by cutaneous C fibre volleys. J Neurophysiol 42:1354–1369.
87. Kenshalo DR, Leonard RB, Chung JM, Willis WT. 1979. Responses of primate spinothalamic neurons to graded and to repeated noxious heat stimuli. J Neurophysiol 42:1370–1389.
88. Emmers R. 1981. Pain — A Spike-Coded Message to the Brain. New York, Raven Press, pp. 1–134.
89. Dirksen R, Rutgers MJ, Coolen JMW. 1987. Cervical epidural steroids in reflex sympathetic dystrophy. Anesthesiology 66:71–73.

5. ENDORPHINS AND NARCOTIC DRUGS: PAIN CONTROL PARADIGMS VS. LEGAL REALITIES

JOSEPH HARRISON

The world we have made as a result of the level of thinking we have done thus far creates problems we cannot solve at the same level at which we created them.

Albert Einstein

Opium is far from being the least of those blessings with which Providence has furnished us for the mitigation of the various sufferings, to which the human form is liable . . . There are specifics, or certain cures for few of our ails, but opium affords some relief to all.

Dr. William Heberden (c.1774)

The control or treatment of severe pain, whether acute or chronic, has understandably long been associated with the utilization of narcotic-containing medications. Yet, our level of thinking about narcotic substances in contemporary American society, other than as short-term treatment for acute, severe pain, is conditioned by perceptions of these substances as representing dangerous external phenomena with adverse medical and legal consequences. Though such perceptions have generally not been supported by convincing scientific evidence, their influence upon governmental and legal controls on narcotic substances has been indubitable. Several administrations in Washington have declared a "war on drugs." It has not been a "successful war" by any standard [1,2].

By focusing attention upon the comparatively new psychopharmacological evidence regarding *endorphins* (a contraction of the term *endogenous morphine*) and through legal analysis of anticipated regulatory issues likely to emerge with the introduction of endorphinlike pharmaceutical products, this chapter offers potential strategies for legal modifications of existent narcotic drug statutes.

The nexus of recent data from neuropharmacology and psychoneuroendocrinology with legal and jurisprudential reasoning is illuminated in such fashion as to scrutinize existing laws and to glean salient arguments for the future judicial or legislative deliberations regarding narcotic regulation that the writer believes to be most likely. Legal and regulatory schemes have not attempted, logically or otherwise, to evaluate or incorporate the new scientific data, despite plausible, if presently theoretical, implications from the evidence about endogenous opiate chemicals that may well have direct relevance for the existing structures and sanctions governing exogenous opiate substances such as heroin or morphine. (*Endo*genous opiates refer to the natural, inbuilt category of opiatelike substances in humans, generically termed endorphins; *exo*genous opiates refer to the external, whether synthetic or natural, varieties of opium and opiatelike drugs, such as heroin, morphine, and codeine.) These implications, in turn, carry profound overlap with the central issue addressed here of treatments for chronic and acute pain.

One important area for consideration involves the matter of logical consistency in legal policy. In a democratic country issues are raised as laws apply severe criminal penalties to exogenous opiumlike chemicals when each human being possesses similar endogenous opiate substances. These logical questions also have implications for the fair, equal application of law within American constitutional guidelines. Consequently, pharmacological discoveries and existent statutory schemes must be studied and likely future developments viewed within the framework of legal and constitutional principles. Specific topics that represent tangible points of departure for serious legal challenges to existent laws should be identified and discussed; chief among these will be the regulatory and legal decisions to emerge when synthetic endorphin products are marketed. The need for a different drug classification scheme becomes apparent as legal challenges to existent statutes are evaluated [3,4].

The social concern with the actions of individuals who are under the influence of narcotic substances or who commit crimes in order to support a habit of narcotic addiction has given rise to substantial regulatory and criminal law designed to limit the use and abuse of such substances. The criminal and regulatory laws have not yet had the full opportunity (or the irresistible impulse) to respond to major new scientific understandings of narcotic addiction and usage gleaned from pharmacological data on the endogenous opioid chemicals, the endorphins. These endogenous opiates are to be distinguished throughout from the exogenous opiates. The term *endorphins* is used in the generic sense to include all endogenous opiates, even though numerous distinct ones have been identified. All the endorphins have characteristics pharmacologically similar to the exogenous opiates, thereby raising issues of legal responsibility, among other questions.

In nature, opium has at least 25 alkaloids that can be extracted. The phenanthrene alkaloids, including morphine and codeine, are used widely as analgesics. The isoquinoline alkaloids, such as papaverine, however, have little influence upon the central nervous system but have marked pharmacological activity on other systems in the body. Morphine is the principal constituent of opium and is a classic painreliever. In the 19th century, the pharmacist Serteurner named the individual narcotic ingredient of opium *morphine* after Morpheus, the greek God of dreams. Endogenously, endorphins produce morphinelike analgesia, physical tolerance, and dependence. The endorphins are addictive and cause tolerance and withdrawal upon discontinuance. Endorphins are cross-tolerant with the exogenous narcotics, such as heroin. Both morphine and endorphins produce acute alpha-EEG activity in humans, indicating that they have similar central nervous system effects. Endorphins cause physical dependence and tolerance, and possess the same addictive potential as exogenous opiates. It is apparent that a degree of tolerance and dependence on endorphins may be the normal state, while drug-induced tolerance and dependence represents only a quantitative deviation from normality [5–7].

Because the narcotic addict seems willing to go to any lengths to obtain a "fix," it is the addition-forming characteristic of the narcotic substances that alarms many observers. As a result, legislatures, responding to these deep social concerns, have created federal and state prohibitions on the use and possession of narcotics, except under medical supervision; selected narcotics, including heroin, are prohibited entirely (in the United States).

Scientific evidence, however, concludes that certain exogenous opiates seem indistinguishable in many of their behavioral effects from those of the opioid peptides (endorphins) and that narcotic-induced tolerance and dependence may represent only a quantitative, rather than a qualitative, deviation from normality. The research data appear to indicate that each individual is biochemically addicted to his or her internal opiumlike substances [8–11]. The relevance of these scientific conclusions to legal issues emerges when one considers the frequency with which the legal system is obligated to judge the responsibility of a particular human being at a specific moment in life — and the purposes to which the criminal and regulatory laws regarding narcotics usage are addressed. For one thing, society's prudential interest in preventing any adverse consequences arising from the use of exogenous narcotics should also include an interest in determining how best to minimize the antisocial actions committed by persons, either in the course of or because of exogenous narcotic usage. Scholars should seek to address the issue of whether it is unfair, as a denial of equal protection and/or due process of law, to punish someone criminally for using amounts of narcotic substances from external sources that differ only in source and quantity from naturally endogenous endorphins. In order to center attention on these questions, matters of constitutional analysis and of regulatory schemes should be examined. The catalyst in the anticipated court challenges for the crux of the legal analysis is the projected legal dilemmas to arise from the classification decisions to be made once synthetic endorphin pharmaceutical products appear in the marketplace. The Food and Drug Administration (FDA) and the Drug Enforcement Administration (DEA) face initially the task of regulating and determining whether and how to include synthetic endorphin products in the existing statutes. The DEA and FDA will find that the synthetic endorphins fit closely within the criteria for scheduling "controlled substances" under the 1970 Federal Comprehensive Drug Abuse and Control Act, 21 U.S.C. Section 801, et seq. (hereinafter referred to as the Controlled Substances Act or CSA) [12], which labels "opiates" as appropriate substances to subject to severe controls.

The Federal Food, Drug, and Cosmetic Act, 21 U.S.C. Section 301–92 (hereinafter referred to as the FD&C Act) [13] also would, under present statutory guidelines, classify synthetic endorphin products as controlled narcotic drugs, thereby raising some overlapping, and some distinct, legal issues, as contrasted with issues raised by CSA classification(s) of future synthesized endorphin products. Since existent CSA and FD&C acts appear to mandate inclusion of synthetic endorphin substances, it would seem inevitable (if one assumes the marketing such products, which is considered a near-certainty) that the classifications of synthetic endorphins as controlled substances will be open to court challenge. There are powerful arguments in the realm of equal protection, due process, and fair, rational application of the laws that may well precipitate a legal impasse.

The requirement that legislative classification of drugs be reasonable is embodied in the Equal Protection Clause of the Fourteenth Amendment. The due process assurance from the Fifth and Fourteenth Amendments relate to the treatment of persons charged with violation of narcotic regulatory and criminal statutes. Courts have also held, under the Eighth Amendment prohibition against cruel and unusual punishment, that one cannot be punished for the mere status of being a narcotic addict [*Robinson v. California*, 370 U.S. 660 (1962)]. Of all likely challenges, it is in the equal protection arena that courts would face the most problematic and significant arguments against what would be termed *irrational* classifications of synthetic endorphins as controlled substances.

The Fourteenth Amendment demands that no state shall deny to its citizens the equal protection of the laws, and the Supreme Court in *Bolling v. Sharpe*, 347 U.S. 497 (1954), held that the equal protection requirements also apply to the Federal government through the Fifth Amendment. Thus, the government *may not use classifications to treat similarly situated persons unequally*. Current evaluations by courts of such classifications search out the purpose as well as the effect of classification schemes and then determine whether equal protection clause protections have been violated. If a fundamental class of rights has been prejudiced by the classification scheme, only a powerful showing by the government may sustain the classifications against a challenge. Otherwise, the courts search for a rational basis (employing the "rational basis test") to determine whether the law or classification scheme has a rational basis; if so, it is sustained (as courts will usually defer to legislative enactments), but *if there is no rational basis in the constitutional law sense of the term, the law or regulation cannot be upheld* [*Shapiro v. Thompson*, 394 U.S. 618, 634 (1969); *McGinnis v. Royster*, 410 U.S. 263, 270 (1973); *Rinaldi v. Yeager*, 384 U.S. 305, 309 (1966)].

The pharmacological evidence may or may not be sufficient to raise immediate equal protection challenges to prosecutions for the sale or possession of exogenous narcotics. It does at least seem valid to consider whether persons now being prosecuted for exogenous narcotic possession and sale are "similarly situated" to individuals who are biochemically addicted to the endogenous opiate substances. *If* persons being prosecuted *are* similarly situated — not an easily arrived at conclusion, but not, for that matter, easily refuted — then (if one assumes that no "fundamental" rights are involved) the issue would be whether the state or federal government can articulate a "rational basis" for the classification scheme as it exists. One may note the logical paradox of courts, following DEA and FDA legislative classifications of synthetic endorphin pharmaceutical substances as controlled substances, attempting to impose punishment for offenses related to — to what, indeed? To external possession of substances already possessed internally? Or to further complicate the matter, if courts decide that they cannot sustain laws prohibiting possession or sale of synthetic endorphins because government(s) are unable to provide any "rational basis" for such classification statutory schemes, then how will courts be able to continue to sustain prosecutions of persons charged with possession or sale of other opiates such as heroin, morphine, meperidine, etc. when these are so chemically similar to the endogenous narcotics?

It is important to keep in one's mind the definition given under the existent CSA statutes of opiates that require severe legal controls: "opiates, with addiction-forming or addiction-sustaining liability similar to morphine." Clearly, endorphins would fall under this categorization, a point of increasing significance as pharmaceutical firms prepare to market synthetic beta-endorphin. Opiate peptides can cause similar euphoria effects as the exogenous narcotics. Receptors in the limbic system, which largely regulates emotion, may explain the emotional or affective component. Respiratory depression, incidentally, is also caused by *both* endorphins and exogenous narcotics. It is the respiratory depression that accounts for the lethal effect of narcotics in overdosage [14–18].

Among the options available to the FDA when it examines a new pharmaceutical product (such as synthetic beta-endorphin) for potential marketing is an initial categorization by type of product. Chemotherapeutic products are designed to inhibit or destroy bacteria, viruses, fungi, tumor cells, etc. Neuropharmacological agents have various impacts upon the central or peripheral nervous system, acting directly on receptors or indirectly through neurotransmitters. Other groups of drugs act on enzyme systems, such as certain diuretics or immunological products; this category includes hormonal substances.

Since the pharmacoloigcal data clearly indicate that endorphins are natural opiates present in the human brain and elsewhere in the body, and that narcotic tolerance to and dependence on such endogenous opiates does occur, how is the criminal law justified in prohibiting exogenous opiates that differ only in source and quantity, but not in quality or characteristics, from endogenous opiates? Because these naturally occurring narcotics are virtually indistinguishable in vivo from exogenous narcotic drugs, the nexus of social and legal controls on exogenous narcotic substances may be utilized as a point of departure for the analysis of the implications for criminal and regulatory laws arising from the recent neuropharmacological findings [2,9]. A principle realm in which such practical and legal effects may come into focus in that of the synthetic manufacture and marketing of endorphinlike pharmaceutical products in the coming years. Endorphins or synthetic endorphin analogues are not found anywhere in the CSA, and to maintain a prosecution against an individual for possession or sale of a controlled substance, that substance must be listed on one of the schedules. However, due to their close similarity to opium derivatives, and high addiction-liability in humans, the inclusion of synthetic endorphin products does not seem avoidable, given existent CSA guidelines and criteria for regulation of opiate substances. In addition to the requirement in the CSA that the U.S. Attorney General evaluate any new drug within the context of CSA schedules for possible inclusion, the CSA does require that the Attorney General and the Secretary of Health and Human Services consider all relevant medical and scientific information regarding any new drug prior to determining its placement within a schedule.

In addition to the CSA, the FD&C Act is likely to play a major role in future regulations governing synthetic endorphin substances; like the CSA, the FD&C Act in its present form lacks the elasticity to categorize rationally the endorphin substances without encountering significant legal and constitutional dilemmas. The scope of the FD&C Act is considerably greater than that of the CSA, though its teeth lack the bite of severe criminal penalties. The FD&C Act defines *drug* in pertinent part as

articles intended for use in the diagnosis, cure, mitigation, treatment, or prevention of disease in man or other animals; and articles (other than food) intended to affect the structure or any function of the body of man or other animals; and articles intended for use as a component of any article specified in [preceding] clauses, but does not include devices or their components, parts or accessories. (Section 321 g).

Consequently, products that are "misbranded" foods or illegal drugs, as well as numerous other categories, come under the jurisdiction of the FD&C Act, as administered by the Food and Drug Administration (FDA).

Of special interest for the immediate focus is that neither the definition of food or the definition of drug appears to capture fully endorphins within their description — even endorphins in synthetic external forms — yet both foods and drugs may have elements pertaining to endorphins or their synthetic equivalents. Perhaps an attempt should be made to describe a possible regulatory scheme to govern synthetic endorphins and other narcotic substances; such a proposal need account for both the "food" and "drug" elements that are characteristic of opiate substances, while further creating a new category along conceptual lines similar to regulations that now govern metabolic supplements and nonessential accessory food factors.

There is precedent for the FDA viewing some products as neither food nor drug, but as "medical food," such as the products used to treat phenylketonuria. Certain individuals have a *metabolic deficiency*, and to those individuals tyrosine, for example, becomes not a "food" but an *essential* "drug" or metabolic supplement to promote life and health. It is normally a nonessential factor because most persons produce enough naturally; in those who do not, however, it becomes essential and is closer to the FD&C Act definition of a "drug." The same may be true for insulin in the instances of diabetics; and, to the point, the pharmacological data indicate that this may also be the case for persons who have a deficiency of naturally produced endorphins — to them, conceivably, supplemental supplies of narcotic substances (whether exogenous morphine or newly synthesized external endorphin products) may indeed represent medically required substances. In any event, the "food" and "drug" categories are not sufficiently inclusive to engage the metabolic individualities [19–21].

There are a number of fundamental precedents and principles that provide an adequate framework to viewing new data on endorphins *vis à vis* narcotics control statutes and regulations for the purpose of predicting a potential legal impasse in the near future. Whatever Supreme Court determinations may be forthcoming in the area of narcotics control laws, the scientific data on endorphins raise new issues and challenges that will most likely be directly confronted by the Court. Though one does not need to take the position that the use of synthetic endorphin products biochemically indistinguishable, in vivo from endogenous, necessary neurotransmitters is a "fundamental" right, it seems reasonable to believe that precisely such an argument would not be dismissed as frivolous. Individual cases determining which rights are fundamental, and therefore in which instances the statute must meet a compelling interest test under "strict scrutiny" (rather than merely the "rational basis" test), have attempted to discuss the parameters of such jurisprudential analyses. One important distinction between equal protection or due process cases in the Supreme Court and potential future challenges to classificatory or scheduling schemes governing narcotic substances is that in a criminal case the state's burden is greater, making a challenge more likely to prevail.

While classification of future synthetic endorphin products on the market as "narcotics" would not be open to question, the relevance and applicability of such a classificatory scheme within criminal constitutional law is most germane to the present inquiry. The issue would be joined at the juncture where the state or federal governments find it within their authority and discretion to classify narcotics within the CSA, despite all available pharmacological data about the endogenous opiates. At this intersection of statutory scheme and logical nexus, a court must go well beyond legalisms to consider analytical challenges and the constitutional baggage they bring, albeit based on equal protection criteria.

There are, it would seem, several legal dilemmas posed by the new psychopharmocological data. First, how can the state or federal government regulate with criminal penalties affixed substances that are not pharmacologically different in vivo from the constantly present endorphins? Is this a denial of a "right" and would the right be recognized as a "fundamental" one? In either event, what is the "rational basis" (or, if it is a fundamental right, what is the "compelling interest") held by the state or federal government that justifies such an interference in personal liberty? Secondly, even if the state or federal government presently can offer a rational basis for its present scheduling and regulatory functions based on arguable differences between exogenous and endogenous narcotic substances (which differ in source and quantity), how will such a rational basis hold up when the regulated substances are synthetic beta-endorphin or similar products, which mimic the human body's natural supply of opiate peptides?

Even medical researchers not directly involved in drug policy politics "urge lawmakers, law enforcement agencies and health care workers to distinguish between the [narcotic] addict . . . and the psychological healthy patient who takes [narcotics] only to relieve pain" [1].

"You are call wrong, but one of you is less wrong than the rest," announced Lord Peter Wimsey in Dorothy L. Sayers' *Five Red Herrings*. "Still none of you has got the right murderer, and none of you has got the method right," he continued, " . . . though some of you have got bits of it." In suggesting certain logical outcomes within legal spheres to the apparent regulatory paradox governing narcotic substances, one feels somewhat like those who made attempts to solve Lord Peter Wimsey's murder mystery; the almost daunting but vital search for solutions cannot conceivably arrive at all the implications of all recent scientific findings regarding endogenous and exogenous opiates. It is worthwhile, however, to speculate coherently upon several paths of analysis that might lead to useful statutory revisions. The realistic chances of courts taking the initiative in decriminalizing and deregulating narcotic substances (whether of the synthetic endogenous or of the current exogenous variety) are not considerable. Certain changes that remove the dramatic elements of discriminatory treatment for those persons who possess external endorphins as compared with the rest of us who possess these substances only endogenously would probably still permit major regulatory functions to be maintained under the CSA, FD&C Act, or related statutes. The first and most essential modification in existing statutes concerns the categorization of narcotic substances.

In nutritional pharmacology, *essential nutrients* are divided between those that cannot be manufactured within the body, those that can be manufactured within the body, and those that can be manufactured, though not always in amounts adequate to meet the needs of most healthy individuals. Their manufacture within the body is inadequate for the prevention of known deficiency diseases, such as pernicious anemia resulting from inadequate vitamin B12. *Nonessential nutrients* or accessory food factors are materials that are manufactured within the human body at levels that for most persons would be considered adequate to maintain health, or freedom from disease. However, in individual cases, one or more of these accessory metabolites may not be maintained at optimal levels to maintain or promote health. This may be due to any number of causes, perhaps genetic deficiencies, injuries, metabolic diseases, etc.

In such cases, it is often appropriate to use *exogenous sources* of such "metabolic factors." Whereas the therapeutic use of such accessory metabolic factors, derived from exogenous sources (e.g., dietary sources or their synthesized equivalents), is now common practice in clinical nutritional medicine, what may be suggested in the present context is that narcotic substances be similarly viewed as accessory metabolic factors, with appropriate therapeutic uses in the maintenance of health. Whereas most individuals manufacture within their own bodies sufficient amounts of endorphins to maintain normal health (and possibly a relatively pain-free state), there are individuals who apparently cannot, because of unique health or genetic or environmental states, manufacture within their own bodies sufficient or optimal quantities of endorphins to maintain a state of normal homeostasis. Such individuals appear to require exogenous supplemental sources of narcotic substances, which may be viewed as *accessory narcotic metabolic substances*. Ideally, their supplemental sources of narcotics should be as close in pharmacological form as possible to the body's endorphins; thus, synthetic endorphin pharmaceutical products apparently would be quite appropriate.

This "justification hypothesis" supposes that certain individuals have insufficient endogenous narcotic substances to meet their health requirements. One may envision at least three classes of individuals:

Type A. Those who can, under normal circumstances, barring injury or disease, manufacture within their own bodies sufficient narcoticlike metabolic factors to maintain their optimal health status. These individuals, however, may temporarily lose their unimpaired ability to manufacture within their own bodies sufficient narcotic metabolic factors if they are injured, afflicted with transient disease, or stress, and then larger quantities of narcotics may be required.

Type B. Those individuals who cannot, even under normal circumstances, perhaps due to genetic deficiencies or permanent disease states, manufacture within their own bodies sufficient narcotic substances to maintain homeostasis. Such persons require regular supplementation of narcotic substances, ideally the synthetic duplicates of endorphins.

Type C. Those individuals who are able to manufacture and maintain adequate levels of narcotics endogenously for body homeostasis, but for one reason or another would prefer to have at their disposal certain supplemental sources of narcotics in order to achieve the psychoactive effects that narcotics are capable of producing when taken in larger than normally produced quantities.

Patients with chronic pain may fall into categories A or B. For Type B individuals, what may be considered nonessential accessory narcotic metabolic factors for normal individuals may be regarded as essential narcotic metabolic factors. Denial of these substances (and punishing attempts to buy such substances with fines and prison terms) in these instances would probably be held as "cruel and unusual punishment" by the Supreme Court under Eighth Amendment analysis, and as a denial of due process and equal protection under the Fifth and Fourteenth Amendments. For Type A individuals, the controls on narcotics under the CSA and FD&C Act provisions may be regarded as provisionally permissible, i.e., not permissible in all circumstances under the analysis applicable to Type B individuals. Even under other circumstances, Type A individuals would have strong equal protection challenges to any statute that prohibited the use or possession of synthetic endorphins, since these persons are similarly situated with other individuals who are not being prosecuted. For Type C individuals, the governmental "rational basis" for continued controls and penalty schemes will be most persuasive. Even here, however, it seems unlikely that the statutes could withstand equal protection legal challenges with reference to possession or use of synthetic endorphin products.

Therefore, in order to avoid the legal impasse, the CSA should be modified as follows:

1. The definition of narcotics should be changed to read "narcotics are derivatives of the opium plant, opium poppy, or pharmacological biochemicals, whether endogenous or exogenous, that are the biochemical equivalents of opiates, including any of the opiate alkaloids, synthetics, or duplicates of endorphins."

2. Narcotics, including exogenous ones such as heroin, morphine, methadone, and meperidine, as well as endogenous ones such as beta-endorphin, and the synthetic endorphin equivalents, should be rescheduled in Schedule IV — a schedule designating "some abuse potential" with "fully appropriate and acceptable medical uses." This regulatory compromise would keep narcotics of all kinds under governmental supervision, since dosage

abuse potential is present, while eliminating the constitutionally impermissible severe criminal penalties.

3. The penalties for unauthorized possession or sale of narcotics in any form should be restricted to reporting and accounting procedures. Specifically, the CSA should read as follows: "Persons who wish to obtain supplemental accessory narcotic metabolic substances of any kind may do so on advice or prescription of any authorized physician or medical practitioner. Persons who obtain or sell narcotics without such authorization may be reported to a designated agency (perhaps the DEA), and may be required to appear in court for medical determinations of narcotic levels. In *no* instance may a person be fined or imprisoned *merely* for possession or sale of narcotic substances. However, persons who illegally sell such substances for financial gain may be subject to prosecution under appropriate corrupt racketeering statutes for illegal enterprises.

4. All manufacture of narcotic substances should be supervised for purity and quality by Food and Drug Administration personnel; adulterated or impure narcotic products should be subject to restriction and investigation just as any other misbranded products.

5. The FD&C Act should include a new category of substances, beyond the presently existent "food" and "drug" category. The new category would be termed *synthetic equivalents of endogenous biochemicals*, and would include all exogenous narcotics and synthetic endorphin products.

The element of *pain* has been of critical relevance and focus to the foregoing discussion of endorphins and legal analysis, and a few concluding comments about pain are in order. Initially, one cannot help but notice that both endogenous and exogenous opiates have as their principal physiological function or feature *analgesia*, or pain relief (perhaps relief from suffering is more precise). The narcotic pain relief system in the human body is fascinating by virtue of its very existence as well as its nature. Narcotics, both endorphins and exogenous varieties, such as heroin, act on the central nervous system, and so there is almost no method to separate the pain-relieving qualities of narcotics from their psychological euphoria-inducing effects. Opiate chemicals act to make the pain perceptions qualitatively less affectively distressing, and the evidence appears to indicate that the human endorphin system is in place as an endogenous pain relief system.

In the multidimensional context, then, of a narcotic drug-control strategy that has been ineffective, an illegal enterprise growth rate that is extraordinary due to the profits involved in illegal narcotics traffic, and a growing awareness by neuroscientists and social policymakers that new biochemical understanding of narcotic addiction and use hold great meaning and impact for our narcotic control strategies, the author believes that his legal analysis of anticipated challenges to existing statutory structures serves to crystallize the nature of necessary modifications and changes that judicial tests will bring to completion.

REFERENCES

1. Melzack R. 1990. The tragedy of needless pain. Scient Amer 262:27–33.
2. Harrison J. 1982. A rationale for the use of new data in psychopharmacology as applied to current federal narcotic drug legislation. Contemp Drug Probl: 21–38.
3. Harrison J. 1981. Endorphins and legal issues. J Legal Med 2:543–568.
4. Uelman G, Haddox V. 1983. Drug Abuse and the Law. New York, Clark Boardman Publishers.
5. Milkman H, Sunderwirth S. 1982. Addictive processes. J Psychoactive Drugs 14:177–192.
6. Olson R, Kastin A, Olson G, Coy D. 1980. Behavioral effects after systemic injection of opiate peptides. Psychoneuroendocrinology 5:47–52.
7. Martin W. 1985. Role of agonist-antagonist analgesics in Medicine. Drug Alcohol Depend 14:221–226.
8. Davis J. 1984. Endorphins: New Waves in Brain Chemistry. New York, The Dial Press.
9. Bunney W, Pert C, Klee W, Costa E, Pert A, Davis G. 1979. Basic and clinical studies of endorphins. Ann Inter Med 91:239–250.
10. Basbaum A, Moss M, Glazer E. 1983. Opiate and stimulation produced analgesia. Adv Pain Res Ther 5:323–339.
11. Balster R, Lukas S. 1985. Review of self-administration. Drug Alcohol Depend 14:249–261.
12. Controlled Substances Act, 1970. Public Law 91–513, 84 Stat. 1242, 21 United States Code #801, et seq.
13. Food Drug and Cosmetic Act, 1976, 1938. 52 Stat. 1040, 21 United States Code #301–92.
14. Jaffe J. 1985. Impact of scheduling on the practice of medicine and biomedical research. Drug Alcohol Depend 14:403–418.
15. Johns A, Gossop M. 1985. Prescribing methadone for the opiate addict: A problem of dosage conversion. Drug Alcohol Depend 15:61–66.
16. Wall PD, Melzack R. (eds). 1989. Textbook of Pain, 2nd ed. New York, Churchill Livingstone.
17. Neil A. 1982. Morphine and methadone tolerant mice differ in cross-tolerance to other opiates. Naunyn-Schmiedebergs Arch Pharmacol 320:50–53.
18. Charney D, Sternber D. 1981. Clinical use of clonodine in abrupt withdrawal from methadone. Arch Gen Psych 38:1273–1277.
19. Amir S, Brown Z, Amit Z. 1980. The role of endorphins in stress. Neurosci Biobehav Rev 4:77–86.
20. Snyder S. 1982. A multiplicity of opiate receptors and enkephalin neuronal systems. J Clin Psychiatry 43:9–12.
21. McNamara S. 1982. When does a food become a drug? Food, Drug, Cosmetic Law J 37:222–231.

6. PHARMACOLOGY OF SUBSTANCE P AND RELATED TACHYKININS

B.V. RAMA SASTRY

The occurrence of a hypotensive substance in extracts of equine intestine and brain was first discovered by von Euler and Gaddum [1]. This hypotensive substance caused contraction of the rabbit jejunum in vitro. They prepared a standard preparation in the form of a dry powder (P). In subsequent studies, Gaddum and Schild [2] referred to the dry powder as *substance P*. This term gained acceptance in the literature and has been retained ever since.

The presence of a sialogogic peptide in extracts of bovine hypothalami was discovered by Leeman and Hammerchlag in 1967 [3]. The sialogogic peptide was biologically and chemically indistinguishable from substance P [3]. The amino acid sequence of substance P, its synthesis, and the first radioimmunoassay were accomplished by subsequent investigators [4–6]. Substance P contains 11 amino acids and is a lead peptide to a family of peptides isolated from mammalian and nonmammlian sources (Table 6-1). The pharmacological activities of these mammalian and nonmammalian peptides have been studied extensively and are referred to as *tachykinins*. All tachykinins have similar C-terminal sequences and pharmacological actions.

The nucleotide sequence of cloned cDNA for substance P precursor, protachykinin (PPT) from bovine brain, has been determined [7]. The PPT gene is organized into seven exons and six introns. While exon three encodes for the peptide substance P, exon six encodes for the peptide neurokinin A. RNA transcripts of this gene have been reported to undergo differential splicing to yield two mRNAs, an alpha–PPT mRNA that is missing exon six

Table 6-1. Primary structures of various tachykinins

Tachykinin	Classification	Structural analogue
		0 1 2 3 4 5 6 7 8 9 10 11
Substance P	Mammalian	Arg-Pro-Lys-Pro-Gln-Gln-Phe-Phe-Gly-Leu-Met-NH$_2$
Neurokinin A[a]	Mammalian	His-Lys-Thr-Asp-Ser-Phe-Val-Gly-Leu-Met-NH$_2$
Neurokinin B[b]	Mammalian	Asp-Met-His-Asp-Phe-Phe-Val-Gly-Leu-Met-NH$_2$
Physalaemin	Nonmammalian	pGlu-Ala-Asp-Pro-Asn-Lys-Phe-Tyr-Gly-Leu-Met-NH$_2$
Eledoisin	Nonmammalian	Glu-Pro-Ser-Lys-Asp-Ala- Phe- Ile-Gly-Leu-Met-NH$_2$
Kassinin	Nonmammalian	Asp-Val-Pro-Lys-Ser-Asp-Gln-Phe-Val-Gly-Leu-Met-NH$_2$

[a] Also known as neurokinin alpha, substance K, neuromedin L.
[b] Also known as neurokinin β, neuromedin K.

and a beta–PPT mRNA that contains all seven exons. These observations led
to the possibility of differential synthesis of substance P and neurokinin A in
different tissues. A gene has also been described for neurokinin B. While all
three tachykinins occur in several brain areas, their proportions vary from one
brain region to another. The concentrations of immunoreactive substance P
are higher than those of neurokinin A and neurokinin B in substantia nigra,
striatum, spinal cord, and cerebellum of the rat brain. In the rat cerebral
cortex, the concentration of immunoreactive neurokinin B is higher than that
of substance P. It is not known whether or not different tachykinins play
different roles in different tissues.

Substance P has been more thoroughly investigated than other tachykinins
for its physiological and pharmacological activities. The role of substance P in
1) sensory neurons and pain transmission, 2) neurogenic inflammation, 3)
intrinsic neurons and extrinsic sensory nerves of gastrointestinal tract, 4)
modulation of the release of primary transmitters, acetylcholine, norepinephrine, dopamine, and 5-hydroxytryptamine; and 5) regulation of blood
pressure have been investigated in considerable detail. Some aspects of the
metabolism of substance P, multiple tachykinin receptors, and the significance
of the occurrence of substance P in some non-neuronal tissues have also been
investigated. In several tissues, the functions of substance P and enkephalins
are interrelated.

PAIN TRANSMISSION NEURONS: SITES FOR MODULATION
BY ENKEPHALINS AND SUBSTANCE P

Pain is a sensation that can be described but cannot be defined. Neurochemical
and pharmacological studies have identified many substances that may be
involved in the regulation of pain transmission and perception. Two groups of
endogenous peptides — tachykinins and opioid peptides (enkephalins and
endorphins) — have been identified to process painful stimuli [9–11]. Three
tachykinins — substance P and neurokinins A and B — occur in mammalian
tissues. These three tachykinins have similar C-terminal sequences and pharmacological activities. *Enkephalin* is a term used to describe normally occur-

ring opiatelike substances in the brain or nervous system. The predominant enkephalins in the brain are two pentapeptides: methionine enkephalin and leucine enkephalin. β-endorphin, which contains 31 amino acids, also occurs in the brain. There is considerable evidence that substance P and enkephalins serve as modulators of chemical transmission and regulators of painful stimuli in the spinal cord and central nervous system.

The sensory afferents and descending projections from periaqueductal gray matter in the pons and nucleus raphae magnus in medulla process painful stimuli in the dorsal horn of the spinal cord (Figure 6-1). Painful stimuli from the environment are transmitted by cutaneous receptors through sensory afferents to their cell bodies in the dorsal root and trigeminal ganglia. The projections of the sensory neurons are densest in laminae I, II, and III of the dorsal horn. Unmyelinated C pain fibers from the sensory neurons project

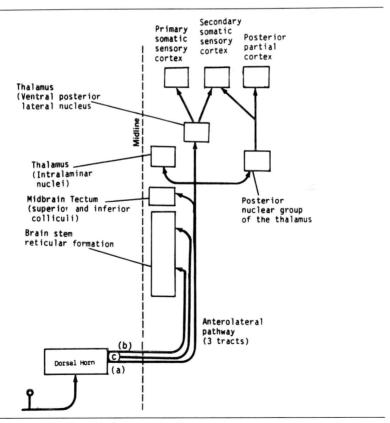

Figure 6-1. A schematic diagram showing major ascending pathways in the anterolateral system: (a) spinothalamic tract, (b) spinoreticular tract, and (c) spinotectal tract. Details of these pathways were described by Martin [9].

mostly into laminae I, and II. These fibers transmit slow pain, which is dull, burning, slow in onset, and long in duration. This type of pain has an emotional component and is often difficult to tolerate. Opiates are effective against slow pain.

Thinly myelinated A-delta fibers of the sensory neurons project to laminae I, II, and III. These fibers mediate fast pain, which is described as sharp and piercing. This type of pain is well localized and is of short duration. It has a weak emotional component. Opiates are not effective against fast pain.

The anterolateral system [9] in the spinal cord mediates pain and temperature sensation. It consists of separate ascending pathways that, together, play a dominant role in pain and temperature sense and only a minor role in tactile sense and limb proprioception. It consists of three major pathways that are distinguishable as follows (Figure 6-1): 1) The spinothalamic (or neospinothalamic) tract originates mainly from cells in lamina I (some from laminae II and III). This tract mediates fast pain, which is relayed from the periphery to the spinal cord by A-delta fibers. 2) The spinoreticular (or paleospinothalamic) tract mediates slow pain, which is relayed from the periphery by C-fibers. Axons of spinoreticular tract cells end on neurons in the reticular formation of the brain stem. From the reticular formation, information is relayed rostrally to the thalamus and other structures in the diencephalon. The spinoreticular tract also transmits information to the mesencephalic periaqueductal grey matter. This area is a part of a descending pathway that regulates pain transmission. Neurons in the periventricular and periaqueductal grey matter excite those in the nucleus raphe magnus in the reticular formation of the medulla. From here, serotonergic fibers descend in the dorsolateral funiculus of the spinal cord to terminate in the substantia gelatinosa, where they activate enkephalinergic inhibitory neurons (Figure 6-2). 3) The spinotectal tract terminates in the tectum of the midbrain (superior and inferior colliculi).

Substance P as a sensory chemical transmitter and/or modulator

The primary sensory neurons are bipolar. The peripheral terminals are linked to many organs, whereas the central terminals transmit information to second-order neurons within the central nervous system. At this first synapse, the incoming message is modulated by other afferent neurons, by interneurons, and by descending neurons. Primary afferent neurons release their neurotransmitters at both their central and peripheral terminals. The transmitters and transmission mechanisms of large-diameter afferent neurons (A-alpha, 13–20 µm; A-beta, 6–12 µm) are not known. There is considerable information available about the function of the various small-diameter neurons containing substance P (A-delta, 5 µm; C, unmyelinated, 0.2–1.5 µm).

Substance P satisfies many of the criteria for a primary neurotransmitter and/or modulator in the small-diameter sensory afferent neurons [11,14,15]: 1) It occurs in 10–20% of spinal neurons of several mammals. 2) It is present in the synaptic vesicles of the neuronal terminals of sensory neurons located in

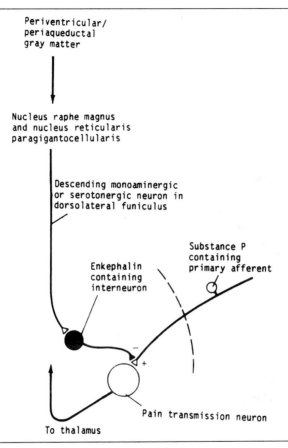

Figure 6-2. A schematic diagram of descending pain modulatory system. Neurons in the periventricular and periaqueductal grey matter stimulate those in the nucleus raphae magnus (NRM) in the reticular formation of medulla. Serotonergic fibers descend from NRM in the dorsolateral funiculus of spinal cord to terminate in the substantia gelatinosa, where they activate enkephalinergic inhibitory neurons. Enkephalinergic neurons may exert presynaptic inhibition over incoming substance P afferent fibers concerned with pain [13]. Details of the descending pathway and modulation by enkephalin were described by Fields and Basbaum [12], Jessell and Iverson [13] and Kelly [10].

laminae I and II of the dorsal horn. 3) It is released into the dorsal horn when C-and A-delta fibers are electrically stimulated. 4) It has an excitatory effect on the dorsal horn that is gradual in onset and prolonged in duration. These observations suggest that substance P may serve as a slow-acting chemical transmitter or modulator. All the well-known chemical transmitters are fast in onset of action and are of short duration. Therefore, a question arises as to whether there is an unidentified fast-acting chemical transmitter the action of which is modulated by substance P.

In sensory neurons containing substance P, it is released from both peripheral and central terminals. Substance P release from afferent terminals is stimulated by antidromic sensory nerve stimulation, capsaicin, irritants, heat, dry ice, anoxia, and antigens. Substance P release is inhibited by somatostatin and opiates. The effects mediated by substance P released from peripheral terminals include vasodilation, plasma extravasation, histamine release, contraction of smooth muscle, and a slow excitatory postsynaptic potential in postganglionic neurons. These responses occur to different degrees in various organs. All these responses are considered in terms of a common denominator — a local defense reaction to various kinds of irritants.

Several studies on the central terminals of substance P neurons have been devoted to the transmission of nociceptive information from the periphery. Central terminals of substance P neurons transmit, in addition to nociceptive messages, information that induces selective reflexes. The various reflexes induced by central terminals of substance P neurons have been discussed by Lembeck [15]. Some examples of these reflexes are listed in Table 6-2. There is no evidence to indicate that the neurons of the central nervous system can stimulate the central terminals of substance P neurons, resulting in an antidromic wave of impulses to the periphery.

Enkephalins as modulators of painful stimuli

Many enkephalin-containing neurons are present in laminae I and II of the dorsal horn [25]. Mu opiate receptors on the neurons and neuronal terminals also occur in the dorsal horn. The distribution of enkephalins and mu opiate receptors parallel one another in the neurons of the dorsal horn. Direct epidural or intrathecal applications of morphine causes intense analgesia. The release of substance P from the sensory and dorsal horn neurons by chemical stimuli is blocked by opioids [13,26]. The blocking effect of exogenous and

Table 6-2. Central terminals of substance P neurons and reflux responses

No.	Reflex	Stimulus	Effect	Ref.
1	Nociception	Intrathecal SP	Scratching	16,17
2	Reflex vasodilation	Mesenteric artery stimulation	Heat dissipation (reflex inhibition of adrenergic tone)	18–20
3	Sneezing reflex	Chemicals	Motor reflex	21
4	Micturition reflex	Bladder distention	Reflex, cholinergic activation	22
5	Decidual response	Cervical stimulation by copulation	Release of progesterone	23
6	Peristalsis	Increase in intraluminal pressure	Activation of various neurons	24

endogenous opioids on substance P release is nullified by the opioid antagonist, naloxone.

Enkephalins are also involved in the descending control of spinal pain transmission. Microinjection of opiates in the area of periaqueductal grey matter of animals causes analgesia. Electrical stimulation of periaqueductal grey matter results in analgesia, possibly due to release of enkephalins, which can be antagonized by naloxone [27]. These observations suggest that the neurons in periaqueductal grey matter are opioid sensitive.

Serotonin in pain pathways and its cooccurrence with substance P

There exists an excitatory connection between the periaqueductal grey matter and the nucleus raphae magnus. The excitatory transmitter is not known. It may be glutamate, aspartate, or neurotensin excitatory transmitters at other sites in the central nervous system.

The nucleus raphae magnus has projections to the dorsal horn, with the highest density of terminals in laminae I, II, and V. Serotonin is the major neurotransmitter associated with the terminal projections of the nucleus raphae magnus [12]. Direct intrathecal application of serotonin decreases the response to noxious stimuli, which is not affected by naloxone. Many of these neurons contain both serotonin and substance P. The significance of the cooccurrence of substance P and serotonin has not yet been clarified. Iontophoretic application of substance P attenuates the excitations of dorsal horn interneurons caused by iontophoretic application of serotonin. It has been demonstrated that substance P displaces serotonin binding from the membranes of the dorsal half of the rat spinal cord [28]. This is a specific effect and substance P probably acts at the SP-P receptor in the interaction with serotonin.

PUTATIVE ROLE OF SUBSTANCE P IN NEUROGENIC INFLAMMATION DUE TO NOXIOUS STIMULI

The role of substane P in inflammation has been studied in several tissues [30]: 1) Substance P is associated with the sensory fibers that are involved in the mechanisms of vasodilation and axon reflex. 2) It is released from peripheral nerve endings of sensory neurons during antidromic stimulation. 3) Local chemical, physical, or mechanical irritants release substance P concomitant with neurogenic inflammation. 4) Topical application or local arterial injection of substance P mimics the effects of antidromic nerve stimulation and local noxious stimuli. These effects include vasodilation, increased vascular permeability and plasma extravasation, and contraction of smooth muscle. 5) Capsaicin, which depletes substance P from primary afferents, and substance P-receptor antagonists block the effects of antidromic nerve stimulation.

In addition to substance P, several other substances are released during inflammation or hyperreactive disorders. The mechanism of inflammation does seem to differ from organ to organ (Table 6-3). Other mediators besides substance P seem to be involved in the inflammation syndrome.

Table 6-3. Role of substance P and other mediators in neurogenic inflammation

Organ	Stimulation for inflammation	Antagonism (A) or stimulation (S)	Release (R) or inhibition (I) of other mediators	Ref.
Skin	Nerve stimulation, noxious stimuli, SP application	Compound 48/80 (A) H1 antagonist (A)	Histamine (R)	31,32
Eye	SP application	Indomethacin (A)	Prostaglandin (PGE1)	33,34
Nasal mucosa	Trigeminal nerve, efferent parasympathomimetics	Substance P release (S)	Acetylcholine (R) substance P (R) VIP (R)	35
Bronchi	Vagal stimulation, local stimuli	Indomethacin (S), substance P release (S)	PG synthesis (I)	36
Dental pulp	Inferior alveolar nerve stimulation	Substance P release (S)	Somatostatin (I)	37

ROLE OF SUBSTANCE P IN GASTROINTESTINAL TRACT

There are two fundamental types of substance P neurons that innervate the digestive tract: intrinsic substance P neurons entirely contained in the intestinal wall and extrinsic sensory nerves from the dorsal root ganglia and sensory ganglia of the vagus nerve. The substance P neuron circuitry is deduced using techniques of 1) surgical lesions of extrinsic and intrinsic nerve pathways, 2) depletion of substance P by capsaicin, and 3) immunohistochemistry. Most of the work has been done in guinea pig, and any extrapolation to other species should be done with caution.

Intrinsic substance P nerve fibers originate from myenteric nerve cell bodies and supply an excitatory input to the longitudinal and circular muscles of the intestine [30,38]. The neurons to the circular muscle are activated when a peristaltic reflex is activated. The physiological conditions in which substance P nerves are activated and the interactions of substance P and cholinergic excitatory nerves, both of which innervate the muscle, have yet to be determined.

Substance P is one of at least 15 substances that have been postulated to have roles in neurotransmission in the intestine. Among these, both acetylcholine (ACh) and norepinephrine are accepted chemical transmitters in the intestine. There is also convincing evidence for substance P and enkephalins as neurotransmitters or neuromodulators in the gut. Among these, ACh and substance P are excitatory substances. There seem to be close interactions between ACh and substance P neurons. Substance P releases ACh from the guinea pig myenteric plexus by acting at the receptors of the soma of the enteric neurons or their nerve terminals [38,39]. There is also evidence that enkephalins inhibit release of ACh from the myenteric plexus [40,41].

There is evidence that substance P is released from the myenteric plexus of the guinea-pig longitudinal ileal muscle. Several other agents — ACh, bombesin, cholecystokinin octapeptide, and neurotensin — release substance P from myenteric neurons. Enkephalins inhibit the release of substance P. Substance P and enkephalins have opposing actions on the release of ACh from myenteric plexus. However, considerable experimental work is necessary to elucidate the role of different neuromodulators on the intestinal function.

MODULATION OF CHEMICAL TRANSMISSION BY SUBSTANCE P AND OPIOID PEPTIDES

Substance P and enkephalins interact with presynaptic receptors and influence the neuronal release of chemical transmitters. Mechanisms of these effects of substance P and enkephalins are not established. However, there is considerable evidence that both substance P and enkephalins influence the neuronal release of acetylcholine, norepinephrine, and dopamine.

Substance P and methionine enkephalin: A credible tandem in the release of cerebral acetylcholine

In order to understand the role of substance P and methionine enkephalin in the release of ACh, Sastry and his collaborators [42–44] measured the simultaneous release of all three from superfused rodent cerebral slices as a function of time. All three were spontaneously released from the cerebral slices. The highest rate of release for substance P preceded those of ACh and methionine enkephalin. The peak release of substance P was followed within 3 minutes by the peak release of ACh. The peak release of ACh was followed by the release of methionine enkephalin, with a broad peak that started within 3 minutes of the peak release of ACh. The release of methionine enkephalin was accompanied by decreases in the amounts of ACh and substance P released. Electrical stimulation of the slices caused an increase in the amouts of ACh and methionine enkephalin released. The time sequence for the evoked release of substance P, ACh, and methionine enkephalin followed the same course as that for their spontaneous release. This time sequence for their release suggests that substance P triggers the release of ACh, which is followed by the release of methionine enkephalin.

The long-acting enkephalin analog, D-ala-enkephalinamide (DALA, 17 nM), depressed the spontaneous ACh release. It did not exhibit any effect in Ca^{2+}-free medium. Naloxone (55 nM) increased the rate of ACh release by about 35%, indicating that endogenously released enkephalins have inhibitory effects on ACh release. Substance P (650 nM) increased the rate of ACh release by about 35%. The effects of DALA, naloxone, and substance P on evoked release of ACh are similar to those effects described above for spontaneous release. DALA (17–350 nM) inhibits Ca^{2+} uptake by cerebral slices by 25–55%, whereas substance P (70–650 nM) enhances Ca^{2+} uptake by 105–165%. Uptake of extracellular Ca^{2+} by nerve terminals is an absolute requirement for the release of ACh.

There seems to be a homeostatic relationship among the rates of release of ACh, methionine enkephalin, and substance P and Ca^{2+} fluxes in the rodent cerebrum [45]. This homeostatic relationship is of significance in the autoregulation of ACh release involving two types of presynaptic muscarinic receptors (Ms and Mi) and the level of ACh in the biophase of the synaptic gap [44–46]. This autoregulation of ACh occurs through the operation of two feedback systems, one positive and one negative. The components of the positive feedback system include an Ms receptor, substance P release, activation of a substance P receptor, and activation of Ca^{2+} influx, and the negative feedback system includes an Mi receptor, methionine enkephalin release, activation of an opiate receptor, and inhibition of Ca^{2+} influx. Low levels of ACh in the biophase of the cholinergic synaptic gap may trigger the positive feedback system, and high levels of ACh may trigger the negative feedback system. These feedback systems are depicted by a schematic model in Figure 6-3.

Methionine enkephalin decreases the rate of release of ACh from mouse cerebral slices. This action is accompanied by a decrease in the uptake of Ca^{2+} by the cerebral slices. Similar to methionine enkephalin, morphine decreases both the release of ACh [47] and Ca^{2+} uptake [48]. The time course for the release of methionine enkephalin and ACh; the effect of the exogenous

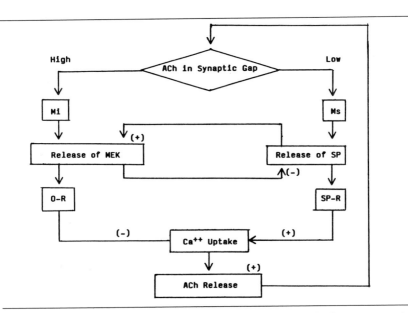

Figure 6-3. A schematic model showing the negative and positive feedback systems postulated to regulate ACh release in the mouse cerebrum. Mi and Ms = presynaptic muscarinic receptors; MEK = methionine enkephalin; SP = substance P; O-R = opiate receptor; SP-R = substance P or tachykinin receptor; (+) = activation; (−) = inhibition.

methionine enkephalin analog, DALA, on the pattern of ACh release; and the effect of naloxone in increasing the rate of ACh release suggest that the rate of methionine enkephalin release is increased in response to the increased rate of release of ACh. These observations support the suggested role of enkephalin as a negative feedback regulator of the release of ACh [42–44].

Substance P increases the rate of ACh release by an action mediated through increased uptake of Ca^{2+} by the cerebral slices. A similar action for substance P on Ca^{2+} uptake was reported for the parotid gland [49]. Further, the increased rate of release of opioid peptides has been reported in response to analgesic doses of substance P [50]. The time course of the simultaneous release of substance P and ACh, and the effect of exogenous substance P on the pattern of ACh release, suggest that ACh is released in response to the preceding high rate of substance P release [42]. These observations indicate a role for substance P as a positive feedback regulator of the release of ACh.

The first step in the negative and positive feedback mechanisms is the activation of two subtypes of presynaptic muscarinic receptors, Mi and Ms, respectively. 5-Hydroxyfurfuryltrimethylammonium (5-HMFT) is a selective agonist for Mi receptors [45,46]. 5-Methoxyfurfuryltrimethylammonium (5-MOFT) is a selective agonist of Ms receptors. 5-MOFT releases ACh at a presynaptic site of action [46]. In low concentrations (1.9 nM), 5-HMFT inhibits both spontaneous and evoked release of ACh. 5-HMFT decreases the rate of release of methionine enkephalin and increases substance P release.

If the rate of release of ACh is regulated by the above feedback mechanisms, they should be affected in conditions producing ACh deficits (e.g., aging and senile dementia). The patterns of release of ACh, methionine enkephalin, and substance P from the cerebral cortical slices of Fischer 344 rats, ages 3–33 months support the above feedback systems [51]. The rates of release of ACh and methionine enkephalin decrease, while the rate of release of substance P increases, as a function of age. Alterations in the release of methionine enkephalin may be a regulatory consequence of the decreased rate of ACh release as a function of age.

Influence of substance P and enkephalins on norepinephrine release

Substance P increases the release of norepinephrine, while enkephalins decrease its release from the mouse and rat vas deferens [52,53]. Decrease in the norepinephrine release from different brain areas of rats, rabbits, and guinea pigs by opioid mu (e.g., rat or guinea pig cortex), kappa (e.g., rabbit cortex), or delta (e.g., guinea pig cortex) agonists have also been reported [54]. The influence of the activation of substance P receptor subtypes on the release of norepinephrine is not yet established.

Influence of substance P and opioid peptides on dopamine synthesis or release

Intranigral injection of substance P increases intraneuronal dopamine metabolism in the rat [55]. It increases levels of dihydroxyphenylacetic acid and homovanillic acid, markers of intraneuronal metabolism of dopamine. Neurokinin A decreases striatal dopamine metabolism in the rat [55]. Delta opioid receptor agonists increase dopamine release, while kappa opioid receptor agonists decrease dopamine release from the rat striatum [54].

SUBSTANCE P AND ENKEPHALINS IN THE REGULATION OF BLOOD PRESSURE

For many years, it was not known which chemical messengers transmitted afferent impulses from the baroreceptors in the aortic arch and carotid sinus to the cardiovascular center in the brain. During the past few years, several peptides, including substance P, enkephalins, and neuropeptide Y, have been found in the afferents [30]. Of these, substance P has been studied in some detail: 1) Substance P has been localized in the adventitia of the aortic arch and carotid sinus, as well as in the vagus and glossopharyngeal nerves by immunofluorescence techniques. 2) Substance P is also present in petrosal and nodosal ganglia, where the cell bodies of sensory afferent neurons that are involved in cardiovascular control are located [56]. 3) The nucleus tractus solitarius (NTS), the terminal for afferent baroreceptor impulses in the medulla oblongata, contains a dense network of substance P nerve terminals surrounding norepinephrine-containing cell bodies [57,58]. When the petrosal or nodosal ganglia are isolated from their central or peripheral branches, substance P disappears from both the central terminals in the NTS and peripheral terminals in the blood vessels [56]. This suggests that substance P is synthesized in the cell bodies in the ganglia and transported to both central and peripheral terminals.

Central injection of substance P 1) stimulates synthesis of catecholamines; 2) raises plasma concentrations of norepinephrine; and 3) raises blood pressure and induces tachycardia, which is accentuated in spontaneously hypertensive rats [59,60]. These central effects are counteracted by the substance P receptor antagonist, D-Pro^2, D-Phe^7, D-Trp^9-SP [61]. It has not been established whether the above effects of substance P are due to sympathetic stimulation or attenuation of the baroreceptor reflex.

Several peptides and catecholamines are not only present in nerve structures located in close proximity to each other, but also coexist in the same population of neurons [62]. The interaction of other peptides, especially enkephalins, with the substance P-induced effects on the baroreceptor system is of interest because enkephalins are known to antagonize substance P-induced effects at some central and peripheral sites.

OPIOID AND TACHYKININ-PEPTIDE SYSTEMS IN MALE GENITAL TRACT

The internal spermic, vesicle, prostatic, and cavernous plexi include components of parasympathetic, sympathetic, and afferent nervous systems. Stimuli for reflex neural pathways for erection, emission, ejaculation, orgasm, and detumescence are coordinated through these plexi. Erection and glandular secretions are regulated by cholinergic impulses, while emission and ejaculation seem to be regulated by adrenergic impulses. The excitation and detumescence of the orgasmic experience is also modified by the neuromodulators of autonomic and sensory nervous systems. Substance P and enkephalins are known to modulate cholinergic and adrenergic transmission. In order to understand the modulation of chemical transmission in the male reproductive tract, the rat epididymis, prostate gland, seminal vesicles, and spermatozoa, and human seminal plasma and spermatozoa were analyzed for substance P, methionine enkephalin, and leucine enkephalin by radioimmunoassays [53,63]. The effects of substance P and enkephalins and their antagonists on chemical transmission in the rat vas deferens [53,64] and human sperm motility [63,65] were determined.

Epididymis is a rich source for substance-P immunoreactivity. Substance P levels in the epididymis are higher by about 2.8 and 19.3 times than those in the prostate and seminal vesicles. Seminal vesicles are a rich source of enkephalins. They have about 2.9 and 2.6 times higher leucine enkephalin than epididymis and prostate, respectively. Human seminal plasma contains about 47 times higher levels of leucine enkephalin than substance P. The split ejaculate technique for semen collection indicates that early fractions of the human ejaculate contain fluids from the prostate (and possibly the epididymis), while later fractions represent seminal vesicle secretions. A low exogenous concentration of substance P (400 nM) increases sperm motility, while leucine enkephalin (100 μM) depresses it. Substance P (1–10 μg/ml) and muscarinic agonists enhance the adrenergic transmission of the rat vas deferens to electrical stimulation. Leucine enkephalin (1–10 μg/ml) depresses adrenergic transmission and antagonizes the effects of substance P and muscarinic agonists. These studies suggest that substance P-like tachykinins may play a role in sperm maturation, expulsion of fluid from epididymis, and initiation of motility, while leucine enkephalinlike peptides may contribute to orgasmic experience and its detumescence. Substance P and leucine enkephalin may exert opposite actions on Ca^{2+} uptake by spermatozoa and thereby regulate sperm motility.

OPIOID AND TACHYKININ PEPTIDE SYSTEMS IN NON-NERVOUS TISSUES

Opioid peptides and several tachykinins are also known to occur in non-mammalian and mammalian tissues. The possible role of substance P and enkephalins in human spermatozoa was discussed in the previous section. The role of opioid peptides in the release of ACh from human placenta, a non-nervous tissue, has been investigated in considerable detail.

Opioid peptides and substance P in human placenta and their role in the regulation of acetylcholine release

Acetylcholine (ACh) occurs in high concentrations in human placenta and is released into maternal and fetal circulations [66]. It has been postulated that ACh released into maternal side stimulates a muscarinic receptor in the trophoblast and regulates the active uptake of amino acids by placenta [67].

Inhibition of ACh synthesis results in the depression of amino acid uptake by isolated human placental villus. ACh may cause relaxation of placental vasculature by interaction at endothelial muscarinic receptors in the presence of vasoactive agents (e.g., 5-hydroxytryptamine) and facilitate diffusion of amino acids from the trophoblast into fetal circulation [68].

The release of ACh from human placental villus resembles that from nervous tissue in several respects [69,70]. The rate of release of ACh is increased by 1) depolarization with high concentrations of K^+ (17–63 mM), 2) increasing concentrations of Ca^{2+} (4.64–9.4 mM), and 3) nicotine [69]. No ACh is released in the absence of extracelluar Ca^{2+}. Depolarizing concentrations of K^+ and nicotine do not increase the rate of release of ACh in the absence of extracellular Ca^{2+}. Cocaine and morphine inhibit ACh release possibly by inhibiting Ca^{2+} influx. Amino acid uptake by placental villus is also depressed in Ca^{2+}-free medium and by cocaine and morphine [71]. Atropine blocks ACh release and amino acid uptake by placental villus, indicating that ACh stimulates a muscarinic receptor and thereby regulates amino acid uptake by the trophoblast.

The presence of several opioid peptides — β-lipotropin, β-endorphin, and methionine enkephalin — in human placenta has been demonstrated by specific radioimmunoassays and bioassays [72–74]. In addition, dinorphin 1–8 has been shown to occur in human placenta [75]. The kappa opiate agonist, ethylketocyclazocine (100 μM), depresses the rate of spontaneous release of ACh from human placental villus by about 50% [76,77]. The kappa antagonist, (−)-2-(3-furylmethyl)-noretazocine (1 mM) enhances the rate of ACh release by about 18-fold. These observations indicate that endogenous methionine enkephalin and β-endorphin downregulate ACh release by a negative feedback mechanism. They may decrease Ca^{2+} influx into the trophoblast and decrease ACh release. Under steady-state conditions, a negative feedback process is the predominant mechanism by which ACh release is regulated. While opiate agonists would enhance the effects of endogenous opiate peptides, opiate antagonists would unmask the downregulation by endogenous peptides and increase ACh release.

The occurrence of substance-P-like activity in human placenta has been demonstrated by specific radioimmunoassays and bioassays [72,73]. However, the role of substance P in the release of ACh from human placenta has yet to be studied. Since ACh synthesis and release are similar in human trophoblast and in the nerve, one may predict that substance P increases ACh release and plays a significant positive feedback role in the regulation of ACh release from placenta.

The physiological role of opioid peptides and tachykinins in human placenta is not established. It has been suggested that the local release of enkephalins and other opioid peptides into maternal circulation by placenta may regulate sensory transmission (or pain impulses) to the central nervous system from the distended uterus and vaginal tract during childbrith [72].

METABOLISM OF SUBSTANCE P AND OTHER TACHYKININS

As there is evidence that substance P and other tachykinins may play roles as chemical transmitters or modulators, there should be mechanisms for the termination of their actions. Three types of mechanisms have been postulated for termination of chemical transmitter action: 1) reuptake by the nerve terminal (e.g., norepinephrine), 2) enzymatic inactivation by hydrolysis (e.g., acetylcholine hydrolysis by acetylcholinesterases, and 3) diffusion of transmitter from receptor sites (e.g., acetylcholine at cholinergic receptors). Although there may be limited possibilities, reuptake mechanisms do not appear to exist for peptide transmitters. It is generally believed that synaptically released peptides are inactivated by hydrolysis of one or more specific peptide bonds by peptidases.

Several criteria have to be satisfied for a peptidase to inactivate a neuropeptide at peptidergic synapses: 1) The products of peptidase hydrolysis must be biologically inactive. 2) Inhibition of the peptidase must protect the synaptically released peptide. 3) Inhibition of the peptidase must prolong the biological action of the peptide. 4) The cellular and subcellular location of the peptidase must be consistent with its action on the synaptically released peptide. 5) The substrate specificity of the peptidase must be compatible with altered biological activity of the peptide analogs. 6) Adaptive peptidase activity may occur in response to alteration in neuronal activity. Not all these criteria are satisfied by any peptidase that inactivates substance P or any of the tachykinins.

Several enzymes have been shown to hydrolyze substance P molecules in vitro at a variety of peptide bonds (Figure 6-4). Dipeptidylaminopepidase B [78], dipeptidylaminopeptidase IV [79], post-proline-cleaving enzyme [80,81], and serum cholinesterase [82] hydrolyze substance P at Pro^2-Lys^3 and Pro^4-Gln^5 bonds. The pharmacological activity of substance P is still retained in the product substance P(5–11) peptide. These enzymes may not play a pharmacological role in inactivating substance P in vivo. Acid proteinase [83], endopeptidase 24.11 [84], and substance P endopeptidase [85] hydrolyze substance P at Gln^6-Phe^7 and Phe^7-Phe^8 bonds. The products may not possess substance P-like activity.

Substance P endopeptidase has been purified from human diencephalon. It is a membrane-bound enzyme and prefers substance P as a substrate (K_m 29 μmol) against a variety of other neuropeptides. Several other substance P analogs serve as inhibitors and prevent hydrolysis of substance P by this enzyme in rat brain slices. This enzyme may therefore play an important role in the physiological inactivation of substance P in the brain. However, more information is necessary on its cellular and subcellular localization to evaluate whether or not this enzyme serves as a synaptic substance P-degrading peptidase.

Endopeptidase 24.11 has been isolated from several tissues [84]. It is membrane bound in synaptosomal membranes of pig caudate. It has a rather broad

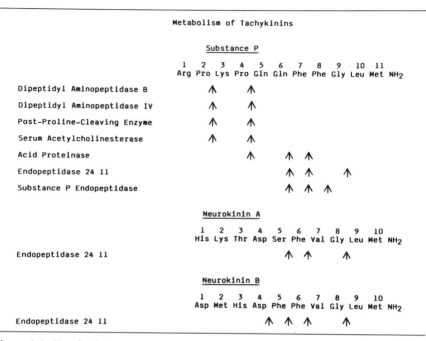

Figure 6-4. Sites for the inactivation of tachykinins by various peptides.

spectrum of substrate specificity and is not peptide specific. It may play a role in physiological inactivation of substance P.

Peptidases may play two other roles besides inactivation of substance P. One of these roles is related to the notion that peptidases (other post-translational enzymes) may be involved in the final step of the expression of the activity of a neuropeptide. The second possible role of peptidases may be to generate a molecule with new biological activity from a peptide of known biological activity. Post-proline-cleaving enzyme may satisfy these roles by its action on substance P [86]. It has a high catalytic efficiency for hydrolysis of substance P. It hydrolyzes substance P into C-terminal heptapeptide amide, substance P(5–11), and N-terminal basic tetrapeptide, Arg-Pro-Lys-Pro. Several activities of substance P are represented in the heptapeptide, substance P(5–11). These include sialogogic activity, vascular effects, smooth-muscle contraction, analgesia, and spinal motor neuron depolarization [87]. There is a high-affinity uptake system for substance P(5–11) in the nerve terminal terminating the action of substance P [88]. Possible roles of N-terminal substance P sequences have also been suggested [87], including enhancement of phagocytosis by mouse macrophages and human polymorphonuclear leucocytes, specific motor effects, and behavioral effects [89,90]. If post-proline-cleaving enzyme has access to substance P in the presynaptic nerve terminals before release or to the extracellular space of the synaptic cleft, then this enzyme could be involved in the production of the synaptically active form of substance P. Evidence is lacking that this happens in situ.

TACHYKININ RECEPTORS

There is considerable evidence that there are multiple classes of receptors for the naturally occurring tachykinins [91–96]. This evidence is based upon the potencies of various tachykinins in different bioassay preparations, pharmacological activities of selective synthetic analogs of substance P, and radioligand studies using ^{125}I-Bolton Hunter conjugates (^{125}I-BH) of tachykinins, phosphatidylinositol hydrolysis by tachykinins, and characterization of functional cDNA encoding the tachykinin receptors. These studies indicate that there are at least three types of tachykinin receptors — SP-P, NK-A, and NK-B — for which the preferred tachykinins are substance P, neurokinin A, and neurokinin B, respectively (Table 6-4). Several authors have used different terminology to indicate subtypes of tachykinin receptors. However, established nomenclature may not adequately explain all the pharmacological actions of all naturally occurring tachykinins. The advent of selective antagonists may serve to explain the postulated differences among subtypes of tachykinin receptors.

The influence of various tachykinins on phosphatidylinositol (PI) hydrolysis has been studied in the hamster urinary bladder, a model tissue for NK-A receptor, and in the rat salivary gland, a model tissue for SP-P receptor. Substance P was the most active tachykinin to stimulate PI hydrolysis in the rat salivary gland, while kassinin and eledoisin were more potent than substance P in stimulating PI hydrolysis in the hamster urinary bladder [95]. These observations indicate that both SP-P and NK-A receptors are coupled to PI hydrolysis.

A complementary DNA (cDNA) encoding the substance P receptor from the rat brain and submandibular gland has been isolated by Hershey and Krause [96]. The distribution of mRNA for this receptor is similar to the distribution of substance P binding sites in urinary bladder, submandibular gland, striatum, and spinal cord. It appears to mediate actions of substance P and may be of the SP-P subtype. NK-A and NK-B receptors have yet to be isolated.

TACHYKININS AND OPIOID PEPTIDES: CLINICAL PHARMACOLOGY SITUATIONS

The widespread distribution of tachykinins in the nervous system and their release in physiological and pathological situations has stimulated the measurement of these peptides in body fluids (plasma, CSF) or tissues. Since opioid peptides and tachykinins regulate one another, both groups of peptides will be affected. Most of the work in this area is limited to the measurement of the immunoreactivities of either substance P or enkephalins (or β-endorphin).

Several clinical situations in which tissue levels of substance P were altered have been discussed by Pernow [99]. It is beyond the scope of this presentation

Table 6-4. Provisional division of tachykinin receptors as three subtypes[a]

Distinguishing features	SP-P	NK-A	NK-B	Ref.
1 Alternate names	NK-P, NK-1, TK-1	SP-E, SP-K, NK-2, TK-3	SP-E, SP-N, NK-3, TK-3	91,97,98
2 Preferred tachykinin	Substance P	Neurokinin A	Neurokinin B	93,94
3 Tachykinin potency	SP > PHY > NKA ≥ NKB ≥ E > KAS	NKA ≥ NKB ≥ KAS ≥ E ≫ SP > PHY	NKB ≫ E ≥ KAS > NKA = PHY > SP	94
4 D-Pro/L-Pro ratio[b]	87–124	0.003	0.3	93,94
5 SPOMe/I-BHSPOMe ratio[c]	0.1–0.3	164–213	1000	93,94
6 Model tissues	Salivary gland (rat), urinary bladder (guinea pig)	Urinary bladder (hamster), vas deferens (rat)	Cerebral cortex (rat), myenteric plexus (rat)	93,94

[a] SP = substance P; E = eledoisin; PHY = physalaemin; KAS = kassinin; NKA = neurokinin A (= neurokinin alpha, neuromedin L, or substance K); NKB = neurokinin B (= neurokinin beta, neuromedin K); TK = tachykinins as a group defined by the C-terminal.
[b] The ratio of IC50s for [Glp^6, D-Pro^9]-SP (6–11) to [Glp^6, L-Pro^9]-SP (6–11).
[c] The ratio of IC50s for SP-O-methyl ester and its iodinated Bolten Hunter conjugate.

to discuss all these situations. The present discussion is limited to three clinical trends as examples of areas where progress is possible for the role of substance P and enkephalins, namely, hypertensive states, chronic pain syndromes, and pregnancy. Leucine enkephalin concentrations at rest and during exercise were lower in the plasma of hypertensive patients than normotensive patients [100,101]. The plasma levels of norepinephrine in hypertensive patients were higher than those in normotensive patients. Enkephalins are known to reduce neuronal release of norepinephrine [102]. Reduced enkephalinergic activity may contribute to development and maintenance of a hypertensive state.

In chronic back pain syndromes, immunoreactive substance P levels decrease in cerebrospinal fluid [103], plasma, and saliva [104]. In cluster headaches, plasma substance P immunoreactivity decreases [105] and methionine enkephalin levels increase. [106,107]. Substance P and opioid peptides are implicated in the pathophysiology of chronic pain syndromes. To obtain direct evidence for this implication, plasma samples from the same groups of patients should be analyzed for both substance P and opioid peptides.

Maternal plasma levels of β-endorphin were significantly elevated during labor and the early postpartum period [108]. It has been suggested that the pain associated with labor and the psychological stress of delivery may serve as potent stimuli for the pituitary release of β-endorphin. Information on the plasma levels of other opioid peptides and substance P during pregnancy are not available. The role of placental production and release of substance P and opioid peptides during pregnancy have yet to be established [72,73].

CONCLUSIONS

Substance P is a key member of the tachykinin family of local peptide hormones/neurotransmitters/neuromodulators. Considerable progress has been made in pharmacological activities of substance P, its synthesis, and metabolism in neuronal tissues. The role of substance P in sensory transmission, inflammation, pain transmission, and modulation of chemical transmission is well established. It functions in concert with other transmitters, especially opioid peptides (enkephalins), to maintain homeostasis of cell or organ functions. Progress has yet to be made in several areas: 1) development of selective antagonists that interact with subtypes of tachykinin receptors; 2) role of substance P antagonists as analgesics; 3) alterations in plasma and salivary concentrations of substance P and enkephalins in various pain syndromes and degenerative diseases; 4) differential functions of various tachykinins and enkephalins in neuronal and non-neuronal cells; and 5) alterations in the plasma and tissue levels of tachykinins and opioid peptides by drugs.

ACKNOWLEDGMENTS

The author's research is supported by United States Public Health Service — National Institutes of Health, The Council for Tobacco Research, Inc., The

Smokeless Tobacco Research Council, Inc., and The Departments of Pharmacology and Anesthesiology, Vanderbilt University.

REFERENCES

1. von Euler VS, Gaddum JH. 1931. An unidentified depressor substance in certain tissue extracts. J Physiol (London) 72:74–87.
2. Gaddum JH, Schild H. 1934. Depressor substance in extracts of intestine. J Physiol (London) 83:1–14.
3. Leeman SE, Hammerschlag R. 1967. Stimulation of salivary secretion by a factor extracted from hypothalamic tissue. Endocrinology 81:803–810.
4. Carroway R, Leeman SE. 1970. The amino acid sequence of bovine hypothalamic substance P. Identity to substance P from colliculi and small intestine. J Biol Chem 254:2944–2945.
5. Tregear GW, Niall HD, Potts JT Jr., Leeman SE, Chang NM. 1971. Synthesis of substance P. Nature New Biol 232:87–89.
6. Powell D, Leeman SE, Tregear GW, Niall HD, Potts JT Jr. 1973. Radioimmunoassay for substance P. Nature New Biol 241:252–254.
7. Nawa H, Kotani H, Nakanishi S. 1984. Tissue specific generation of two preprotachykinin mRNAs from one gene by alternative tissue splicing. Nature 312:729–734.
8. Bonner TI, Young AC, Affolter HU. 1987. Cloning and expression of rat and human tachykinin genes. In JL Henry, et al. (eds), Substance P and Neurokinins. New York, Springer Verlag, pp. 3–4.
9. Martin JH. 1985. Anatomical substrates for somatic sensation. In ER Kandel, JH Schwartz (eds), Principles of Neural Science. New York, Elsevier, pp. 301–330.
10. Kelly DD. 1985. Central representations of pain and analgesia. In ER Kandel, JH Schwartz (eds), Principles of Neural Science. New York, Elsevier, pp. 331–334.
11. Kahn CH, Warfield CA. 1989. The role of neurotransmitters in processing painful stimuli. Hosp Prac 24(1):165–170.
12. Fields HL, Basbaum AI. 1978. Brain stem control of spinal pain-transmission neurons. Ann Rev Physiol 40:217–248.
13. Jessell TM, Iversen LL. 1977. Opiate analgesics inhibit substance P release from rat trigeminal nucleus. Nature 268:549–551.
14. Hokfelt T, Kellerth JO, Nilsson G, Pernow B. 1975. Substance P: Localization in central nervous system and some primary sensory neurons. Science 190:889–890.
15. Lembeck F. 1985. Substance P and sensory neurons. In CC Jordan, P Oehme (eds), Substance P Metabolism and Metabolic Actions. London, Taylor and Francis, pp. 137–152.
16. Yaksh TL, Jessell TM, Gamse R, Mudge AW, Leeman SE. 1980. Intrathecal morphine inhibits substance P release from mammalian spinal cord in vivo. Nature 286:155–157.
17. Murase K, Nedeljkov V, Randic M. 1982. The actions of neuropeptides on dorsal horn neurons in the rat spinal cord slick preparation: An intracellular study. Brain Res 234:170–176.
18. Lembeck F, Skofitsch G. 1982. Visceral pain reflex after pretreatment with capsaicin and morphine. Naunyn-Schmiedebergs Arch Pharmacol 321:116–122.
19. Donnerer J, Lembeck F. 1983. Heat loss reaction to capsaicin through a peripheral site of action. Br J Pharmacol 79:719–723.
20. Dib B. 1982. Effects of intracerebroventricular capsaicin on thermoregulatory behavior in the rat. Pharmacol, Biochem Behav 16:23–27.
21. Lundblad L. 1984. Protective reflexes and vascular effects in the nasal mucosa elicited by activation of capsaicin-sensitive substance P-immunoreactive trigeminal neurons. Acta Physiologica Scand 529(Suppl):1–42.
22. Holzer-Petsche V, Lembeck F. 1984. Systemic capsaicin treatment impairs the micturition reflex in the rat. Br J Pharmacol 83:935–942.
23. Traurig H, Saria A, Lembeck F. 1984. Substance P in primary afferent neurons of the female rat reproductive system. Naunyn-Schmiedebergs Arch Pharmacol 326:343–346.
24. Donnerer J, Bartho L, Holzer P, Lembeck F. 1984. Intestinal peristalsis associated with release of immunoreactive substance P. Neuroscience 11:913–918.
25. Miller RJ, Pickel VM. 1980. The distribution and functions of enkephalins. J Histochem Cytochem 28:903–917.
26. Mudge AW, Leeman SE, Fischbach GD. 1979. Enkephalin inhibits release of substance P

from sensory neurons in culture and decreases action potential duration. Proc Natl Acad Sci USA 76:526–530.

27. Akil H, Meyer DJ, Leibeskind JC. 1976. Antagonism of stimulation-produced analgesia by naloxone, a narcotic antagonist. Science 191:961–962.

28. Ward RA, Roberts MHT. 1985. The effects of substance P and related peptides on 5-hydroxytryptamine binding in the dorsal half of the rat spinal cord. In CC Jordan, P Oehme (eds), Substance P. Metabolism and Biological Actions. London, Taylor & Francis, p. 217.

29. Ward RA, Roberts MHT. 1983. The possible role of substance P coexisting with 5-hydroxytryptamine in central neurones. Regul Pept 7:306.

30. Pernow B. 1985. Substance P: Present status and future prospects. In CC Jordan, P Oehme (eds), Substance P. Metabolism and Biological Action. London, Taylor & Francis, pp. 187–196.

31. Hagermark O, Hokfelt T, Pernow B. 1978. Flare and itch induced by substance P in human skin. J Invest Dermatol 71:233–235.

32. Lembeck F, Holzer P. 1979. Substance P as neurogenic mediator of antidromic vasodilation and neurogenic plasma extravasation. Naunyn-Schmiedebergs Arch Pharmacol 310:175–183.

33. Bill A, Stjernschantz J, Mandahl A, Brodin E, Nilsson G. 1979. Substance P: Release on trigeminal nerve stimulation, effects in the eye. Acta Physiol Scand 106:371–373.

34. Mandahl A, Bill A. 1983. In the eye (D-Pro^2, D-Trp^{7,9})-SP is a substance P agonist, which modifies the responses to substance P, prostaglandin E_1 and antidromic trigeminal nerve stimulation. Acta Physiol Scand 117:139–144.

35. Lundblad L, Anggard A, Lundberg JM. 1983. Effects of antidromic trigeminal nerve stimulation in relation to parasympathetic vasodilation in cat nasal mucosa. Acta Physiol Scand 119:7–13.

36. Lundberg JM, Brodin E, Hua Y, Saria A. 1984. Vascular permeability changes and smooth muscle contraction in relation to capsaicin-sensitive substance P afferents in the guinea-pig. Acta Physiol Scand 120:217–227.

37. Brodin E, Gaxelius B, Olgart L, Nilsson G. 1981. Tissue concentration and release of substance P-like immunoreactivity in the dental pulp. Acta Physiol Scand 111:141–149.

38. Costa M, Furness JB, Llewellyn-Smith IJ, Murphy R, Bornstein JC, Keast JR. 1985. Functional roles for substance P-containing neurones in the gastrointestinal tract. In CC Jordan, P Oehme (eds), Substance P. Metabolism and Biological Actions. London, Taylor & Francis, pp. 99–120.

39. Gallacher DV, Petersen OH. 1981. Substance P: Indirect and direct effects of parotid acinar cell membrane potential. Pflügers Arch Eur J Physiol 389:127–130.

40. Sastry BVR, Rowell PP, Ochillo RF, Chaturvedi AK. 1977. 5-Hydroxymethylfurfuryltri-methylammonium, a muscarine analog with novel pharmacological action. Pharmacologist 19:220.

41. Sastry BVR, Owens LK, Chaturvedi AK. 1978. The role of presynaptic muscarinic receptors and enkephalins for release of acetylcholine in the guinea pig longitudinal ileal muscle. In Absts 7th Int Cong Pharmacol, Paris, p. 173.

42. Sastry BVR, Tayeb OS. 1982. Regulation of acetylcholine release in the mouse cerebrum by methionine enkephalin and substance P. Adv Biosci 38:165–172.

43. Sastry BVR, Janson VE, Jaiswal N, Tayeb OS. 1983. Changes in enzymes of the cholinergic system and acetylcholine release in the cerebra of aging male Fischer rats. Pharmacology 26:61–72.

44. Tayeb OS, Sastry BVR. 1987. Release of substance P, acetylcholine, and methionine enkephalin from mouse cerebral slices: Effects of nicotine. In JL Henry, et al. (eds), Substance P and Neurokinins. New York, Springer-Verlag, pp. 350–352.

45. Sastry BVR, Jaiswal N, Tayeb OS. 1986. Regulation of acetylcholine release from rodent cerebrum by presynaptic receptors, methionine enkephalin and substance P. Adv Behavioral Biol 30:1047–1056.

46. Sastry BVR, Owens LK, Ochillo RF. 1990. Two furan analogs of muscarine as selective agonists at the presynaptic muscarinic receptors of the guinea pig longitudinal ileal muscle. Ann NY Acad Sci. 604:566–568.

47. Yaksh TL, Yamamura HI. 1977. Depression by morphine of the resting and evoked release of [^{3}H]-acetylcholine from the cat caudate nucleus in vivo. Neuropharmacol 16:227–233.

48. Munoz FG, Guerraro MDL, Way EL. 1979. Effect of β-endorphin on calcium uptake in the

brain. Science 206:89–91.

49. Putney JW, Van de Walle CM, Leslie BA. 1978. Receptor control of calcium influx in parotid aciner cells. Mol Pharmacol 14:1046–1053.
50. Malik JB, Goldstein JM. 1978. Analgesic activity of substance P following intracellular administration in rats. Life Sci 23:835–844.
51. Sastry BVR, Tayeb OS. 1988. Autoregulation of acetylcholine release. Modulation by substance P and methionine enkephalin as a function of age. Regul Pept 22:168.
52. Segawa T, Murakami H, Ogawa H, Yajima H. 1977. Effect of enkephalin and substance P on sympathetic nerve transmission in mouse vas deferens. Jpn J Pharmacol 28:13–19.
53. Sastry BVR, Janson VE, Owens LK, Tayeb OS. 1982. Enkephalin and substance P-like immunoreactivities of mammalian sperm and accessory sex glands. Biochem Pharmacol 31:3519–3522.
54. Jakisch J, Geppert M, Lupp A, Huang HY, Illes P. 1988. Types of opioid receptors modulating neurotransmitter release in discrete brain regions. In P Illes, C Farsang (eds), Regulatory Roles of Opioid Peptides. Weinheim, FRG, VCH, pp. 240–258.
55. Quirion R, Dam T-V. 1985. Multiple tachykinin receptors. In CC Jordon, P Oehme (eds), Substance P. Metabolism and Biological Actions. London, Taylor & Francis, pp. 45–64.
56. Gillis RA, Helke CJ, Hamilton BL, Norman WP, Jacobowitz DM. 1980. Evidence that substance P is a neurotransmitter of baro- and chemoreceptor afferents in nucleus tractus solitarius. Brain Res 181:476–481.
57. Cuello AC, Kanazawa I. 1978. The distribution of substance P immunoreactive fibers in the rat central nervous system. J Comp Neurol 178:129–156.
58. Ljungdahl A, Hokfelt T, Nilsson G. 1978. Distribution of substance P-like immunoreactivity in the central nervous system of the rat — I. Cell bodies and nerve terminals. Neuroscience 3:861–943.
59. Unger T, Rockhold RW, Yajimura T, Rettig R, Ganten D. 1980. Blood pressure and heart rate responses to centrally administered substance P are increased in spontaneously hypertensive rats. Clin Sci 59:299S–302S.
60. Unger T, Rascher W, Schuster C, Pavlovitch R, Schomig A, Dietz R, Ganten D. 1981. Central blood pressure effects of substance P and angiotensin II: Role of the sympathetic nervous system and vasopressin. Eur J Pharmacol 71:33–42.
61. Fuxe K, Agnati LF, Rosell S, Harfstrand A, Folders K, Lundberg JM, Andersson K, Hokfelt T. 1982. Vassopressor effects of substance P and C-terminal sequences after intracisternal injection to alpha-chloralose-anaesthetized rats: Blockade by a substance P antagonist. Eur J Pharmacol 77:171–176.
62. Hokfelt T, Johansson O, Ljungdahl A, Lundberg JM, Schulzberg M. 1980. Peptidergic neurones. Nature 284:515–521.
63. Sastry BVR, Janson VE. 1987. Substance P in human spermatozoa and modulation of sperm motility by substance P and its antagonists. In JL Henry, et al. (eds), Substance P and Neurokinins. New York, Springer-Verlag, pp. 179–181.
64. Sastry BVR, Janson VE, Owens LK. 1990, Significance of substance P and enkephalin-peptide systems in male genital tract. Ann NY Acad Sci. in press.
65. Sastry BVR, Janson VE. 1987. Opioid-like peptides in human semen and their effects in sperm motility. Ann NY Acad Sci 513:586–588.
66. Sastry BVR, Sadavongvivad C. 1979. Cholinergic systems in non-nervous tissues. Pharmacol Rev 30:65–132.
67. Sastry BVR, Barnwell SL, Moore RD. 1983. Factors affecting the uptake of alpha-amino acids by human placental villus: acetylcholine, phospholipid methylation, Ca^{2+} and cytoskeletal organization. Trophoblast Res 1:81–100.
68. Sastry BVR, Owens LK. 1987. Regional and differential sensitivity of umbilico-placental vasculature to 5-hydroxytryptamine, nicotine, and ethyl alcohol. Trophoblast Res 2:289–304.
69. Sastry BVR, Olubadewo J, Boehm FH. 1977. Effects of nicotine and cocaine on the release of acetylcholine from isolated placental villi. Arch Int Pharmacodyn Ther 229:23–36.
70. Olubadewo JO, Sastry BVR. 1978. Human placental cholinergic system: Stimulation-secretion coupling for release of acetylcholine from isolated placental villus. J Pharmacol Exp Therap 204:433–445.
71. Barnwell SL, Sastry BVR. 1983. Depression of amino acid uptake in human placental villus by cocaine, morphine and nicotine. Trophoblast Res 1:101–120.

72. Sastry BVR, Barnwell SL, Tayeb OS, Janson VE, Owens LK. 1980. Occurrence of methionine enkephalin in human placental villus. Biochem Pharmacol 29:475–478.
73. Sastry BVR, Tayeb OS, Janson VE, Owens LK. 1981. Peptides from human placenta: Methionine enkephalin and substance P. Placenta (Suppl. 3):327–337.
74. Odagiri E, Sherrell BJ, Mount CD, Nicolson WE, Orth DN. 1979. Human placental immunoreactive corticotropin lipotropin and beta-endorphin: Evidence for a common precursor. Proc Natl Acad Sci USA 76:2027–2031.
75. Ahmed MS, Randall LW, Sibai B, Dass C, Fridland G, Desiderio DM, Tolun E. 1987. Identification of dynorphin 1–8 in human placenta. Life Sci 40:2067–2076.
76. Ahmed MS, Horst MA. 1986. Opioid receptors of human placental villi modulate acetylcholine release. Life Sci 39:535–540.
77. Sastry BVR. 1988. Role of opioid peptides in human placenta. A comparative study on the down regulation of acetylcholine release in human placental villus, guinea pig Auerbach plexus and mouse cerebrum. In Y Tomada, et al. (eds), Placental and Endometrial Proteins. Utrect, Netherlands, VSP Press, pp. 357–360.
78. Kato T, Hama T, Nagatsu T, 1980. Separation of two dipeptidyl aminopeptidases in the human brain. J Neurochem 34:602–608.
79. Heymann E, Mentlein R. 1978. Liver dipeptidyl aminopeptidase IV hydrolyzes substance. P. FEBS Lett 91:360–364.
80. Kato T, Nakano N, Kojima K, Nagatsu T, Sakikibara S. 1980. Changes in prolyl endopeptidase during maturation of rat brain and hydrolysis of substance P by the purified enzyme. J Neurochem 35:527–535.
81. Wilk S, Orlowski M. 1980. Cation-sensitive neutral endopeptidase: Isolation and specificity of the bovine pituitary enzyme. J Neurochem 35:1172–1182.
82. Lockridge O. 1982. Substance P hydrolysis of human serum cholinesterase. J Neurochem 39:106–110.
83. Akopyran TN, Arutunyan AA, Lajtha A, Galoyan AA. 1978. Acid proteinase of hypothalamus: Purification, some properties, and action of somatostatin and Substance P. Neurochemical Res 3:89–99.
84. Matsas R, Fulcher IS, Kenny AJ, Turner AJ. 1983. Substance P and [leu]enkephalin are hydrolyzed by an enzyme in pig caudate synaptic membranes that is identical with the endopeptidase to kidney microvilli. Proc Natl Acad Sci USA 80:3111–3115.
85. Lee CM, Sandberg BEB, Hanley MR, Iversen LL. 1981. Purification and characterization of a membrane-bound substance-P-degrading enzyme from human brain. Eur J Biochem 114:315–327.
86. Krause JE. 1985. On the physiological metabolism of substance P. In CC Jordan, P Oehme (eds), Substance P. Metabolism and Biological Actions. London, Taylor & Francis, pp. 13–33.
87. Blumberg S, Teichberg V. 1982. The role of the N-terminal sequence in the biological activities of substance P. In CE Trabucchi (ed), Regulatory Peptides: From Molecular Biology to Function. New York, Raven Press, pp. 445–452.
88. Nakata Y, Yajima H, Segawa T. 1981. Active uptake of substance P carboxy-terminal heptapeptide (5–11) into rat brain and rabbit spinal cord slices. J Neurochem 37:1529–1543.
89. Hall ME, Stewart JM. 1983. Substance P and behavior: Opposite effects of N-terminal and C-terminal fragments. Peptides 4:763–768.
90. Stewart JM, Hall ME, Harkins J, Frederickson RCA, Terenius L, Hokfelt T, Krivoy W. 1982. A fragment of substance P with specific central activity: SP(1–7). Peptides 3:351–357.
91. Lee CM, Iversen LL, Hanley MR, Sandberg BEB. 1982. The possible existence of multiple receptors for substance P. Naunyn Schmiedebergs Arch Pharmacol 318:281–287.
92. Iversen LL. 1985. Multiple receptors for tachykinins. In R Hakanson, F Sundler (eds), Tachykinin Antagonists. Amsterdam, Elsevier, pp. 291–304.
93. Iversen LL, Foster AC, Watling KJ, McKnight AT, Williams BJ, Lee CM. 1987. Multiple receptors and binding sites for tachykinins. In JL Henry, et al. (eds), Substance P and Neurokinins. New York, Springer-Verlag, pp. 40–43.
94. Lee CM, Campbell NJ, Williams BJ, Iversen LL. 1987. Multiple tachykinin binding sites in rat brain and peripheral tissues. In JL Henry, et al. (eds), Substance P and Neurokinins. New York, Springer-Verlag, pp. 44–46.
95. Watling KJ, Suman-Chanham, Bristow DR. 1987. Tachykinin-induced phosphatidylinositol

turnover in hamster urinary bladder. In JL Henry, et al. (eds), Substance P and Neurokinins. New York, Springer-Verlag, pp. 56–59.

96. Hershey AD, Krause JE. 1989. Molecular characterization of a functional cDNA encoding the rat substance P receptor. Science 247:958–962.
97. Buck SH, Burcher E, Shults CW, Lovenberg W, O'Donohue TL. 1984. Novel pharmacology of substance K-binding sites: A third type of tachykinin receptor. Science 226:987–989.
98. Regoli D, D'Orleans-Juste P, Drapeau G, Dion S, Escher E. 1985. Pharmacological characterization of substance P antagonists. In: R Hakanson, F Sundler (eds), Tachykinin Antagonists. Amsterdam, Elsevier Science.
99. Pernow B. 1987. Research on tachykinins: Clinical trends. In JL, Henry, et al. (eds), Substance P and Neurokinins. New York, Springer-Verlag, pp. 372–379.
100. Esler M, Jennings G, Biviane B, Lambert G, Hasking G. 1986. Mechanism of elevated plasma noradrenaline in the course of essential hypertension. J Cardiovasc Pharmacol 8(Suppl. 5):S39–S43.
101. Kraft K, Kokorsch F, Diehl J, Kolloch R, Stumpe KO. 1990. Altered plasma leucine-enkephalin concentrations in patients with established hypertension. Prog Clin Biol Res 328:367–370.
102. Gaddes RR, Dixon W. 1982. Presynaptic opiate receptor-mediated inhibition of endogenous norepinephrine and dopamine-beta-hydroxylase in the cat spleen. J Pharmacol Exp Therap 223:77–83.
103. Almay BGL, Johansson F, Von Knorring L, Le Greves P, Terenius L. 1988. Substance P in CSF of patients with chronic pain syndromes. Pain 33:3–9.
104. Parris WCV, Kambam JR, Naukam RJ, Sastry BVR. 1990. Immunoreactive substance P is decreased in saliva of patients with chronic back pain syndromes. Anesth Analg 70:63–67.
105. Sicuteri F, Renzi D, Geppetti P. 1986. Substance P and enkephalins: A credible tandem in the pathophysiology of cluster headache and migraine. Adv Exp Med Biol 198:142–152.
106. Mosnaim AD, Chevesich J, Wolf ME, Freitag FG, Diamond S. 1986. Plasma methionine enkephalin. Increased levels during a migraine episode. Headache 26:278–281.
107. Mosnaim AD, Diamond S, Freitag F, Chevesich J, Wolf ME, Solomon G. 1987. Plasma and platelet methionine enkephalin levels in chronic cluster patients during an acute headache episode. Headache 27:325–328.
108. Hoffman DL, Abboud TK, Hasse HR, Hung TT, Goebelsman U. 1984. Plasma beta-endorphin concentrations prior to and during pregnancy, in labor, and after delivery. Am J Obstet Gynecol 150:492–496.

7. SOMATOSTATIN AND CHRONIC PAIN MANAGEMENT

JOACHIM CHRUBASIK

There is increasing information that nonopioid peptides in the central nervous system play a role in pain physiology and pathophysiology. Among these neuropeptides, somatostatin is apparently one of the most significant. The tetradecapeptide (Figure 7-1) is present in high concentrations in several regions of the brain and in the spinal cord [1,2]. In the latter, the neuropeptide is mostly localized in the dorsal horn (Figure 7-2) [2,3]. The somatostatin concentration in rexed laminae II and III of the dorsal horn suggests that somatostatin has important functions in modulating the transmission of soma-tosensory information. Consistent with this hypothesis, are animal experiments indicating that somatostatin transmits painful stimuli within the spinal cord. While it was demonstrated that the neurotransmitter substance P was released from the rabbit dorsal horn by noxious stimuli (pinching), it was also shown that somatostatin was released by radiant heat (Figure 7-3) [4]. Moreover, administration of somatostatin close to the central nervous system in rats resulted in caudally directed bites and scratches, probably due to a painful sensation [5].

However, intrathecal somatostatin also resulted in naloxone-reversible respiratory depression in rats [6,7] and urinary retention in cats [8], indicating that mu opiate receptors are involved in the mediation of the somatostatin effect. Inconsistent with this finding is the failure of this neuropeptide to produce analgesia in rats, cats, and mice [8–10]. Increasing somatostatin doses ($\geqslant 100\,\mu g/kg$) and concentrations of the somatostatin solutions (up to 1%)

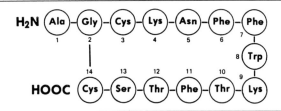

Figure 7-1. Amino acid sequence of the tetradecapeptide somatostatin.

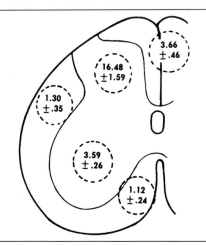

Figure 7-2. Dorsoventral distribution of somatostatin (pmole/mg protein) in rat spinal cord. Modified from Stine et al. [3], with permission.

even produced toxic reactions, such as motor disturbances, paraplegia, and inflammatory and necrotic changes of the spinal cord [8–10]. In contrast, intrathecal administration of somatostatin doses <100 g/kg of somatostatin solutions up to 0.1% had no neurobehavioral or neurotoxic effects in mice, rats, or monkeys [9–11], and in these doses seemed to have no side effects at all.

Prior to clinical use of epidural somatostatin, animal experiments had been carried out to determine whether epidural somatostatin has adverse effects. In one trial, the spinal cord, dura, and two spinal ganglia of 12 dogs after epidural somatostatin exposure (6 mg/day over 672 hours in 10 dogs, 10 mg/hr over 5 hours (one dog) and 7 hours (one dog), of one dog after intrathecal somatostatin exposure (10 mg/hr over 3 hours), and of four controls (epidural saline over 672 hours in three dogs, over 7 hours in one dog) were examined histologically for signs of neurological damage, inflammatory response, or demyelination [12]. The pathologist had no knowledge of the identity of the

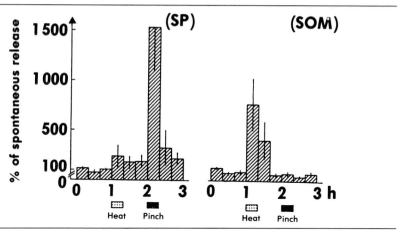

Figure 7-3. Effects of noxious stimuli on the release of substance P (SP) and somatostatin (SOM) from the rabbit spinal dorsal horn in situ. Modified from Kuraishi et al. [4], with permission.

histological specimen. The results after decoding revealed signs of varying degrees of acute inflammation and hematoma in different stages of organization (epidural, subdural, and subarachnoid) attributed to the prolonged epidural catheter placement. In one instance, suppurative encephalitis was also noted. Nonspecific damage was less pronounced in the controls. No other pathological changes were found in the brain, spine, ganglia, or nerves. There was agreement between Prof. B. Volk (Chairman of Neuropathology, University of Freiburg, Freiburg, FRG) and Prof. Rosenmann (Chairman of Pathology, Hebrew University, Hadassah Medical School, Jerusalem, Israel) that epidural somatostatin in the dosage used did not have any neuropathological effects on the dog spinal cord. Perfusion of the intrathecal space of dogs with saline and the collection of the perfusate after epidural somatostatin administration revealed that only small amounts of somatostatin might bypass the dura mater and reach the intrathecal space [13]. Based on these preliminary results, the Human Ethics Committee approved the use of epidural somatostatin in postoperative pain patients.

Although none of the studies in animals predicted somatostatin antinociception, a dermatomal distribution of analgesia could be demarcated in humans after epidural administration of 1 mg somatostatin [14]. In contrast to local anesthetics, however, the limit of this dermatomal analgesia is independent of the injected volume and can be maintained with low-dose epidural infusion of somatostatin (0.125 mg/hr following 0.25 mg initially) (Figure 7-4). Moreover, an increase in the dose of epidurally applied somatostatin (1 mg/hr following 0.5 mg initially) produced a total-body negative pin-prick response [15]. The fact (contrary to what is seen in humans) that administration of somatostatin close to the central nervous system is devoid of analgesic effects in cats, rats,

Catheter placement L2/L3	Epidural Somatostatin 1 mg/2 ml		Epidural Somatostatin 1 mg/10 ml		Epidural Somatostatin 0.25 mg + 0.125 mg/h
Analgesia					
TH Superior	5.3	ns	5.2	ns	6.3
Segm. Level					
TH Inferior	12.3	ns	12.3	ns	11.2
Duration (min)	69 ± 19	ns	68 ± 11		1 h

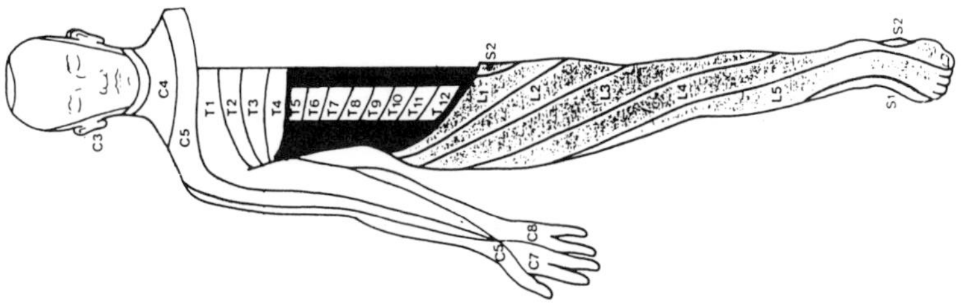

Figure 7-4. Limits of dermatomal analgesia and duration of analgesia following epidural somatostatin administration. Modified from Carli et al. [14], with permission.

Table 7-1. Respiratory variables (mean ± SD) obtained before, 30, and 90 minutes after epidural somatostatin injection

	Before	After 30 min	After 90 min
	1 mg epidural somatostatin		
R-$PETCO_2$ mmHg	37.5 ±4.1	37.7 ±5.2	38.1 ±3.1
R–RR breath/min	17 ±6	16 ±5	17 ±3
R–VE l/min	8.7 ±4.3	9.3 ±2.0	9.8 ±1.5
Slope VE / $PETCO_2$ l/min/mmHg	2.74 ±0.99	2.63 ±0.83	2.85 ±0.54

Modified from Carli et al. [14], with permission.

and mice [8,10] therefore suggests that the spinal animal models are inadequate or inapproriate for studying the analgesic effects of somatostatin. Furthermore, similar animal studies have failed to reveal the analgesic effect of opiate agonist-antagonists, e.g., pentazocine and butorphanol, known to be potent

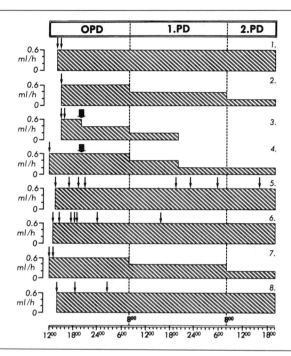

Figure 7-5. Individual epidural somatostatin consumptions (bolus injections of 250 μg, infusions of 250 μg/ml) for constant pain relief after abdominal surgery on the day of operation (OPD) and on the first and second postoperative days (PD). Administration of naloxone, 0.4 mg i.v., 0.8 mg i.m. Modified from Chrubasik et al. [20], with permission.

analgesics in humans [16,17]. It is assumed that due to evolutionary processes, central receptor subtype occupations might differ for nonopioid peptides and opiate agonist-antagonists in animals and humans.

Despite the somatostatin respiratory depressive effect in rats [7], ventilation while breathing room air and during carbon dioxide stimulation is not affected by epidural somatostatin (Table 7-1) [14]. It is therefore unlikely that epidural somatostatin, in contrast to epidural opiates, carries the risk of respiratory depression. Moreover, somatostatin analgesia was not reversed by naloxone (Figure 7-5) and did not demonstrate other central effects, e.g., euphoria or sedation [18–20]. In humans, somatostatin should therefore act on its own mu opiate receptor-different receptor sites within the central nervous system [21,22].

Although an antinociceptive effect of epidural somatostatin in all patients was evident using the pin-prick test [4,5], in two studies about 40% of patients given epidural somatostatin did not develop complete postoperative analgesia [15,18]. Effective doses of epidural somatostatin in the management of acute postoperative pain therefore remains to be determined, as only a small number

Table 7-2. Biometrical data of terminal cancer patients suffering from intractable pain and analgesic effectiveness of intrathecal somatostatin subsequent to intrathecal morphine

Patient	1	2	3	4	5	6	7	8	9	10
Site of the carcinoma	Kidney	Colon	Tongue	Cervix	Rectum	Colon	Bladder	Bladder	Esophag.	Cervix
Age (years)	69	60	64	44	61	58	62	61	51	36
Size (cm)	163	169	172	161	180	169	158	170	172	168
Weight (kg)	74	68	54	51	66	68	45	40	48	52
Sex	Female	Female	Male	Female	Male	Male	Female	Male	Male	Female
Subj. pain before morphine treatment (VAS 1-10)	10	10	10	10	10	10	10	10	10	10
Intrathecal morphine dosage (mg/24^h)	6	1	1	3	2	3	1	3	4	3
Subj. pain under morph.	0-2	0	0-1	0-1	0	1	3	0	4	5
Subj. pain before somatostatin bolus	10	8	10	8			10		10	10
Dose of intrathecal somatostatin (μg)	250	250	250	250			250		250	250
Side effects	Flush. emesis vomiting			Flush.						
Subj. pain at 15 min	0	0	0-1	0-1			4		4	3
Duration of analgesia (hr)	12	2	4	6			(3)		(3)	(2)
Subj. pain before somatostatin infusion				10	6	5		10	10	10
Intrathecal somatostatin dosage: bolus (μg)				250	250	250		250	250	250
infusion (μg/hr)				10	10	10		10	50	50
Subj. pain under somatostatin treatment over 24 hours				0-1	0	1		0	4	5

Modified from Chrubasik et al. [18], with permission.

of patients have received postoperative epidural somatostatin to date, and in those cases the studies were carried out under varying experimental conditions (premedication, anesthetic technique, type of surgery etc.) [18–20].

With institutional review board approval, 15 terminal cancer patients suffering from intractable pain were investigated [18]. In ten patients receiving intrathecal morphine, the analgesic effectiveness of intrathecal somatostatin was evaluated. When complaints of pain became severe, seven patients received a bolus intrathecal injection of 250 µg somatostatin instead of the morphine bolus (Table 7-2). Within 15 minutes, subjective pain decreased in four patients. These patients were free of pain over a period of 2–12 hours. In three patients who suffered moderate pain despite the intrathecal morphine therapy, intrathecal somatostatin was not more effective than morphine (Table 7-2). Six [10] patients received a continuous intrathecal somatostatin infusion (10 µg/hr) following a bolus intrathecal somatostatin injection of 250 µg. In the patients who responded to the morphine treatment, analgesia could be maintained during the continuous intrathecal somatostatin infusion treatment, which lasted 24 hours. In those patients whose pain in pretreatment was not successfully alleviated with intrathecal morphine, somatostatin was not more effective (Table 7-1).

Long-term epidural somatostatin infusion treatment (3 mg/day) over 7 days following an initial bolus of 250 µg [23] resulted in sufficient analgesia and did not reveal any undesirable side effects due to the peptide (Table 7-3). Similarly, intrathecal somatostatin infusion treatment titrated to the patient's individual need for analgesics provided sufficient analgesia and was well tolerated in two patients for up to 8 weeks (Table 7-4) [24]. No toxic effects were found in the postmortem histopathological examination of the spinal cord in one of them, whose death was caused by progression of the disease [24]. One patient suffering from terminal carcinoma of the tongue, who could be maintained pain-free with intraventricular morphine (0.5 mg/day) from a reservoir under the scalp, received a bolus intraventricular injection of 250 µg when complaining of severe pain [25]. Within 5 minutes, the patient attained analgesia that lasted 4 hours. An intraventricular infusion of 10 µg/hr after an initial bolus of 250 µg kept the patient pain-free for 6 hours. When the patient's pain returned, the intraventricular infusion rate was increased to 25 µg/hr after a bolus of 250 µg. Analgesia could be maintained over 5 days. Twenty-seven hours after the intraventricular infusion had been stopped, the patient complained of severe pain.

In summary, it was demonstrated that analgesia can be maintained in patients suffering from intractable cancer pain through administration of somatostatin close to the central nervous system. These preliminary investigations indicate that patients who did not respond to morphine failed to have better analgesia under intrathecal somatostatin. It remains to be established whether the increase in somatostatin consumption in some of the patients was caused by tachyphylaxis or by deterioration of the patient's condition. The

Table 7-3. Biometrical data of two terminal cancer patients suffering from intractable pain and analgesic effectiveness of epidural somatostatin treatment over 7 days

Patient	1	2
Site of the carcinoma	Rectum	Rectum
Age (years)	52	61
Size (cm)	159	181
Weight (kg)	52	82
Sex	Female	Male
Subj. pain before somatostatine treatment	7	10
Epidural somatostatin		
Bolus (μg)	250	250
Infusion (μg/hr)	125	125
Subj. pain over 7 days of treatment	0–1	0–1

Modified from Chrubasik [23], with permission.

Table 7-4. Biometrical data of two terminal cancer patients suffering from intractable pain and weekly intrathecal somatostatin (Som) consumption for constant pain relief until the patient's death (*died on day 25)

Patient		1	2
Site of carcinoma		Rectosigmoid	
Age (years)		61	71
Size (cm)		180	181
Weight (kg)		66	100
Sex		male	male
Som (mg/week)	1	1.75	2.3
	2	1.75	2.8
	3	1.75	1.7
	4	1.75	1.0*
	5	1.75	
	6	1.75	
	7	3.75	
	8	3.75	

From Meynadier et al. [24], with permission.

complete lack of somatostatin euphoria and sedation suggests that treatment with somatostatin might not result in addiction. Chronic pain, however, has many origins and is affected to a great extent by psychological factors, which can conceal or distort the analgesic effect of a drug. Thus, further investigations are necessary to examine the somatostatin analgesic effectiveness of epidural/intrathecal/intraventricular treatment of chronic pain. Side effects that might occur under the somatostatin treatment close to the central nervous system include flushing, emesis, and vomiting following the bolus injection or an increase in blood glucose in maturity-onset diabetes under infusion of the peptide [19].

REFERENCES

1. Patel YC, Rao K, Reichlin S. 1977. Somatostatin in human cerebrospinal fluid. N Engl Med J 296:529–533.
2. Massari VJ, Tizabi J, Park CH, Moody TW, Helke CJ, O'Donohue TL. 1983. Distribution and origin of bombesin, substance P and somatostatin in cat spinal cord. Peptides 4:673–681.
3. Stine SM, Yang H-Y, Costa E. 1984. Role of somatostatin in rat spinal cord: Comparison with substance P and metenkephalin. In I Hanin (ed), Dynamics of Neurotransmitter Function. New York, Raven Press, pp. 159–168.
4. Kuraishi Y, Hirota N, Sato Y, Hino Y. Satoh M, Takagi H. 1985. Evidence that substance P and somatostatin transmit separate information related to pain in the spinal cord. Brain Res 325:294–298.
5. Wiesenfeld-Hallin Z. 1985. Intrathecal somatostatin modulates spinal sensory and reflex mechanisms: Behavioral and electrophysiological studies in the rat. Neurosci Lett 62:69–74.
6. Ackerman E, Chrubasik J, Weinstock M, Wünsch E. 1985. Effect of intrathecal somatostatin on pain threshold in rats. Schmerz Pain Douleur 6:41–42.
7. Härfstrand A, Kalia M, Fuxe K, Laijser L, Agnati LF. 1984. Somatostatin-induced apnea: Interaction with hypoxia and hypercapnea in the rat. Neurosci Lett 50:37–42.
8. Gaumann DM, Yaksh TL, Post CM, Wilcox, Rodriguez M. 1989. Intrathecal somatostatin in cat and mouse. Studies on pain, motor behavior, and histopathology. Anesth Analg 68:623–632.
9. Mollenholt P, Post C, Rawal N, Freedman J, Hökfelt T, Paulsson I. 1988. Antinociceptive and neurotoxic actions of somatostatin in rat spinal cord after intrathecal administration. Pain 32:95–105.
10. Gaumann DM, Yaksh TL. 1988. Intrathecal somatostatin in rats: Antinociception only in the presence of toxic effects. Anesthesiology 68:733–742.
11. Leblanc R, Gauthier S, Gauvin M, Quirion R, Palmour R, Masson H. 1988. Neurobehavioral effects of intrathecal somatostatinergic treatment in subhuman primates. Neurology 38:1887–1890.
12. Chrubasik J, Volk B, Meynadier J, Berg G, Wünsch E. 1986. Observations in dogs receiving spinal somatostatin and calcitonin. Schmerz Pain Douleur 7:10–12.
13. Chrubasik J, Bonath K, Cramer H, Rissler K, Wünsch E. 1986. Permeability of epidural somatostatin and morphine into the intrathecal space of dogs. Regul Peptides 13:119–124.
14. Carli P, Ecoffey C, Chrubasik J, Benlabed M, Gross JB, Samii K. 1986. Spread of analgesia and ventilatory response to CO_2 following epidural somatostatin. Anesthesiology 65(Suppl.): 216.
15. Hügler P, Mendl G, Landgraf R, Madler C, Martin E. 1987. First experience using epidural somatostatin in extracorporeal-schock-wave-lithotrypsy. Anaesthesist 36:388.
16. Schmauss C, Doherty C, Yaksh TL. 1983. The analgetic effects of an intrathecally administered partial opiate agonist, nalbuphine hydrochloride, Eur J Pharmacol 86:1–7.
17. Yaksh TL, Rudy TA. 1978. Narcotic analgetics: CNS sites and mechanisms of action as revealed by intracerebral injection techniques. Pain 4:299–359.
18. Chrubasik J. 1988. Intrathecal somatostatin. Ann NY Acad Sci 531:133–146.
19. Chrubasik J, Meynadier J, Scherpereel P. 1985. Somatostatin versus morphine in epidural treatment after major abdominal operations. Anesthesiology 63(Suppl.):237.
20. Chrubasik J, Meynadier J, Scherpereel P, Wünsch E. 1985. The effect of epidural somatostatin on postoperative pain. Anesth Analg 64:1085–1088.
21. Reubi JC, Cortes R, Maurer R, Probst A, Palacios JM. 1986. Distribution of somatostatin receptors in the human brain: An autoradiographic study. Neuroscience 18:329–346.
22. Tran VT, Uhl GR, Perry DC, Manning DC, Vale WW, Perrin MH, Rivier MH, Martin JB, Snyder SH. 1984. Autoradiographic localization of somatostatin receptors in rat brain. Eur J

Pharmacol 101:307–309.
23. Chrubasik J. 1985. Spinal Infusion of Opiates and Somatostatin. Oberursel, FRG, Hygiene Press.
24. Meynadier J, Chrubasik J, Dubar M, Wünsch E. 1985. Intrathecal somatostatin in terminally ill patients: A report of two cases. Pain 23:9–12.
25. Chrubasik J, Meynadier J, Blond S, Scherpereel P, Ackerman E, Weinstock M, Bonath K, Cramer H, Wünsch E. 1984. Somatostatin, a potent analgesic. Lancet 1:13–17.

8. PERSPECTIVES OF CAPSAICIN-TYPE AGENTS IN PAIN THERAPY AND RESEARCH

JANOS SZOLCSANYI

There is a "painfully" absent chapter in pharmacological textbooks, which could be entitled: "Drugs acting on sensory neurons" or "Sensory neuron-blocking analgesics." For over 100 years, varieties of narcotic analgesics, analgesic-antipyretics, and local anesthetics have provided the repertoire of drugs used for pain management. In contrast to effector neurons (particularly their peripheral neurotransmission processes, which have become multiple targets for drug development), sensory neurons and their receptors have remained almost unexplored as sites for the selective action of drugs in clinical practice. The main reason for this situation resides in a very simple fact. In the field of neuroeffector transmissions, delicate molecules produced by nature, such as curare, ergot alkaloids, or atropine, had served as excellent guides by highlighting special features of each neural mechanism as suitable sites for selective blockade and possible starting points for further drug development. Similar approaches in sensory pharmacology, however, have received less attention.

It is remarkable that a potential selective drug action on sensory nerves was discovered around that period of the last century when initial progress towards the understanding of the pharmacology of the autonomic nervous system was being made [1]. Endre Hogyes, the ingenious Hungarian pathophysiologist, published a paper in 1878 in which he analyzed the effects of the extract of red pepper "capsicol" and postulated that its principal action was on sensory nerves with considerable selectivity [2]. The crucial evidence that sensory nerve endings subserving pain cannot only be stimulated, but also put out of action, has been established by other pioneers of capsaicin research, such as Miklos (Nicholas) Jancso and his wife Aranka (Aurelia) Jancso-Gabor after World War II, whom I joined in the early 1960s. Detailed description of the "capsaicin story" has already been described [1]. It is worth mentioning, however, that from 1967, when the first full paper on capsaicin desensitization was published in a well-circulated journal, not much interest was raised by this new trend of "afferent pharmacology" for more than 10 years [1].

SOMATOSENSORY EFFECTS OF CAPSAICIN

Sensory effects on human subjects

Stimulation

It is common experience that capsaicin in paprika induces a hot or burning sensation in the mucous membranes of the mouth. Detection threshold on the tongue [16,24] or in the oral cavity [25] is around 0.2 micrograms/ml (range = 0.09–0.35 g/ml), and in this low concentration, capsaicin provokes a simple warmth sensation on the tongue. Sharp, prickly sensations are elicited in the throat, and pain without a definite thermal component occurs as a response to intracutaneous capsaicin injection or when it is applied to the blister base. These responses indicate that a variety of pain sensation qualities can be evoked by this agent [4,16,24,26]. Furthermore, capsaicin can provoke itching sensation on the skin, sneezing from the nasal mucosa, and coughing from the respiratory airways [4,16,27–30]. Intravenous injection of capsaicin (0.5–4 micrograms/kg has evoked "hot-flushing" sensations in the chest, face, rectum, and extremities [31]). On the other hand, tactile sensations (tapping, pressure, vibration, paresthesia, numbness tickling, pulsating, stroking, etc.), which are characteristic of activation of low-threshold mechanoreceptors [32], or irritant sensation with a cold component, as well as paresthesia or numbing, have never been reported. Cooling of the capsaicin-treated skin area to 26–28°C abolished not only the burning pain but the hyperalgesia evoked by gentle rubbing the skin. Warming had an opposite effect. This thermodependence can be demonstrated also by recording action potentials from sensory nerves in animal experiments [16,24] or in human skin under pathological conditions [33].

These observation on humans indicate that the receptors stimulated by capsaicin can provoke various qualities of pain sensation. Receptors subserving other types of chemically induced sensations or reflexes are also excited by capsaicin. Regional differences as well as concentration and time-dependent factors due to different methods of drug application might produce qualitatively different results. For example, topical capsaicin application on the skin could induce an itching sensation [27]. This does not occur when the drug is injected intracutaneously, although histamine is highly effective [26] in the latter situation.

Desensitization

In several studies, topical application of capsaicin in high concentration (1%) desensitized the receptors of the treated area (tongue, skin, blister base, nasal mucosa) to subsequent stimuli applied to the area for several hours or days [16,24,34–38]. Chemically induced pain was strongly inhibited, but pain induced by potassium chloride on the blister base or by means of a pin prick on the tongue or skin was not reduced. The threshold of noxious heat was enhanced by 9°C or more if short-lasting test stimuli (2's) were applied [16]. Long duration of heating might affect also deeper structures that are less accessible for the drug by percutaneous diffusion. Therefore, under the latter conditions the measured change in noxious heat threshold is less pronounced.

In one study, the discrimination threshold became broader and the estimation of magnitude of warmth sensation was impaired [16]. Itching upon histamine or antigen challenge was prevented [35,37]. On the other hand, the following innocuous testings produced unaltered perception in skin or mucosal areas desensitized by capsaicin. The discrimination threshold in the cold range (23–24°C) in the tongue, the magnitude estimation of cold stimuli in the skin, tactile threshold, and the tactile discrimination limen in both areas remained unimpaired. Furthermore, the recognition thresholds on the tongue for quinine, glucose, sodium chloride, ascorbic acid, and menthol also did not change, indicating that specific taste receptors and the chemical excitability of cold receptors also remained unaltered. It is worth mentioning that capsaicin over 500 times concentration range did not evoke any sensation after this desensitization procedure [16,24].

These observations clearly show the selective effect of capsaicin among receptor populations. It is not related to the chemical excitability of the receptor. For example, desensitization of the tongue by capsaicin blocked the irritant effect of mustard oil, but when its concentration was raised 10–25 times higher, it was felt to be sweet without any irritant character [24]. Consequently, the effect of mustard oil was prevented on receptors responsible for pain but not on taste receptors. The fact that, after desensitization, similar conversion of the pungent sensation induced by capsaicin and piperine was not observed underlines their selective action among sensory receptors. In the light of these findings, it is highly misleading to use the terms *chemosensitive* or *capsaicin-sensitive* sensory neurons as alternative synonyms [39].

Nociceptive and antinociceptive effect in animal experiments

Solutions of capsaicin, piperine, and their congeners elicit protective nocifensor reactions when applied to exteroceptive mucosal areas of the rat, guinea pig, and other mammals [4,16,40,41]. Subcutaneous, intraarterial, intrathecal injections are also effective in this respect [8,11,16]. Phylogenetically lower species, such as bird, pigeon, and chicken, for example, are extremely insensitive to the stimulatory and desensitizing effect of the drug [42,43], although they do have "chemosensitive nociceptors." In fact, the threshold dose of bradykinin or KCL given intraarterially was the same in pigeon, chicken, and guinea pig. It has been concluded that the presence of a pharmacological receptor [41] for capsaicin is required for the selective action of the drug.

The antinociceptive effect of high doses of capsaicin has been analyzed by different groups of authors and has been summarized [5,11,16], with various aspects discussed [4,7,8,9,12] in several reviews. The structure-activity relationship of capsaicin and piperine congeners [44] and the effectiveness of resiniferatoxin [22,23] suggest that the desensitizing, antinociceptive effect is not due to the irritant potency of the drug. The excitatory and blocking effects of the compounds did not run parallel. Furthermore, desensitization can be achieved even if capsaicin is applied under the effect of local anesthetics [1,9,16,17].

Characteristics of the antinociceptive effect of capsaicin after topical, systemic, perineural, intracisternal, epidural application to adult animals, as well as the special aspects of systemic treatments of neonatal rats and mice, have been recently reviewed [16]. Therefore, only some major issues of therapeutic relevance are summarized here.

1. The *time course* of desensitization is determined by the type of application. Topical application to the skin and mucosal areas results in reversible local analgesia lasting for days. Some months after systemic pretreatment of the rat, the recovery of chemonociception is still not complete, while thermonociception recovers faster in a matter of days or weeks, depending on the dose [11,16,40]. Intrathecal, intracisternal, or perineural administration induces dose-dependent analgesia and the effect is practically irreversible [16,45–47].

2. *Type of nociceptive stimulus.* The marked desensitizing effect induced by different routes of capsaicin pretreatments against chemonociceptive stimuli has been invariably verified. The noxious heat threshold was shown to be increased by local, systemic, perineural, or intrathecal application [11,16]. Earlier conflicting results were attributed to methodical factors (application of suprathreshold stimulations, discarding the time course of the analgesic effect to different stimuli, etc.). Another source of contradiction originated from the less selective effect of neonatal treatment [11,16,48,49].

Nocifensor reactions to mechanical stimuli were variably influenced by capsaicin treatment [11]. It is worth mentioning that perineural capsaicin around the sciatic nerve did not induce autotomy of the leg in rats and guinea pigs, nor was there any impairment of tactile and noxious cold sensitivity in the rat [50]. These data are in line with the selective sensory loss induced by capsaicin in human subjects. Injection of tissue-damaging chemicals, such as formalin, could produce nociception through activation of mechanonociceptors either directly or indirectly by the extreme swelling of the injected paw. Therefore, the analgesic effect of capsaicin pretreatment against tissue-damaging chemical stimuli is less pronounced [51].

SELECTIVE ACTION OF CAPSAICIN AMONG SENSORY NEURONS

Neurophysiological results

Selective action of capsaicin on cutaneous C-polymodal nociceptors was shown by the collision technique in the saphenous nerve of the cat [24] and subsequently by recording single unit activity from peripheral nerves of the rat, rabbit, and human subjects [16,48,49,52,54].

Some characteristics of the excitatory and desensitizing effects of capsaicin on two polymodal nociceptive units of the rabbit ear can be seen in Figure 8-1: 1) Repeated injections of capsaicin into the main artery of the ear in the lower dose range 20 micrograms) evoked a similar number of discharges, but the highest instantaneous frequencies (bursting character) declined (B,C). 2) The higher the dose, the more pronounced the desensitizing effect (B,D). 3) Desensitization against its own effect is accompanied by a decreased respon-

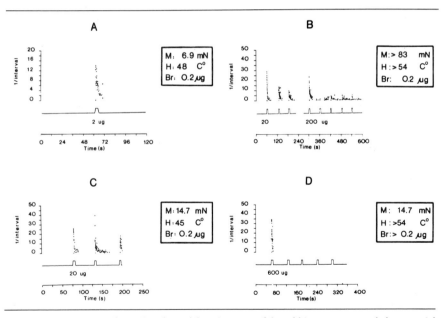

Figure 8-1. Response of two C-polymodal nociceptors of the rabbit ear to repeated close arterial injections of capsaicin. Records A and B are from one unit and C and D from the other. Ordinate: Interval between discharges (instantaneous frequency). The marks below the graphs indicate the duration and dose of capsaicin injection. Within the inserts are depicted the threshold stimuli that evoked discharges 10–30 minutes after the injections. The values were identical before and after the first panels (A and C). M = mechanical threshold (von Frey hair); H = noxious heat threshold; Br = threshold dose of bradykinin injected into the artery. Note various degrees of desensitization to different stimuli. Unpublished details from Szolcsanyi [48].

siveness of these nociceptors to natural stimuli (see inserts). 4) It is remarkable that, although excitability of the receptors to mechanical, noxious heat and chemical (bradykinin) stimuli was decreased or prevented, the inhibitions were not parallel to all types of stimulation in a given unit. Pronounced desensitization to the capsaicin effect and to noxious heat was not accompanied by threshold changes in one unit to bradykinin (B), nor in the other to mechanical stimulation (D). Consequently, the effect is not due to blockade of axonal conduction, because in that case all types of stimulation would be blocked. Furthermore, these nonparallel shifts in thresholds might indicate that the excitatory processes in a single terminal are different in each case of stimulation. The other possibility is that the polymodal nociceptive unit is composed of terminal arborizations of unimodal nociceptive endings. In this case, the difference in degree of desensitization might be due to their variant positions and accessibilities through the microcirculation. On the average, however, capsaicin desensitization altered responses to thermal, chemical, and mechanical stimuli without afferent selectivity.

These data clearly show that capsaicin is a unique tool to study the function of receptive terminals of the polymodal nociceptors.

In addition to the C-polymodal nociceptors, A-delta mechanoheat-nociceptors in the rat [49], two examples of warm units [16], and some mechanically insensitive C-nociceptors of the skin [26,48], were excited by capsaicin. On the other hand, A-delta mechanonociceptors, C- and A-delta cold receptors, and all types of low-threshold mechanoreceptors, including the C-mechanoreceptors, were insensitive to the effects of capsaicin [16,48,49,52,54]. This high selectivity was observed in the rat, both in respect to receptor stimulation after topical, intraarterial, and intradermal applications, or when chronic desensitizing effects induced by systemic or perineural treatments were investigated. Consequently, in adult animals, capsaicin acts on functionally well-defined groups of sensory units and the agent cannot be considered as a general C-fiber sensory neurotoxin.

It is important to note that *neonatal treatment of the rat* induced neurotoxic degenerations in which the expected and often referred similar neuroselectivity [20,39,55] was not verified. After this treatment, single-unit studies of adult subjects revealed an indiscriminate loss of afferent C-fibers [52,54,56], and morphological evidence indicates a dose-dependent spectrum of degeneration of A-delta afferents and some neurons with A-beta fibers [8,12,16,57,58]. Autonomic C-efferents, however, were not impaired [8,12,16]. This method is therefore useful in determining whether or not peptidergic fibers originate from sensory neurons. However, it could be the source of misleading conclusions when the functional role of polymodal nociceptors or other capsaicin-sensitive receptors are intended to be investigated. It should also be kept in mind that during several months of maturation after the pretreatment, secondary changes and reorganization develop in the central nervous system [59], in the immunological picture [60], and in nociception [61]. It seems also likely that degeneration of myelinated afferent fibers is also the result of secondary changes [61].

In vitro electrophysiological and ion flux studies on cranial and spinal sensory ganglia have provided further evidence of the existence of a distinct capsaicin-sensitive subpopulation of sensory neurons [62–68]. Capsaicin and bradykinin in nanomolar concentrations induced depolarization on C-type neurons, but not on A-type cells or sympathetic neurons of the rat [62–65]. Depolarization induced by capsaicin can be attributed to an increase in calcium, sodium, and potassium conductance, while the chloride conductance seems to remain intact [66,68]. This apparently new type of cation channel opened by capsaicin is not influenced by tetrodotoxin or calcium-channel blockers, but seems to be blocked by ruthenium red [66,67,69]. This neuroselective and channel-selective actions of capsaicin should be distinguished from the local anesthetic effect induced by higher concentrations in the micromolar range under in vitro conditions [9,16,64]. This latter response is elicitable in all types of neurons obtained also from species in which capsaicin does not produce irritant or analgesic effects. Furthermore, under in vitro conditions, the blocking action of capsaicin on C-type neurons and on their processes cannot be reversed by washing out the drug, while the nonselective action is fully reversible.

This local anesthetic effect manifests itself in vivo when capsaicin is applied around the nerve trunk of the rat, [47,52,70] guinea pig, ferret, rabbit [70], cat [71], and monkey [72]. The conduction blockade might explain some conflicting results made within hours vs. days after perineural capsaicin application. Figure 8-2. compares the elevation of noxious heat threshold 3–4 days after perineural capsaicin treatment around the sciatic nerve [11,16] with the acute decrease in compound action potential of C-fibers under identical conditions [70]. Capsaicin was 30 times more effective in the rat on axonal conduction while the antinociceptive effect was more pronounced in the guinea pig, from a few days up to 2 months after the treatment [16]. Therefore the long-term analgesic effect cannot be predicted on the basis of efficacy in the acute blocking effect on axonal conduction.

Morphological evidence

Selective action of capsaicin on small, dark B-type sensory neurons was discovered in the 1960s [73]. These neurons of the nodosal, trigeminal, and dorsal root ganglia comprise the cell body of unmyelinated C-afferents and are denoted as C-type cells by electrophysiological characterization. The ultrastructural changes induced by capsaicin after topical or systemic application to adult rats are illustrated on Figure 8-3. It can be seen that in the trigeminal ganglion 5 days after systemic pretreatment (90 + 125 mg/kg s.c.), the mitochondria of B-type neurons (F) are swollen with disorganized christae, and some of the nerve terminals (Axl) in the cornea show degenerative dilatation (E). Mitochondria and other ultrastructural features of a light, A-

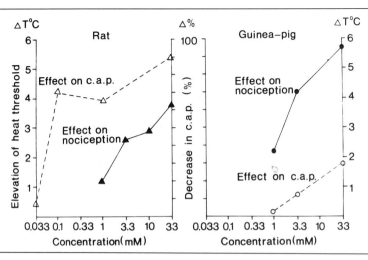

Figure 8-2. Comparison of the effectiveness of perineural capsaicin application on the height of compound action potential (c.a.p.) of C-fibers (acute experiments, see ref. 70), and on nociception (1–3 days after the treatment, see ref. 16). Capsaicin was applied in different concentrations around the sciatic nerve of rats and guinea pigs, and noxious heat threshold was determined by the paw immersion method [11].

type cell (G) and neural cell body and nerve terminals in the superior cervical ganglia (H) remain intact. After topical application into the eye (five times instillation of a 1% capsaicin solution 1 day before the animal was killed), swollen mitochondria can be seen in an intraepithelial nerve terminal (A–D are serial sections), but not in the epithelial cells, the ultrastructure of which remained intact.

On the basis of these illustrations and subsequent studies on adult animals, [20,39,40,52,65,74–80], the following conclusions can be drawn:

1. Repeated topical application of 1% capsaicin solution produces ultrastructural changes, but there is no evidence to support the assumption that fiber degeneration would result if the drug were to diffuse through epithelia.

2. In vitro exposure of nodosal ganglia to 10 micromole capsaicin for 30 minutes [65] elicits similar ultrastructural changes in B-type cells, as does systemic pretreatment. Longer exposure (overnight) selectively destroys these neurons [67,68].

3. Systemic pretreatment in rats and guinea pigs induces degeneration of central and peripheral terminals and unmyelinated axons of the sensory neurons [75–79]. Evidence that a special subpopulation of B-type sensory neurons is degenerated (cell death) in this way [79] is not conclusive [16]. Instead, the dominant feature is the large number of B-type neurons that show ultrastructural alterations for remarkably long duration (42–60 days) [40,73,74].

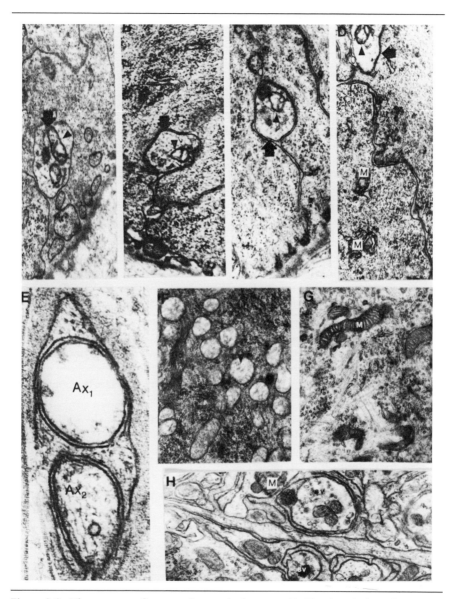

Figure 8-3. Ultrastructure of nervous elements in the cornea (A–E), trigeminal ganglion (F, G), and superior cervical ganglion (H) of the rat after capsaicin treatment. A–D: Serial sections of a sensory nerve ending (arrows) in the capsaicin-treated cornea. A 1% solution of capsaicin was instilled into the eye five times over 5–46 hours before the animal was killed. E–H: Ultrastructural features after systemic pretreatment (90 + 125 mg/kg s.c. 5 and 6 days before killing). E: dilated degenerating (AX$_1$) and normal (AX$_2$) axons in the cornea. F: Part of a B-type sensory neuron. G: Detail of an A-type sensory neuron. H: Pre- and postsynaptic elements in the sympathetic ganglion. Triangles point to swollen mitochondria. M = intact mitochondria; SV = synaptic vesicles. Magnifications: A: ×40000; B,C,H: ×32000; D,F,G: ×26000; E: ×65000. Unpublished details from Szolcsanyi et al. [40], with permission.

4. Perineural capsaicin application (1%) induces a selective loss of C-fibers in the rat [39,80], but causes no degeneration, only substance P depletion in the rabbit [80]. This species is 20 times less sensitive to capsaicin than the rat [4,16].

In newborn rats and mice, systemic capsaicin treatment [39,55] induces degeneration of a larger population of neurons, including some of the A-types [57,58,61] and the spectrum of degenerated afferent fibers is dose- [16,81] and time- [61] dependent.

SOME NEW CONCEPTS AND FUTURE PERSPECTIVES EMERGING FROM RECENT CAPSAICIN RESEARCH

Capsaicin-sensitive (CS) neural system with dual sensory-efferent function

Since the Cartesian reflex principle was formulated more than three centuries ago, the peripheral nervous system has been thought to be composed of separate afferent and efferent elements. According to my concept [4,9,16,36,82], a substantial portion of primary afferent neurons form a third type of neural organization. Peripheral terminals of these capsaicin-sensitive (CS) neurons operate not only as receptive (afferent) structures, but also as a source from where tissue responses are elicited in the efferent direction.

It has been known for some time that antidromic stimulation of the dorsal roots elicits cutaneous vasodilatation [83–85] and, as demonstrated recently, plasma extravasation in the skin, mucosae, and in various internal organs [36]. These proinflammatory responses can be attributed to the release of neuropeptides (substance P, other tachykinins, and calcitonin gene-related peptide) from the activated peripheral terminals of the CS primary afferent neurons. Systemic or local capsaicin treatments stop the release of these mediators and prevent these vascular responses evoked either by antidromic nerve stimulation or by orthodromic excitation of the receptors by irritants [1,3,9,13–15, 86,87].

Nerve fibers of the dorsal roots originate exclusively from neurons of the dorsal root ganglia and are all sensory in nature [88]. In the skin, plasma extravasation to antidromic stimulation can be elicited only when the C-polymodal nociceptors are activated [9,89–91]. Some A-delta fibers also appear to contribute to vasodilatation [92]. The selective effect of capsaicin on cutaneous polymodal nociceptors (see Neurophysiological results), along with its lack of effect on autonomic efferent neurotransmission processes [9,14,15], provides firm evidence for the exclusion of autonomic efferent fibers in mediation of antidromic vasodilatation and neurogenic inflammation.

CS sensory neurons also have important direct influences on the function of a variety of internal organs independently of the above-mentioned vascular events. The first example of this new type of innervation has been described in the guinea-pig isolated ileum [4,93] and taenia coli [95]. subsequently, visceromotor responses to capsaicin have been revealed in a number of isolated organs, including the gastrointestinal tract, tracheobronchial tree, heart, genitourinary tract, and iris [14]. In most cases, the putative peptide mediators have been identified, and the neural site of action has been verified by capsaicin desensitization and by chronic denervation. Furthermore, the responses were reproduced by electrical nerve stimulation and blocked by capsaicin desensitization. On the other hand, smooth muscle responses of the same preparation, evoked by excitation of autonomic efferent neural structures, remained completely unaffected after similar capsaicin pretreatment [9,14,15].

Under in vivo conditions, some of the CS visceromotor changes have already been demonstrated and further CS sensory-efferent responses have been discovered, e.g., the protective effect against gastric ulceration [96,97] and other trophic influences [98]. It seems that the CS sensory-efferent mechanisms are particularly suitable for microregulation of the tissues at localized sites where chemical or other stimuli excite these endings. This local response, as well as distant reflex changes triggered by the same set of CS afferents, are certainly related to nociception and form a kind of defensive "nocifensor system" [99,100]. Nevertheless, subsequent section of this chapter indicates that at threshold stimulation the effector role of CS endings might cover a wider range of physiological regulation (e.g., modulation of peristalsis, participation in regulation of cutaneous microcirculation).

Reevaluation of the axon reflex theory

According to the classical concept [15,37,84,85,101,102], the mediators of antidromic vasodilatation are not released from the receptors. Instead, involvement of an axon reflex arrangement with a hypothetical nerve terminal specialized for efferent function has been suggested (Figure 8-4A): " . . . fibres divide near their peripheral terminations, one branch supplying the sensory endorgan in skin, muscle etc., while the other ends as an efferent inhibitory endorgan on the muscular coat of the arterioles . . . " [84].

The following data and considerations contradict this traditional view and support the bidirectional axon reflex concept [1,9,16,36,103,104], according to which CS receptors themselves (e.g., polymodal nociceptors) are the sites from where the mediators are released (Figures 8-4B–8-4D).

1. Neurogenic inflammation provoked by irritants is not inhibited at sites where axonal conduction is blocked by tetrodotoxin or local anesthetics [1,9,103]. Criticism [1] of earlier conflicting findings, which formed the basis of the classical axon reflex theory, have been raised on procedural grounds.
2. In the presence of tetrodotoxin, efferent responses (neurogenic inflammation, in vitro bronchoconstriction, etc.) evoked by capsaicin-type agents are related to their sensory stimulant potency [9,17].
3. Capsaicin and bradykinin in nanomolar concentrations evoke depolarization and discharges in one set of neurons in dorsal root and trigeminal

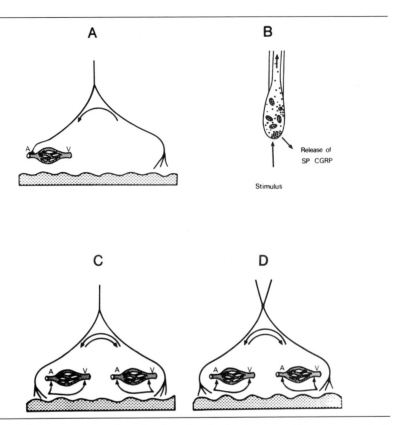

Figure 8-4. Schematic representation of various theories for the axon reflex arrangement. A: Classical unidirectional axon reflex theory of Lewis [101]. B: Dual sensory-efferent function of a polymodal nociceptor [9,36]. C,D: Two versions of bidirectional axon reflex arrangement [36] with polymodal nociceptors from where the mediators diffuse to the arterioles (A) and venules (V). C: Axonal arborization of a single fiber. D: Coupling between two fibers.

ganglia in vitro [62,63,64]. Depolarization is accompanied by release of the putative neuropeptide transmitter (CGRP) from these cell bodies [105]. Therefore, it seems very unlikely that, at the periphery, these two functions might be separated into different nerve endings.

4. Calcitonin gene-related peptide and substance P-like immunoreactive perivascular varicosities of sensory fibers are localized not in the media, but in the adventitia of arterioles. Membrane specialization for synaptic nature and predilection for receptor binding sites of the mediators has not been found [106,107].

5. The long latency and slow time course of the vasodilatation [9,36,108,109] or the hyperpolarization of vascular smooth muscle cells [110] to antidromic

nerve stimulation indicate that the mediator reaches the vessels by diffusion and not through a neuroeffector junction.

6. In the rat, antidromic stimulation of single fibers of polymodal nociceptors elicits spotlike plasma extravasation localized to the receptive field [89,90]. In the human skin, where polymodal nociceptive units often have multiple receptive fields [111,112], axon reflex flare can be elicited. "Cross-talk" or coupling between polymodal nociceptive fibers has been established in primates but not in other species [113]. Therefore, axon reflex flare is not necessarily evoked through axonal arborizations of a single fiber (Figure 8-4C), but could be mediated by axonal interaction between two polymodal nociceptive units (Figure 8-4D).

7. Flare reaction is absent in human skin desensitized by capsaicin. No difference in the time course of functional recovery of the receptive and effector terminals was observed [36] (see Figure 8-5).

It can be concluded that, in the human skin, the flare reaction is due to axon reflex but at both ends of the reflex arc are polymodal nociceptors (Figures 8-4C and 8-4D).

The receptive field of a single polymodal nociceptive unit often covers a skin area of $1 \, cm^2$ in the hand supplied by the superficial radial nerve [111,112]. If we suppose that side branches of four units with large receptive fields extending in all four directions are stimulated by intracutaneous injection, then a flare

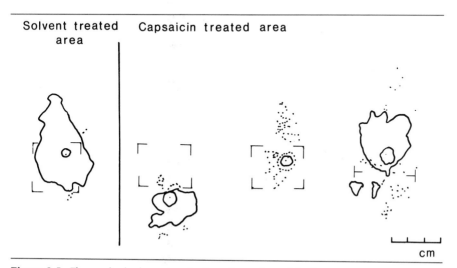

Solvent treated area   **Capsaicin treated area**

cm

Figure 8-5. Flare and wheal reactions in the volar surface of the forearm elicited by intracutaneous injection of substance P (5 ng). Skin areas marked by faint lines were painted five times with 1% capsaicin solution or the solvent (96% ethanol) 10 days before the injections. The linear strip was painted at the right side of the figure. Unpublished results from Szolcsanyi [36], with permission. For more details see the text.

area of $3-4\,cm^2$ could be expected. In fact, the flare area measured after capsaicin i.c. injection (50 microliter, 100 microgram/ml) was $3.52 \pm 0.39\,cm^2$ in the dorsum of the hand and $2.03 \pm 0.22\,cm^2$ at the first phalanx of the second finger (n = 6). These figures are well within the predicted limits.

Recently, a cascade theory of flare reaction was suggested [100]. This concept coincides with the postulation [1,103] that the mediator is released from the receptive terminals themselves. It further hypothesizes that histamine and noxious chemical agents excite the preterminal axons and the endings are antidromically activated. According to this theory, spreading the flare is not mediated through axonal conduction but by cascade release of humoral agents from nerve endings and mast cells. Therefore, the term *axon response* has been proposed instead of the conventional *axon reflex*.

On this ground, it is difficult to reconcile why the flare prevented by local anesthetics but not the neurogenic reddening induced by axonal stimulation of capsaicin at the site of contact [103]. Furthermore, flare reaction could "jump" through skin area that is desensitized by capsaicin, (Figure 8-5) or when diffusion is prevented [36,102]. These experiments indicate a spread without humoral cascade transmission. If capsaicin is applied to one side of the midline of the forehead, it provokes unilateral flare corresponding to the innervation area [114]. Furthermore, the onset of flare at a distance of 15 mm from the site of transcutaneous electrical stimulation of the forearm is 5 seconds [109]. These findings also contradict the theory of a slow humoral spreading of the flare reaction.

It is concluded that involvement of mast cells [87,100] and excitation of polymodal nociceptors by the released histamine might operate during flare reaction, but the size of the flare is principally determined by axonal arborization or by coupling between polymodal nociceptive fibers.

Theory for multiple functions of cutaneous polymodal nociceptors

The premise that activation of *polymodal nociceptors produces sensory pain* has been tested in human beings by comparing single-unit activity with the perceived sensation. Percutaneous recordings from several hundred single C-fibers of conscious subjects showed a rather good correlation between discharges of polymodal nociceptors and pain sensation when natural stimuli were applied [111,112,115–118]. Furthermore, intraneural electrical microstimulation at threshold intensity for identified polymodal nociceptive units elicited dull, burning, or pricking pain referred to the receptive field, i.e., to the skin spot from where the unit could be excited by mechanical stimulation [115,119]. Intraneural microstimulation at threshold intensity for a variety of tactile units did not evoke pain [32,116].

These data together with animal experiments in which single-unit recordings were compared with behavioral responses of the same species under identical stimulation conditions provide firm evidence that polymodal nociceptors initiate impulses for pain and nociception [118]. On the other hand, it can be deduced from these studies that few impulses at low frequencies transmitted by the units do not evoke pain sensation.

1. Intraneural microstimulation of polymodal nociceptive fibers for several seconds at 1 or 0.5 Hz frequencies is not painful [115, personal observation as subject in the series of ref. 119].
2. Thermal threshold of these nociceptors is often in the innocuous range of 40–43°C, and 0.2 Hz frequency of discharges is not accompanied by pain perception [111,112,115,120]. Irritant chemicals initiate activity of the fibers several seconds before the onset of any sensation [117]. Furthermore, the mechanical threshold of polymodal nociceptors is in most cases within the non-noxious range [111,112,115,117].
3. Animal experiments are in line with observations on humans. For example, in the rat's paw, a substantial number of polymodal nociceptors have lower thermal threshold [121] than is required to elicit a nocifensive reaction [11].

It is generally assumed that temporal summation of signals initiated by polymodal nociceptors is necessary for pain perception [115,117,120]. Nevertheless, the average firing rate evoked by very painful stimuli (e.g., temperatures above 50°C) seldom exceed three to four impulses per second [116].

An interesting picture appears if we compare the above characteristics of input messages to the number and frequency of antidromic discharges that are necessary to elicit effector responses by activation of these nerve terminals.

Antidromic stimulation of the saphenous nerve of the rat evoked plasma extravasation in the innervated area of the paw. The frequency optimum was around 2 Hz, and the amount of accumulated Evans blue tracer evoked by a given number of pulses was less when 0.5-Hz or 8-Hz stimulation frequencies were applied. Thirty impulses at 2 Hz were sufficient to induce a detectable effect [1,9]. These quantitative characteristics correspond to those of ongoing discharges that are required to provoke pain sensation. Therefore, it is tempting to assume that when environmental changes become noxious and the tissue injury signals pain through the polymodal nociceptors, these nerve terminals release a sufficient amount of mediators to initiate a local inflammatory reaction. The pathophysiological relevance of this dual function of these sense organs seems plausible.

Further interesting aspects emerged when blood flux changes evoked by antidromic stimulation of the dorsal roots were measured in the glabrous skin of the rat's hind paw. It became clear that one or two impulses were sufficient to evoke vasodilatation, and the response lasted for several minutes. Furthermore, the frequency optimum was extremely low (0.025–0.2 Hz), and at this frequency range stimulation for 30 minutes induced sustained enhancement of cutaneous microcirculation without exhaustion. These responses were prevented or strongly inhibited by perineural or systemic capsaicin pretreatments, indicating that the mediator is released from CS nerve endings [16,36,108].

Antidromic stimulation of A-beta fibers of the saphenous nerve induced no blood flux changes, and the slight effect produced by excitation of A-delta fibers had a frequency optimum in the range of 5–10 Hz [92]. Consequently, the highly efficient stimulation of the dorsal roots is due to activation of capsaicin-sensitive C-afferents, i.e., polymodal nociceptive fibers.

All these findings support the hypothesis that near-threshold excitation of polymodal nociceptors (which elicits few spikes at low frequencies) results in the discharge of mediators from these nociceptors in amounts sufficient to provoke an efferent response (vasodilatation), while the afferent information transmitted in this way is subliminal for evoking pain, nociception, or any sensation [36,108].

Evidence that few impulses are able to evoke antidromic vasodilatation or a flare reaction has been obtained in other species as well, for example, in the rabbit [122,123], pig [124], and human subjects [109]. In these experiments, however, peripheral nerves with admixed autonomic fibers were stimulated, and the type of units characterized by their capsaicin sensitivity was demonstrated only in the case of human skin [109]. In this context, it is worth noting that ultraviolet irradiation of the rabbit ear initiates low-frequency discharges of polymodal nociceptors within 30 minutes [48]. This might explain the common observation that after sunburn injuries, reddening of the skin begins earlier than the onset of burning sensation. Flare reaction could also be elicited without pain sensation.

The following question might well be asked. Is there any evidence that these sensory nerve endings might participate in cutaneous microcirculation under physiological conditions? Preliminary experiments support this notion. After perineural capsaicin pretreatment of the sciatic nerve in the rat, skin blood flow of the paw was reduced [125]. It can be concluded that this physiological effector role of polymodal nociceptors forms the basis of "trophic effects" that have been shown to be impaired by capsaicin desensitization [98,126].

A final point deserving of comment is the sensation of itching, which is also mediated by polymodal nociceptors [127] and can be prevented by capsaicin desensitization [35,128]. Studies with iontophoretic application of histamine combined with laser Doppler recordings have already begun. The relationship between the onset of vasodilatation, however, and pruritus has not yet been evaluated [129]. The issue of the specific relationship between different sensations [27] and the messages initiated by the group of polymodal nociceptors is still an open question. It should be also considered that, provided that they form a homogenous receptor population with respect to excitability characteristics, subgroups of these units might have different connections in the spinal cord causing perceptual differences.

CLINICAL RELEVANCE AND PERSPECTIVES IN PAIN THERAPY

Among a large number of irritant extracts, ointments, and liniments, capsaicin-containing preparations have been used over centuries as counterirritants

[1,4,130]. When local irritation and hyperemia developed after these treatments, a beneficial effect on pain stemming from internal organs (e.g., muscles, joints, intestines) was observed.

There have been attempts to clarify the mechanism of this therapeutic agent, but the explanations have remained on a speculative basis [131]. Revival of interest in capsaicin-type agents in clinical practice has recently emerged. On the basis of experimental results accumulated during the last two decades, a much broader field of therapeutic approaches has developed. A critical survey of these first attempts as well as further perspectives are summarized in this section.

Response stages of nociceptive afferents to capsaicin-type agents

Capsaicin has excitatory, sensory neuron blocking, and neurotoxic effects on polymodal nociceptors and other capsaicin-senstive (CS) chemoreceptors. All these stages of capsaicin effects can be utilized in therapy. Nevertheless, in order to use them in a rational way, it should be decided which of these effects has the desired beneficial value with respect to a particular disease. Four stages of the neuroselective action of capsaicin have been characterized [11,16].

Stage 1. Excitation

The first response of polymodal nociceptors and other CS sensory receptors to capsaicin-type agents is excitation [41]. The effect is reproducible if capsaicin is applied either topically [16,40,44] or intraarterially [4,8,49,132] in near-threshold concentrations.

Stage 2. Sensory neuron blocking effect

This stage of drug action is characterized by functional desensitization of the affected sensory receptors (Figure 8-1) without neurotoxic nerve degeneration. Ultrastructural changes may occur (Figures 8-3A–8-3D). Local or systemic administration of capsaicin in severalfold higher doses than the threshold is required for this effect. Nevertheless, the blocking action of capsaicin and their congeners is not due to excessive stimulation of the receptors [12,40,44]; the blocking action develops also under the effect of local anesthesia [1]. Both the sensory and the mediator-releasing functions of the nerve endings are inhibited. The blockade is reversible, but could last for several days. Substance P is depleted after perineural application [80], but desensitization without depletion was observed after topical treatment [133].

Stage 3. Selective neurotoxic impairment

The loss of function is due to degeneration of the peripheral and central terminals and axons of the capsaicin-sensitive primary afferent neurons. The cell body is preserved with swollen mitochondria. Its neuropeptide content is depleted. The effect is practically irreversible, but signs of recovery in function and neuropeptide levels [5,11,12,15,16,134] indicate a certain degree of regeneration.

Stage 4. Irreversible cell destruction

This severe stage of neurotoxicity is induced by capsaicin in neonatal rats and mice. The evidence that similar complete cell destruction may occur in adult animals is not convincing [16]. Therefore, it has probably no clinical relevance.

Capsaicin in clinical practice

Application of capsaicin as an irritant or counterirritant

When capsaicin is used as a counterirritant in the treatment of myositis, arthritis, tenosynovitis, and similar afflictions, the beneficial effect can be attributed to the excitatory (Stage 1) effect of the drug. This is indicated by the fact that irritants without desensitizing potency (e.g., mustard oil) have also been used for this purpose. Theoretically, the therapeutic effect could be due either to the mediators released from the sensory nerve endings or to changes in the reflexes and sensations initiated by these receptors through the central nervous system. Experimental evidence for the former possibility has already been obtained. Antidromic stimulation of capsaicin-sensitive afferent fibers in the rat inhibited neurogenic inflammation in skin areas that were not innervated by the stimulated nerves [135].

Recently, the reproducible irritant effect of capsaicin has been used to elicit the cough reflex in humans for evaluation of the antitussive action of drugs [136,137].

Application of capsaicin as a desensitizing agent

Topical treatment of the skin or blister base with capsaicin solution induces local analgesia and blocking of flare response [16,24,35,36,109,138–140] and thermal hyperemia [141]. The loss of function of nociceptive nerve endings lasts for days, but it is fully reversible, indicating that the desensitization is probably due to Stage 2 action of the irritant.

Capsaicin in ointments has been used in the treatment of painful diabetic neuropathy [142] and postherpetic neuralgia [143–145]. Capsaicin solution applied in desensitizing concentration (10 mM) to the nasal mucosa was beneficial for several weeks in patients having cluster headache [38,146] or in hyperactive rhinopathy and vasomotor rhinitis [147,148]. It is worthy to mention that stimulation of capsaicin-sensitive perivascular afferents in the rat evokes neurogenic inflammation in the dura mater. Ergot alkaloids that may be operative in human headaches, such as migraine and cluster headache, inhibited this response [149]. Capsaicin applied to the receptive field induces an inhibition of axonal flow for several months [150] and could affect sensory neurons that have axon collaterals both in the nasal mucosa and in the dura mater. Intravesicular instillations of capsaicin (10 mM) showed signs of desensitization and attenuated the symptoms of hypersensitive disorders of the urinary bladder [151]. There are, however, many open questions about how to use capsaicin in the clinical practice and which mechanisms cause the observed effects.

The following guidelines for topical treatments with capsaicin-type agents are suggested:

1. Randomized, double-blind, parallel trials are needed by using nondesensitizing irritants as controls (mustard oil, homovanilloyl octyl ester, xylene, zingerone).
2. Desensitization procedure can be made under the effect of local anesthetics.
3. The desensitizing effect should be checked during the treatment by monitoring the threshold concentration of irritants that elicit sensation. In the skin, axon reflex flare is also a good indicator.
4. The excitatory (stage 1) and desensitizing (stages 2 and 3) effects of capsaicin could both produce pain relief. In order to introduce an appropriate schedule for the treatment, a differentiation should be made.
5. When capsaicin is used in a mucosal area that has not tested before, a careful increase in concentrations in the first trials is needed. Circulatory and other autonomic reflexes elicited by local irritation should be considered besides the pain sensation.
6. The neurotoxic (stage 3) effect of capsaicin seems to be a promising approach in the treatment of intractable pain. Perineural application is a powerful means of inducing selective degeneration of polymodal nociceptive units [152] and can elicit analgesia over a year [16]. Subperineural injection is also effective.

The first steps in using the desensitizing effect of capsaicin in pain management have been made. The results with topical treatments are promising. The fact that the sensory stimulant and desensitizing effects of capsaicin congeners do not run parallel [44] has raised the possibility of developing congeners of capsaicin that might be useful analgesics in systemic treatments. In any case, with the aid of capsaicin, polymodal nociceptors and other capsaicin-sensitive interoceptors have become new targets for drug development in pain management.

ACKNOWLEDGMENTS
This work was supported by research grants OTKA and TKT. The author is indebted to his coworkers listed as coauthors in the references.

REFERENCES

1. Szolcsanyi J. 1984. Capsaicin and neurogenic inflammation: History and early findings. In LA Chahl, J Szolcsanyi, F Lembeck (eds), Antidromic Vasodilatation and Neurogenic Inflammation. Budapest, Akademiai Kiado, pp. 7–26.

2. Hogyes A. 1878. Beitrage zur physiologischen wirkung des bestandteile des *capsicum annuum*. Arch Exp Pathol Pharmakol 9:117–130.
3. Jancso N, Jancso-Gabor A, Szolcsanyi J. 1967. Direct evidence for neurogenic inflammation and its prevention by denervation and by pretreatment with capsaicin. Br J Pharmacol 31:138–151.
4. Szolcsanyi J. 1982. Capsaicin-type pungent agents producing pyrexia. In AS Milton (ed), Handbook of Experimental Pharmacology, Vol. 60. Pyretics and Antipyretics. Berlin, Springer-Verlag, pp. 437–478.
5. Nagy JI. 1982. Capsaicin: A chemical probe for sensory neuron mechanism. In LL Iversen, SD Iversen, SH Snyder (eds), Handbook of Psychopharmacology, Vol. 15. New York, Plenum Press, pp. 185–235.
6. Monsereenusorn Y, Kongsamut S, Pezalla PD. 1982. Capsaicin — A literature survey. CRC Crit Rev Toxicol 10:321–339.
7. Fitzgerald M. (1983). Capsaicin and sensory neurons — a review. Pain 15:109–130.
8. Russell LC, Burchiel KJ. (1984). Neurophysiological effects of capsaicin. Brain Res Rev 8:165–176.
9. Szolcsanyi J. 1984. Capsaicin-sensitive chemoceptive neural system with dual sensory-efferent function. In LA Chahl, J Szolcsanyi, F Lembeck (eds), Antidromic Vasodilatation and Neurogenic Inflammation. Budapest, Akademiai Kiado, pp. 27–56.
10. Hori T. 1984. Capsaicin and central control of thermoregulation. Pharm Ther 26:389–416.
11. Szolcsanyi J. 1985. Sensory receptors and the antinociceptive effects of capsaicin. In R Hakanson, F Sundler (eds), Tachykinin Antagonists. Amsterdam, Elsevier, pp. 45–54.
12. Buck SH, Burks TF. 1986. The neuropharmacology of capsaicin: Review of some recent observations. Pharmacol Rev 38:179–226.
13. Lembeck F. 1988. Substance P: From extract to excitement. Acta Physiol Scan 133:435–454.
14. Maggi CA, Meli A. 1988. The sensory-efferent function of capsaicin-sensitive sensory neurons. Gen Pharmacol 19:1–43.
15. Holzer P. 1988. The local effector function of capsaicin-sensitive sensory nerve endings: Involvement of tachykinins, and other neuropeptides. Neuroscience 24:739–768.
16. Szolcsanyi J. 1989. Capsaicin, irritation, and desensitization: Neurophysiological basis and future perspectives. In BG Green, JR Mason, MR Kare (eds), Chemical Senses, Vol. 2: Irritation. New York, Marcel Dekker, pp. 141–169.
17. Szolcsanyi J. 1983. Tetrodotoxin-resistant non-cholinergic neurogenic contraction evoked by capsaicinoids and piperine on the guinea-pig trachea. Neurosci Lett 42:83–88.
18. Hayes AG, Oxford A, Reynolds M, Shingler AHS, Skingle M, Smith C, and Tyers MB. 1984. The effects of a series of capsaicin analogues on nociception and body temperature in the rat. Life Sci 34:1241–1248.
19. Hayes AG, Hawcock AB, Hill RG. 1984. The depolarizing action of capsaicin on rat isolated sciatic nerve. Life Sci 34:1561–1568.
20. Jancso G, Ferencsik M, Such G, Kiraly E, Nagy A, Bujdoso M. 1985. In R Hakanson, F Sundler (eds), Tachykinin Antagonists. Amsterdam, Elsevier, pp. 35–44.
21. Sietsema WK, Berman EF, Farmer RW, Maddin CS. 1988. The antinociceptive effect and pharmacokinetics of olvanil following oral and subcutaneous dosing in the mouse. Life Sci 43:1385–1391.
22. Szallasi A, Blumberg PM. 1989. Resiniferatoxin, a phorbol-related diterpene, acts as an ultrapotent analog of capsaicin, the irritant constituent in red pepper. Neuroscience 30:515–520.
23. Szallasi A, Joo F, Blumberg P. 1989. Duration of desensitization an ultrastructural changes in dorsal root ganglia in rats treated with resiniferatoxin, an ultapotent capsaicin analog. Brain Res 503:68–72.
24. Szolcsanyi J. 1977. A pharmacological approach to elucidation of the role of different nerve fibers and receptor endings in mediation of pain. J Physiol (Paris) 73:251–259.
25. Sizer F, Harris N. 1985. The influence of common food additives and temperature on threshold perception of capsaicin. Chem Senses 10:279–286.
26. La Motte RH, Simone DA, Baumann TK, Shain CN, Alreja M. 1988. Hypothesis for novel classes of chemoreceptors mediating chemogenic pain and itch. In GF Gebhart, MR Bond (eds), Proc. Vth World Congress on Pain. Amsterdam, Elsevier Press, pp. 529–535.
27. Green BG Flammer LJ. 1988. Capsaicin as a cutaneous stimulus: Sensitivity and sensory qualitics on hairy skin. Chem Senses 13:367–384.

28. Gepetti P, Fusco BM, Marabini S, Maggi CA, Fanciullacci M, Sicuteri F. 1988. Secretion, pain and sneezing induced by the application of capsaicin to the nasal mucosa in man. Br J Pharmac 93:509–514.

29. Barnes PJ, Chung KF, Lammers J-WJ, McCusker M, Minette P. 1988. Non-adrenergic bronchodilator mechanism in man. J Physiol 396:179.

30. Collier JG, Fuller RW. 1984. Capsaicin inhalation in man and the effects of sodium cromoglycate. Br J Pharmac 81:113–117.

31. Winning AJ, Hamilton RD, Shea SA, Guz A. 1986. Respiratory and cardiovascular effects of central and peripheral intravenous injections of capsaicin in man: Evidence for pulmonary chemosensitivity. Cin Sci 71:519–526.

32. Torebjork HE, Vallbo AB, Ochoa JL. 1987. Intraneural microstimulation in man: Its relation to specificity of tactile sensations. Brain 110:1509–1529.

33. Ochoa J. 1986. The newly recognized painful ABC syndrome: Thermographic aspects. Thermology 2:65–107.

34. Carpenter SE, Lynn B. 1981. Vascular and sensory responses of human skin to mild injury after topical treatment with capsaicin. Br J Pharmacol 73:755–758.

35. Toth-Kasa I, Jancso G, Bognar A, Husz S, Obal F Jr. 1986. Capsaicin prevents histamine-induced itching. Int J Clin Pharm Res 6:163–169.

36. Szolcsanyi J. 1988. Antidromic vasodilatation and neurogenic inflammation. Agents Actions 23:4–11.

37. Lundblad L, Lundberg JM, Anggard A, Zetterstrom O. 1987. Capsaicin-sensitive nerves and the cutaneous allergy reaction in man. Allergy 42:20–25.

38. Sicuteri F, Fusco BM, Marabini S, Fanciullacci M. 1988. Capsaicin as a potential medication for cluster headache. Med Sci Res 16:1079–1080.

39. Jancso G, Kiraly E, Such G, Joo F, Nagy A. 1987. Neurotoxic effect of capsaicin in mammals. Acta Physiol Hung 69:259–313.

40. Szolcsanyi J, Jancso-Gabor A, Joo F. 1975. Functional and fine structural characteristics of the sensory neuron blocking effect of capsaicin. Naunyn-Schmiedebergs Arch Pharmacol 287:157–169.

41. Szolcsanyi J, Jancso-Gabor A. 1975. Sensory effects of capsaicin congeners. I. Relationship between chemical structure and pain producing potency of pungent agents. Arzneim Forsch (Drug Res) 25:1877–1881.

42. Szolcsanyi J, Sann H, Pierau F-K. 1986. Nociception in pigeons is not impaired by capsaicin. Pain 27:247–260.

43. Sann H, Harti G, Pierau F-K, Simon E. 1987. Effect of capsaicin upon afferent and efferent mechanisms of nociception and temperature regulation in birds. Can J Physiol Pharm 65:1347–1354.

44. Szolcsanyi J, Jancso-Gabor A. 1976. Sensory effect of capsaicin congeners II. Importance of chemical structure and pungency in desensitizing activity of capsaicin-type compounds. Arzneim-Forsch (Drug Res) 26:33–37.

45. Yaksh TL, Farb D, Leeman S, Jessell T. 1979. Intrathecal capsaicin depletes substance P in the rat spinal cord and produces prolonged thermal analgesia. Science 206:481–483.

46. Jancso G. 1981 Intracisternal capsaicin: Selective degeneration of chemosensitive primary sensory afferents in the adult rat. Neurosci Lett 27:41–45.

47. Jancso G, Kiraly E, Jancso-Gabor A. 1980. Direct evidence for an axonal site of action of capsaicin. Naunyn-Schmiedebergs Arch Pharmacol 313:91–94.

48. Szolcsanyi J. 1987. Selective responsiveness of polymodal nociceptors of the rabbit ear to capsaicin, bradykinin and ultra violet irradiation. J Physiol 388:9–23.

49. Szolcsanyi J, Anton F, Reeh PW, Handwerker HO. 1988. Selective excitation by capsaicin of mechano-heat sensitive nociceptors in rat skin. Brain Res 446:262–268.

50. Coderre TJ, Abbott FV, Melzack R. 1984. Behavioral evidence in rats for a peptidergic-noradrenergic interaction in cutaneous sensory and vascular function. Neurosci Lett 47: 113–118.

51. Abbott FV, Grimes RW, and Melzack R. 1984. Single nerve capsaicin. Effects on pain and morphine analgesia in the formalin and foot-flick tests. Brain Res 295:77–84.

52. Handwerker HO, Holzer-Petsche, U, Heym C, Welk E. 1984. C-fibre functions after topical application of capsaicin to a peripheral nerve and after neonatal capsaicin treatment. In LA Chahl, J Szolcsanyi, F Lembeck (eds), Antidromic Vasodilatation and Neurogenic Inflammation. Budapest, Akademiai Kiado, pp. 57–82.

53. Konietzny F, Hensel H. 1983. The effect of capsaicin on the response characteristic of human C-polymodal nociceptors. J Therm Biol 8:213–215.
54. Lynn B, Carpenter SE, Pini A. 1984. Capsaicin and cutaneous afferents. In LA Chahl, J Szolcsanyi, F Lembeck (eds), Antidromic Vasodilatation and Neurogenic Inflammation. Budapest, Akademiai Kiado, pp. 83–92.
55. Jancso G, Kiraly E, Jancso-Gabor A. 1977. Pharmacologically induced selective degeneration of chemosensitive primary sensory neurone. Nature 270:741–743.
56. Welk E, Fleischer E, Petsche U, Handwerker HO. 1984. Afferent C-fibers in rats after neonatal capsaicin treatment. Pflügers Arch 400:66–71.
57. Lawson SN. 1978. The morphological consequences of neonatal treatment with capsaicin on primary afferent neurons in adult rats. Acta Physiol Hung 69:315–321.
58. Lawson SN, Harper AA. 1984. Neonatal capsaicin is not a specific neurotoxin for sensory C-fibres or small dark cells of rat dorsal root ganglia. In LA Chahl, J Szolcsanyi, F Lembeck (eds), Antidromic Vasodilatation and Neurogenic Inflammation. Budapest, Akademiai Kiado, pp. 111–118.
59. Rethelyi M, Salim MZ, Jancso G. 1986. Altered distribution of dorsal root fibers in the rat following neonatal capsaicin treatment. Neuroscience 18:749–762.
60. Nillson G, Alving K, Lundberg JM, Ahlstedt S. 1989. Effect of neonatal or later capsaicin treatment on bronchial reactivity in sensitized rats: Relation to humoral changes. Int Arch Allergy Appl Immunol 88:234–236.
61. Hiura A, Ishizuka H. 1989. Changes in features of degenerating primary sensory neurons with time after capsaicin treatment. Acta Neuropathol 78:35–46.
62. Baccaglini PJ, Hogan PG. 1983. Some rat sensory neurons in culture express characteristic of differentiated pain sensory cells. Proc Natl Acad Sci USA 80:594–598.
63. Heyman I, Rang HP. 1985. Depolarizing responses to capsaicin in a subpopulation of rat dorsal root ganglion cells. Neurosci Lett 56:69–75.
64. Bevan SJ, James IF, Rang HP, Winter J Wood JN. 1987. The mechanism of action of capsaicin: A sensory neurotoxin. In P Jenner (ed), Neurotoxins and their Pharmacological Implications. New York, Raven Press, pp. 261–277.
65. Marsh SJ, Stansfeld CE, Brown DA, McCarthy D. 1987. The mechanism of action of capsaicin on sensory C-type neurons and their axons in vitro. Neuroscience 23:275–289.
66. Wood JN, Winter J, James IF, Rang MP, Yeats J, Bevan S. 1988. Capsaicin-induced ion fluxes in dorsal root ganglion cells in culture. J Neurosci 8:3208–3220.
67. Wood JN, Coote PR, Minhas A, Mullaney J, McNeil M, Burgess GM. 1989. Capsaicin-induced ion fluxes increase cyclic GMP but not cyclic AMP levels in rat sensory neurons in culture. J Neurochem 53:1203–1211.
68. Maggi CA, Patacchini R, Santicioli P, Guiliani S, Gepetti P, Meli A. 1988. Protective action of Ruthenium red toward capsaicin desensitization of sensory fibers. Neurosci Lett 88:201–205.
69. Maggi CA, Patacchini R, Santicioli P, Giuliani S, Gepetti P, Meli A. 1988. Protective action of Ruthenium red toward capsaicin desensitization of sensory fibers. Neurosci Lett 88:201–205.
70. Baranowski R, Lynn B, Pini A. 1986. The effect of locally applied capsaicin on conduction in cutaneous nerves in four mammalian species. Br J Pharmacol 89:267–277.
71. Jancso G, Such G. 1983. Effects of capsaicin applied perineurally to the vagus nerve on cardiovascular and respiratory function in the cat. J Physiol 341:359–370.
72. Chung JM, Lee KH, Hori Y, Willis WD. 1985. Effect of capsaicin applied to a peripheral nerve on the responses of primate spinothalamic tract cells. Brain Res 329:27–38.
73. Joo F, Szolcsanyi J, Jancso-Gabor A. 1969. Mitochondrial alterations in the spinal ganglion cells of the rat accompanying the long-lasting sensory disturbance induced by capsaicin. Life Sci 8:621–626.
74. Chiba T, Masuko S, Kavano H. 1986. Correlation of mitochondrial swelling after capsaicin treatment and substance P and somatostatin immunoreactivity in small neurons of dorsal root ganglion in the rat. Neurosc Lett 64:311–316.
75. Palermo NN, Brown HK, Smith DL. 1981. Selective neurotoxic action of capsaicin on glomerular C-type terminals in rat substantia gelatinosa. Brain Res 208:506–510.
76. Hoyes AD, Barber P. 1981. Degeneration of axons in the ureteric and duodenal nerve plexuses of the adult rat following in vivo treatment with capsaicin. Neurosci Lett 25:19–24.

77. Papka RE, Furness JB, Della NG, Murphy R, Costa M. 1984. Time course of effect of capsaicin on ultrastructure and histochemistry of substance P-immunoreactive nerves associated with the cardiovascular system of the guinea pig. Neuroscience 12:1277–1292.
78. Chung K, Schwen RJ, Coggeshall RE. 1985. Ureteral axon damage following subcutaneous administration of capsaicin in adult rats. Neurosci Lett 53:221–226.
79. Jancso G, Kiraly E, Joo I, Such G, Nagy A. 1985. Selective degeneration by capsaicin of a subpopulation of primary sensory neurons in the adult rat. Neurosci Lett 59:200–214.
80. Lynn B, Shakhantseh J. 1988. Substance P content of the skin, neurogenic inflammation and numbers of C-fibers following capsaicin application to a cutaneous nerve in the rabbit. Neuroscience 24:769–776.
81. Nagy JI, Iversen LL, Goedert M, Chapman D, Hunt SP. 1983. Dose-dependent effect of capsaicin on primary sensory neurons in the neonatal rat. J Neurosci 3:399–406.
82. Szolcsanyi J. 1990. Capsaicin-sensitive chemoceptive B-afferents: A neural system with dual sensory-efferent function. Behav Brain Sci 13:316.
83. Stricker S. 1876. Untersuchungen uber die gefasserwurzeln des Ischiadicus. S-B Kaiserl Akad Wiss Wien 3:173–185.
84. Bayliss WM 1923. The Vaso-motor System. London, Longsman, Green.
85. Langley JN. 1923. Antidromic action. J Physiol (London) 57:428–446.
86. Kowalski ML, Kaliner MA. 1988. Neurogenic inflammation, vascular permeability, and mast cells. J Immun 140:3905–3911.
87. Chahl L. 1988. Antidromic vasodilatation and neurogenic inflammation. Pharmac Ther 37:275–300.
88. Coggeshall RE. 1980. Law of separation of function of the spinal roots. Physiol Rev 60:716–755.
89. Kennins P. 1984. Electrophysiological and histological studies on vascular permeability after antidromic sensory nerve stimulation. In LA Chahl, J Szolcsanyi, F Lembeck (eds), Antidromic Vasodilatation and Neurogenic Inflammation. Budapest, Akademiai Kiado, pp. 175–188.
90. Lisney SJW, Bharali LAM. 1989. The axon reflex: An outdated idea or a valid hypothesis? News Physiol Sci 4:45–48.
91. Chahl LA, Ladd RJ. 1976. Local oedema and general excitation of cutaneous sensory receptors produced by electrical stimulation of the saphenous nerve in the rat. Pain 2:25–31.
92. Janig W, Lisney SJW. 1989. Small diameter myelinated afferents produce vasodilatation but not plasma extravasation in rat skin. J Physiol 415:477–486.
93. Bartho L, Szolcsanyi J. 1978. The site of action of capsaicin on the guinea pig isolated ileum. Naunyn-Schmiedebergs Arch Pharmacol 305:75–81.
94. Szolcsanyi J, Bartho L. 1978. New type of nerve-mediated cholinergic contractions of the guinea pig small intestine and its selective blockade by capsaicin. Naunyn-Schmiedebergs Arch Pharmacol 305:83–90.
95. Szolcsanyi J, and Bartho L. 1979. Capsaicin-sensitive innervation of the guinea pig taenia caeci. Naunyn-Schmiedebergs Arch Pharmacol 309:77–82.
96. Szolcsanyi J, Bartho L. 1981. Impaired defense mechanism to peptic ulcer in the capsaicin-desensitized rat. In G Mozsik, O, Hanninen, T Javor (eds), Gastrointestinal Defense Mechanisms. Advances in Physiological Science, Vol. 15. Oxford and Budapest, Pergamon Press and Akademiai Kiado, pp. 39–51.
97. Holzer P, Lippe JT. 1988. Stimulation of afferent nerve endings by intragastric capsaicin protects against ethanol-induced damage of gastric mucosa. Neuroscience 27:981–988.
98. Maggi CA, Borsini F, Santicioli P, Gepetti P, Abelli L, Evangelista S, Manzini S, Theodorsson-Norheim E, Somma V, Amenta F, Bacciarelli C, Meli A. 1987. Cutaneous lesions in capsaicin-pretreated rats. A trophic role of capsaicin-sensitive afferents? Naunyn-Schmiedebergs Arch Pharmacol 336:538–545.
99. Lewis T. 1937. The nocifensor system of nerves and its reactions. Br Med J 194:431–435, 491–494.
100. Lembeck F. 1983. Sir Thomas Lewis' nocifensor system, histamine and substance-P-containing primary afferent nerves. Trends Neuro Sci 6:106–108.
101. Lewis T. 1927. The Blood Vessels of the Human Skin and their Responses London, Shaw.
102. Izumi H. Karita K. 1988. Investigation of mechanisms of the flare and wheal reactions in human skin by band method. Brain Res 449:328–331.

103. Jancso N, Jancso-Gabor A, Szolcsanyi J. 1968. The role of sensory nerve endings in neurogenic inflammation induced in human skin and in the eye and paw of the rat. Br J Pharmacol 33:32–41.
104. Szolcsanyi J, Sebok B, Bartho L. 1985. Capsaicin, sensation and flare reaction. The concept of bidirectional axon reflex. In: CC Jordan, P Oehme (eds), Substance P Metabolism and Biological Actions. London, Taylor and Francis, p. 234.
105. Peterfreund RA, Vale WW. 1986. Local anesthetics inhibit veratridine-induced secretion of calcitonin gene-related peptide (CGRP) from cultured rat trigeminal ganglion cells. Brain Res 380:159–161.
106. Gulbenkian S, Merighi A, Wharton J, Varndell IM. 1986. Ultrastructural evidence for the coexistence of calcitonin gene-related peptide (CGRP) and substance P (SP) in secretory vesicles of peripheral nerves in the guinea pig. J Neurocytol 15:535–542.
107. Kruger L. 1988. Morphological features of thin sensory afferent fibers: A new interpretation of "nociceptor" function. In W Hamann, A Iggo (eds), Progress in Brain Research, Vol. 74. Amsterdam, Elsevier Press, pp. 253–257.
108. Szolcsanyi J, Westerman RA, Magerl W, Pinter E. 1988. Capsaicin-sensitive cutaneous sense organs: Nerve terminals with multiple functions. Regul Peptides 22:38.
109. Magerl V, Szolcsanyi J, Westerman RA, Handwerker HO. 1987. Laser Doppler measurements of skin vasodilatation elicited by percutaneous electrical stimulation of nociceptors in humans. Neurosci Lett 82:349–354.
110. Kreulen DL. 1986. Activation of mesenteric arteries and veins by preganglionic and postganglionic nerves. Am J Physiol. 251:H1267–H1275.
111. Torebjork HE. 1980. Activity in C nociceptors and sensation. In DR Kenshalo (ed), Sensory Functions of the Skin of Humans. New York, Plenum, pp. 313–323.
112. Van Hees J, Gybels J. 1981 C nociceptor activity in human nerve during painful and non-painful skin stimulation. J Neurol Neurosurg Psychiatry 44:600–607.
113. Meyer RA, Raja SN, Campbell JN. 1985. Coupling of action potential activity between unmyelinated fibers in the peripheral nerve of monkey. Science 227:184–187.
114. Helme RD, McKernan S. 1984. Flare responses in man following topical application of capsaicin. In LA Chahl, J Szolcsanyi, F Lembeck (eds), Antidromic Vasodilatation and Neurogenic Inflammation. Budapest, Akademiai Kiado, pp. 303–315.
115. Torebjork E. 1985. Nociceptor activation and pain. Phil Trans R Soc London B308:227–234.
116. Hallin RG. 1984. Human pain mechanisms studied with percutaneous microneurography. In B Bromm (ed), Pain Measurement in Man. Neurophysiological Correlates of Pain. Amsterdam, Elsevier, pp. 39–53.
117. Handwerker HO, Adriaensen HFM, Gybels JM, Van Hees J. 1984. In B Bromm (ed), Pain measurement in Man. Neurophysiological Correlates of Pain. Amsterdam, Elsevier, pp. 55–64.
118. Perl ER. 1984. Pain and nociception. In JM Brookhart, VB Mountcastle (eds), Handbook of Physiology, Nervous System III. Bethesda, MD, pp. 915–975.
119. Konietzny F, Perl ER, Trevino D, Light A, Hensel H. 1981. Sensory experience in man evoked by intraneural electrical simulation of intact cutaneous afferent fibers. Exp Brain Res 42:219–222.
120. Wall PD, McMahon SB. 1985. Microneuronography and its relation to perceived sensation. A critical review. Pain 21:209–229.
121. Fleischer E, Handwerker HO, Joukhadar SH. 1983. Unmyelinated nociceptive units in two skin areas of the rat. Brain Res 267:81–92.
122. Holton P, Perry WLM. 1951. On the transmitter responsible for antidromic vasodilatation in the rabbit's ear, J Physiol (London) 114:240–251.
123. Lynn B, Sckakhanbeh J. 1988. Neurogenic inflammation in the skin of the rabbit. Agents Actions 25:228–230.
124. Pierau F-K, Szolcsanyi J. 1989. Neurogenic inflammation; Axon reflex in pigs. Agents Actions 26:231–232.
125. Sann J, Pinter E, Szolcsanyi J, Pierau F-K. 1988. Peptidergic afferents might contribute to the regulation of the skin blood flow. Agents Actions 23:14–15.
126. Kjartansson J, Dalsgaard C-J, Jonsson C-E. 1987. Decreased survival of experimental critical flaps in rats after sensory denervation with capsaicin. Plast Surg 79:218–222.
127. Tuckett RP, Wei JY. 1987. Response to an itch-producing substance in cat. II. Cutaneous receptor populations with unmyelinated axons. Brain Res 413:95–103.

128. Westerman RA, Magerl E, Handwerker HO, Szolcsanyi J. 1985. Itch sensation evoked by percutaneous microiontophoresis of histamine on human hairy skin. In Proc. Australian Physiology and Pharmacology Societys Vol. 16:70.

129. Magerl W, Handwerker HO. 1988. A reliable model of experimental itching by iontophoresis of histamine In GF Gebhart, MR Bond (eds), Proc. Vth World Congress on Pain. Amsterdam, Elsevier Press, pp. 536–540.

130. Lembeck F. 1987. Columbus, capsicum and capsaicin: Past, present and future. Acta Physiol Hung 69:263–273.

131. Bonta IL. 1978. Endogenous modulators of the inflammatory response. In JR Vane, SH Ferreira (eds), Handbook of Experimental Pharmacology, Vol. 50(1). Inflammation. Berlin, Springer-Verlag, pp. 523–567.

132. Donnerer J, Lembeck F. 1983. Capsaicin-induced reflex fall in rat blood pressure is mediated by afferent substance P-containing neurons via a reflex centre in the brain. Naunyn-Schmiedebergs Arch Pharmacol 324:293–295.

133. Lembeck F, Donnerer J. 1981. The time course of capsaicin-induced functional impairment in comparison with changes in neural substance P content.

134. Gamse R, Lackner D, Gamse G, Leeman SE 1981. Effect of capsaicin pretreatment on capsaicin-evoked release of immunoreactive somatostatin and substance P from primary sensory neurons. Naunyn-Schmiedebergs Arch Pharmacol 316:38–41.

135. Pinter E, Szolcsanyi J. 1988. Inflammatory and antiinflammatory effects of antidromic stimulation of dorsal roots in the rat. Agents Actions 25:240–242.

136. McEwan JR, Choudry N, Street R, Fuller RW 1989. Change in cough reflex after treatment with enalapril and ramipril. Br Med J 299:13–16.

137. Choudry NB, Fuller RW, Pride NB. 1989. Sensitivity of the human cough reflex: Effect of inflammatory mediators prostaglandin E_2, bradykinin, and histamine. Am Rev Resp Dis 140:137–141.

138. Bernstein JE, Swift RM, Soltani K, Loricz AL. 1981. Inhibition of axon reflex vasodilatation by topically applied capsaicin. J Invest Dermatol 76:394–395.

139. Anand P, Bloom SR, McGregor GP. 1983. Topical capsaicin pretreatment inhibits axon reflex vasodilatation caused by somatostatin and vasoactive intestinal polypeptide in human skin. Br J Pharmac 78:665–670.

140. McCusker MT, Chung KF, Roberts NM, Barnes PJ. 1989. Effect of topical capsaicin on the cutaneous responses to inflammatory mediators and to antigen in man. Allergy Clin Immunol 83:1118–1123.

141. Neeck G, Rusch D, Schmidt KL. 1987. Uber die hemmung von erythemen durch capsaicin. 1. Ein beitrag zum entstehungsmechanisms von hautrotungen durch physikalisch-medizinische massnahmen am beispiel des hitzeerythems. Physik Med Balneol Med Klimatol 16:383–388.

142. Ross DR, Varipapa RJ. 1989. Treatment of painful diabetic neuropathy with topical capsaicin. N Engl J Med 321:474–475.

143. Bernstein JE, Korman NJ, Bickers DR, Dahl MV, Millikan, LE. 1989. Topical capsaicin treatment of chronic postherpetic neuralgia. J Am Acad Dermatol 21:265–270.

144. Bucci FA Jr, Gabriels CF, Krohel GB. 1988. Successful treatment of postherpetic neuralgia with capsaicin. Am J Ophthamol 106:758.

145. Watson CP, Evans RJ, Watt VR. 1988. Postherpetic neuralgia and topical capsaicin. Pain 33:333–340.

146. Sicuteri F, Fusco BM, Marabini S, Campagnolo V, Maggi CA, Geppetti P, Fanciullacci M. 1990. Beneficial effect of capsaicin application to the nasal mucosa in cluster headache. Clin J Pain, in press.

147. Marabini S, Ciabatti PG, Polli G, Fusco BM, Geppetti P, Maggi CA, Fanciullacci M, Sicuteri F. 1988. Effect of topical nasal treatment with capsaicin in vasomotor rhinitis. Regul Peptides 22:121.

148. Stammberger H, Wlf G. 1988. Headaches and sinus disease: the endoscopic approach. Ann Otol Rhinol Laryngol 97(Suppl. 134):3–23.

149. Saito K, Markowitz S, Moskowitz MA. 1988. Ergot alkaloids block neurogenic extravasation in dura mater: proposed action in vascular headaches. Ann Neurol 24:732–737.

150. Taylor DCM, Pierau F-K, Szolcsanyi J. 1984. Long-lasting inhibition of horseradish peroxidase (HRP) transport in sensory nerves induced by capsaicin pretreatment for the receptive field. Brain Res 298:45–49.

151. Maggi CA, Barbanti G, Santicioli P, Beneforti P, Misuri D, Meli A, Turini D. 1989. Cystometric evidence that capsaicin-sensitive nerves modulate the afferent branch of micturition reflex in humans. J Urol 142:150–154.
152. Lynn B, Pini A, Baranowski R. 1987. Injury of somatosensory afferents by capsaicin. Selectivity and failure to regenerate. In LM Pubols, BJ Sessle, (eds), Effective of Injury on Trigeminal and Spinal Somatosensory Systems. New York, Alan R. Liss, pp. 115–124.

9. PAIN MEASUREMENT

JONATHAN J. LIPMAN

Pain is the perception of noxious sensation. Its measurement is confounded, therefore, by the act of perception. In the manner of love, hate, or anger, it is an intensely personal experience that defies ready communication. As a cognitive process, pain may be described by language, and a sophisticated lexicon has been developed to achieve this. Such description does not measure pain, however, only the opinion one has regarding its perception. The map is not the territory.

The definition of *pain* according to the International Association for the Study of Pain (IASP) is "an unpleasant sensory and emotional experience associated with actual or potential tissue damage and described in terms of such damage." This comes close to providing the rules for such language, but falls short of providing the operational rules for pain's measurement.

As a "perception," pain does not bear a direct relationship to the intensity of the noxious stimulus that elicits it. The individual perceiving the pain does so from within a psychological set that incorporates the experiential background and contextual emotionality of the perception.

Both set and setting influence the act of perception. It is reasonable to suppose that perception of an acute pain administered to a healthy experimental research subject differs in terms of imputed "meaning" from that perceived as a result of injury in an otherwise healthy individual, which also differs from that experienced by the chronic pain sufferer. The emotional import of the pain is inextricably woven into the fabric of the overall perception. As a perception, then, pain cannot be separated from its experiential matrix. In the mind's eye, it is viewed through the lens of experience, projected onto a screen composed of our judgement of its significance.

In attempting to measure pain in humans, the clinical scientist must first decide from which viewpoint he or she will observe the phenomenon. As in the case of the blind men describing the elephant, no one viewpoint can provide a complete view of the phenomenon, yet it is necessary to select a viewpoint in order to avoid syncretism.

The phenomenology of pain resides exclusively within the domain of the nervous system. On the afferent arm of the phenomenon lies *nociception*, the sensory detection of dangerously intense stimuli. It is generally agreed by biologists that nonverbal, infrahuman, species experience nociception. Nociception engenders reflex *behaviors*, and these are measurable: They can be observed. The unicellular paramecia experience nociception; they move away from a noxious stimulus — we call this phobotaxis. Paramecia do not call it anything. In humans, and only in humans, is the *perception* of nociception called pain. This is the behaviorist's dilemma. We cannot *know* whether nonverbal species experience pain as we do. We cannot know, that is, whether they "perceive."

This chapter is about the measurement of pain. It deals, therefore, with the human experience.

In common with nonverbal species, the human pain sufferer, in detecting the nociceptive stimulus, undergoes *physiological* changes, both on the afferent arm of the sensory detection experience and within the central nervous system (CNS) and its efferent limbs. These changes occur at the spinal and autonomic levels of nervous system organization. They manifest as *reflex behaviors*, and they can be observed and measured.

In attempting to measure this phenomenon in our fellow humans, however, we naturally rely on language. This is reasonable: Language is the operational difference between nociception and pain. Underlying the outward manifestations of behavior lie the neurophysiological correlates of perception. Underlying these are the biochemical bases of nerve function. Each is accessible to measurement.

BEHAVIOR

At the behavioral level, pain is manifest to the observer through the *voluntary* behaviors of language and of motor activity, and through the *involuntary* behaviors that are both specific to pain and general to suffering. These are the characteristic guarding, facial expression, and body postures of the pain-suffering individual. The expression of organized locomotor activity is affected also, with guarded gait, restriction of movement, and both the acquisition of certain pain-related behaviors (such as taking medication) and the extinction of normal movements. Such behaviors may represent strategies for both *pain relief* and *analgesia*, but a distinction between these must be made [1–3].

Pain relief is the process by which the perceived intensity of an ongoing pain is attenuated. Analgesia (more correctly, hypalgesia, but we shall follow the convention and use the term *analgesia*) is the state whereby sensibility to noxious stimulation is diminished. Analgesia can only be measured by the application of an external noxious stimulus, and it makes its presence known by a reduction in perceived noxiousness [4]. In the context of the modification of movements by the pain state, then, these modifications may serve the purpose of relieving the perceived intensity of a pain or of avoiding nociceptive stimulation.

BEHAVIORAL ASSESSMENT INSTRUMENTS

Behavioral assessment of pain is conducted at the verbal and nonverbal levels. At the verbal level, the information that is captured is the patient's self-report of the applicable language of pain. Instruments for its capture range from simple unidimensional measures to complex instruments that attempt to capture opinions of (or poll) more than one dimension of the pain experience. So much reliance is placed on these instruments, and their veracity, accuracy, reproducibility, and internal and external validity — described below — that it is sobering to remember that they are no more veridical than the patient's own descriptive choice of language. To make this obvious point more forcefully, if the patient were lying we could not detect this.

UNIDIMENSIONAL VERBAL DESCRIPTOR AND CATEGORY SCALES

Verbal rating scales

The simplest method of obtaining information on the patient's perceived pain intensity is to ask. Typically, the patient is asked to choose a number between zero and 100 that "best describes the intensity of their pain." This method, which has been termed the *101 point numerical rating scale* or NRS-101, is fraught with difficulty. The voice, tone, facial expression, and demeanor of the questioner are inevitably communicated to patients and influences their opinions. This face-to-face method is so capable of engendering bias that it has been used by investigators studying the placebo response as a means of provoking the subliminal expectation of pain relief [5].

Visual analog scales

In an attempt to place distance between the conscious or unconscious expectations of the questioner and the response of the patient, printed questionnaires are commonly preferred. A printed form of the NRS-101 has, for instance, been used. The visual analog scale (VAS) is another simple questionnaire method. A 10 cm line is printed having two extreme descriptors at either end, thus:

NO PAIN ———————————————————————————— MAXIMUM POSSIBLE PAIN

The VAS may also be interrupted by index lines, thus:

NO
PAIN ─ ─ ─ + ─ ─ ─ + ─ ─ ─ + ─ ─ ─ + ─ ─ ─ + ─ ─ ─ + ─ ─ ─ + ─ ─ ─   MAXIMUM
POSSIBLE
PAIN

   The subject is asked to rate the intensity of his or her pain by marking the line at some appropriate distance along its length. The marked line is then removed from the patient's sight so that it does not influence the scoring of subsequent presentations of the VAS, which may be at hourly or shorter intervals. For simplicity, some investigators use measurements of the reciprocal of the VAS for "pain intensity" as a "pain relief" scale in the assessment of pain-relieving and analgesic effects of drugs. Within certain limitations, the VAS is a reliable way of polling opinion on a unidimensional axis, and it has the advantage of being quick and easy to do, is easily understood by the patient, is readily scored by measuring the distance of the patient's mark along the line, and has been validated against other polling methods [6–10].

Limitations of analog methods

Apart from the obvious limitation that pain is not an unidimensional experience, and from the consequences of representing the pain experience as an ordinal continuum when it is not, the VAS methods suffer from peculiar disadvantages. Patients vary in their predilection toward "clumping" and "splitting" of their responses. Chronic pain patients tend to use only the right-hand side of the VAS, whereas cancer patients may use both ends and make relatively little use of the middle. The instructions given to the patient are also critical. There are additional problems with the way in which the VAS may be analyzed. One patient's "7.5 cm" may be another patient's "4.0 cm." These scores are not ordinal numbers, each patient's pain dimension is his or her own, and it is incorrect to treat different patients' scores as co-ordinal, by, for instance, averaging them. The precision with which the line can be measured also tends to give a false impression of precision to the VAS's meaning. There is, in addition, a tendency among investigators to treat the data so acquired as an ordinal scale subject to analysis by parametric statistics. This is clearly wrong. A more honest, and yet still uncertain, method of treating such data is to normalize it relative to each patient's own response range. The data are thus trnasformed to a ratio scale that can be analyzed by nonparametric methods.

Category scales

Whereas the NRS-101 and the VAS methods purport to represent pain as an undivided continuum, category scales seek to limit the patient's response to one of several predetermined choices in a single dimension. A numerical category scale is the simplest form, such as the category version of the VAS called the 11 point box scale (BS-11) [8]:

NO PAIN	0	1	2	3	4	5	6	7	8	9	10	MAXIMUM POSSIBLE PAIN

The majority of category scales permit the patient to choose from among a ranked list of verbal descriptors, the accepted meanings of which punctuate the range of the dimension that they describe and delimit. Category scales are used to poll patients' reports of pain relief (having elements of: NONE, A LITTLE, SOME, A LOT, COMPLETE), of pain intensity (e.g., NONE, A LITTLE, SOME, A LOT, TERRIBLE), or of the emotional aspects of pain [11].

Category scales have entered widespread use in the assessment of pain and pain-relief therapies. In use, the patient marks the category that best describes his or her opinion of the dimension being measured. This rating is repeated at intervals of time. Each category is assigned a numerical value by the investigator (e.g., NONE = 0, A LITTLE = 1, etc.), and the numerical sum of each time interval's category score is obtained for the entire measuring period. When used with a "pain relief" scale, this has been called the total pain relief (TOTPAR) score. Such a method, using a five-category pain relief scale (NONE, SLEIGHT, MODERATE, LOTS, and COMPLETE) has been used by Wallenstein, et al. [12] to compare the analgesic efficacy of Zomepirac® and morphine. These same investigators report that in a large population of cancer patients, this category scale is sensitive enough to detect dosage, age, and ethnic differences in response to morphine administration.

Category scales do not necessarily have to be limited to ranked scales of words or numbers. Frank et al. [13] used eight "cartoon faces" drawn to represent a ranked continuum of facial expressions representing the range extending from tears and misery to smiles and laughter. They found good correlation between patients' cartoon choices and their VAS and verbal descriptor scale responses.

Limitations of category methods

As with the analog scales described above, problems surround the validity of quantified category scales. The assignment of equally spaced integers to a rank order of verbal descriptors gives the appearance of an ordinal distribution that is, in fact, not real. Since the numerical assignments are ranked, they are perhaps more ordinal than nominal, yet the ordinal distribution is unknown. The "distances," that is, between the word–values, are unknown. Consider, for instance, the series of pain intensity scores such as 4,2,2,1,0, which may represent the opinion of a patient who starts out with "terrible" pain and who responds to the administration of morphine by recording "some," "some," "a little," and then "none" at 15-minute intervals. It is invalid to state that the patient's average pain intensity is "1.8," there is no such rank as 1.8. Heft and Parker [14] have shown experimentally that commonly used pain descriptors are unequally spaced along the intensity continuum. They propose that category scale quantification should reflect this with a weighting scale that corrects for unequal spacing. This argument has merit.

MULTIDIMENSIONAL REPORT SCALES

Insofar as unidimensional pain scales represent the overall intensity of pain as existing on a single axis, these methods fail to describe its qualities.

A number of questionnaires have been devised that attempt to give respondents a range of qualitative dimensions over which to describe their perceived pain. Such instruments are particularly useful in polling the opinions of the chronic pain patient over time and in response to treatment. In substance, multidimensional questionnaires are made up of batteries of analog and category scales, completed at a single time. Several of these instruments have been reviewed recently by Chapman and Syrjala [15], the most well known of which are perhaps the McGill Pain Questionnaire (MPQ) devised by Melzack [16] and the Wisconsin Brief Pain Inventory [17].

The Memorial Pain Assessment Card

The Memorial Pain Assessment Card (MPAC) [18] is the simplest of the multidimensional assessment tools. It is a single sheet of paper containing a battery of three visual analog scales (for pain intensity, pain relief, and mood), and a set of eight adjectives describing pain intensity (no pain, just noticeable, mild, severe, etc.), which the respondents mark to indicate their perceived pain status at the moment of completing the test. The test takes seconds to complete and the questionnaire is arranged in such a way that it can be folded, so that respondents can see only one scale at a time. The MPAC — and similar scales of this type — are ideal for the assessment of pain relief following analgesic drug administration or other therapies. It has the advantages of the unidimensional VAS methods, including simplicity and ease of use, with the added benefit that more than one dimension is polled.

The McGill Pain Questionnaire (MPQ)

This questionnaire attempts to poll the report of three dimensions of the pain experience: sensory, affective, and evaluative [16]. There are four parts to the MPQ. In the first part, the patient is asked to mark a picture of the human form so as to indicate the location of pain and whether it is external or internal. In the second part, the patient is presented with 20 sets of adjectives, each set composed of a ranked list of words in increasing order of severity (e.g., pinching, pressing, gnawing, cramping, crushing). The most appropriate single word in each set is to be circled. Ten of the sets describe sensory qualities of the pain, and five describe affective qualities. One set, referred to as "evaluative," lists "annoying, troublesome, miserable, intense, and unbearable." Four additional sets described as "miscellaneous" are primarily sensorial in nature. The third part of the MPQ polls the patient's opinion regarding what factors exacerbate or relieve his or her pain. Three sets of related words are provided from which the patient chooses to describe the temporal qualities of his or her pain (continuous, rhythmic, transient, etc.). The fourth part of the MPQ provides the patient with a ranked list of five pain intensity descriptors, category choices from which to answer six questions regarding his or her pain history.

Arising from the work of Melzack and Torgerson [11], the MPQ has been subjected to widespread application and testing in a variety of clinical pain states. To quantify its responses, the investigator scores the ranked adjectives and computes the total rank of chosen words, either as a global total or as a total within each dimension. Factor analysis studies of the responses to the MPQ tend to support the dimensional assignments of descriptors [19,20] and for the grouping of words into semantically homogenous sets [21], although there is evidence that the scaling of ranks within sets might differ across different groups of pain patients [19].

Unique patterns of MPQ responses have been associated with different types of chronic pain state, including those of arthritis, cancer pain, and low back pain [21–23]. Despite its widespread application in chronic pain assessment and of pain relief, the MPQ is time consuming to perform (about 15 minutes) and does not readily lend itself to the assessment of analgesic drug effects, where measurements must be polled at 10- or 15-minute intervals. Perhaps its most serious drawback is its requirement that the respondent possess a fairly sophisticated vocabulary.

The Wisconsin Brief Pain Inventory

The Wisconsin Brief Pain Inventory (BPI) is a multidimensional pain measure, the reliability and validity of which has been demonstrated in the assessment of pain of various types. These include the pain of cancer, chronic orthopedic pain, and arthritis pain [17,24]. It has also been used to assess procedural pain [25]. Using a scale of 0–10, patients report on the intensity of their pain as they perceived it at its worst, least, and average during the preceding week, as well as at the time they are filling out the questionnaire. They report on analgesic medications and pain relief obtained, qualitative descriptions of pain, location of pain, and areas of interference with quality of life. When the questionnaires were applied cross-culturally, cancer patients in Wisconsin and (using a Vietnamese translation) in Vietnam demonstrated comparable factor loadings in their patterns of response in the "pain severity" and "pain interference" scales of this instrument. The utility of the BPI thus appears to generalize across cultural and linguistic barriers [26].

West Haven-Yale Multidimensional Pain Inventory (WHYMPI)

Introduced by Kerns, Turk, and Rudy [27] as a briefer alternative to the MPQ, the WHYMPI is more well founded in classical psychological theory, with a strong cognitive-behavioral orientation. It is principally designed to assess self-reported behaviors relevant to the chronic pain population. It is a 52-item questionnaire, and is arranged in three parts comprised of 12 scales. The first assesses the impact of pain on the patient's life, the second assesses the patient's opinions regarding the responses of others to the patient's communications of pain. The third scale polls the opinion of the patient regarding the extent to which he or she participates in the activities of daily living.

Because of its cognitive-behavioral orientation, the WHYMPI may be considered a form of behavioral activity self-report, the general limitations of which are considered more fully below. It does not lend itself to the assessment of pain relief or analgesic effects in the acute setting.

ASSESSMENT OF BEHAVIORAL ACTIVITIES
The rather clumsy term *behavioral activities* is used here to denote those non-verbal activities associated with everyday life, such as eating, walking, sleeping, and social interaction, that may be affected by the pain state. The modification of behavioral activities is seen by many investigators as being "more objective" than verbal self-estimates of pain intensity and quality. It is the experience of most investigators in the field, for instance, that many chronic pain patients, unlike acute pain patients [26], misjudge their own pain intensity in relation to its history [28]. In an attempt to capture this report of behavioral activity, investigators either solicit it from the patient themselves (self-report) or rely on external observers. The disadvantage of the former is that self-reports of activity suffer the same inaccuracies and misestimations as do those of pain intensity [29,30]. Despite this major limitation, many investigators poll this information as an estimate of the patient's own opinion of his or her physical disability.

Self-report of behavioral activity
Several of the multidimensional assessment tools cited above, including the WHYMPT and the BPI, include a behavioral dimension by which the patient may score — as a category scale — the extent to which his or her pain state interferes with activity. Thus, on the BPI, patients are asked on the "pain interference" axis the extent to which their pain has influenced their general activity: walking, work, relations with others, and sleep.

Perhaps the simplest category scale for behavioral self-report is the six-item behavior rating scale of Budzynski et al. [31], termed the *BRS-6* by Jensen et al. [32]. It has the elements of:

( ) No pain
( ) Pain present, but can easily be ignored
( ) Pain present, cannot be ignored, but does not interfere with everyday activities
( ) Pain present, cannot be ignored, interferes with concentration

( ) Pain present, cannot be ignored, interferes with all tasks except taking
    care of basic needs such as toileting and eating
( ) Pain present, cannot be ignored, rest or bedrest required

A major reason for seeking nonverbal assessment of pain behavioral activity is to ascertain the extent of the patient's incapacity when not in the clinic. There is a well-known class of chronic pain patients — many without obvious organic pathology — who tend to overemphasize their reported pain and disability. Measures such as the BPI detect this easily, yet their measurement is compromised thereby [26].

The pain diary
To the extent that such overemphasis is a characteristic of the poor historian rather than the dissimulator, more accurate self-reports can be obtained by the use of a contemporary pain diary. A pain diary is a log of daily activities in which the respondent records, at intervals of 1 hour or less, every day, the amount of time spent sitting, standing, walking, or reclining. It may also be used to record contemporaneously the subjective pain intensity at those times and the medication consumed. The pain diary is extremely useful in chronic pain assessment, yet it will not overcome the problem of dissimulation. Ready et al. [33] have found, for instance, that certain chronic pain patients report medication consumption that is 50–60% below actual consumption. Similarly Kremer [29], who compared patient self-report records with staff observations, found major discrepancies. For this reason, many investigators have sought "objectivity" in behavioral activity assessment by the use of standardized observer reports and automatic motion detection.

OBSERVATIONAL ASSESSMENT OF BEHAVIOR
Immune to self-reporting errors, observational assessment by trained observers detects the objective impact of pain behavior — and to an extent the underlying disease state engendering the pain — on controlled and free responding of the patient.

Controlled behavior
As recently reviewed by Keefe [34], the "specific" behaviors that elicit pain and the behavioral modifications that the pain patient enacts in order to avoid pain, differ among the different pain syndromes. For this reason, several investigators have instituted standardized test situations to exert control over the pain behaviors emitted. These tests have certain common features. Richards [35], who developed the University of Alabama at Birmingham (UAB) Pain Behavior Scale, uses the following simple method: The patient is asked to walk a short distance, stand for a brief time, then transfer to a sitting, and again to a standing position. Trained observers estimate the severity of ten

behaviors characteristic of pain by using a three-point rating scale. Inter-observer reliability is high, 95%, and scores correlate well with self-assessed pain rating at discharge, though not with the MPQ score. A recently revised version of the scale using eight categories has been found to correlate better with the MPQ [36]. Keefe and Block [37] have also used a standardized test situation to elicit controlled behavioral responding. These authors recommend that the sequence in which the tests are carried out be randomized, with the duration of each task held constant to prevent order effects in the study of populations [34]. They report that quantitative indices of pain behaviors in their test subjects (guarding, grimacing, rubbing the painful area, etc.), scored at regular 30-second intervals, provides an accurate measure of low back pain. To the observational measurements of Keefe and Block [37] have been added four additional behavioral categories by Follick, Ahern, and Aberger [38]. These authors report that the four behavioral categories: partial movement, limitation statements, sounds, and position shifts, correctly classified 94% of the patients and 95% of the controls.

Free behavioral responding

Behavioral observations in the natural setting have significant advantages over controlled responding in formal test situations. In general, such methods use the same or similar checklist items to which is added a pain-diary type of dimension, often called the activities of dialy living (ADL). Appropriate only to the in-patient setting, these observations may be conducted by the nursing staff during the course of their daily duties [39]. An earlier study by Cinciripini and Floreen [40] used trained observers to observe patients for 5 minutes in each half-hour throughout a 12- to 15-hour day. The behavioral elements that they scored included nonverbal pain behavior, pain talk, nonpain complaints, pro-health talk, and assertion. They found, as might be expected or hoped, dramatic increases in "well behavior" and reduction in "pain behavior" over the course of treatment.

Particularly in the chronic pain patient population, time spent walking and moving about ("up time") is considered an index of therapeutic progress. It is generally realized, as found by Linton [41], that there is no relationship between activity level and pain intensity report, yet increased "up time", even with no reduction in pain intensity, is a behaviorally desirable therapeutic goal. Since the use of trained observers in an outpatient setting is impractical, several investigators have examined the use of automatic activity monitors to capture this information. Such electromechanical and electronic devices are of various degrees of sophistication. Keefe and Hill [42] have found that chronic pain patients differ from normals in terms of gait parameters as measured by pressure transducers placed in the heels of their shoes. Patients are found to take smaller steps and to have asymmetrical gait. Their method could even distinguish patients receiving disability payments from those not so blessed! The former had a longer stride length. Some success has been obtained with simpler devices that indiscriminately record "up time" by means of inertial measurement or orientation sensors. In the manner of Keefe and Hills' pressure transducers [42], they are relatively expensive and unsuitable for general outpatient use, however [30,43]. Cheaper methods such as the "actometer," which is a pedometerlike instrument modified from a mechanical watch [44], appear to fail in reliability over time when used in the general pain population, possibly as a result of gait constraints [45]. Automated procedures for gross monitoring of behavioral activity may thus show future promise, but do not currently appear to be applicable to the chronic pain patient — the population in which such measurements are most needed.

As recently reviewed by Keefe [34], specific facial expressions are highly characteristic of the pain experience. Insofar as these are largely unconscious primitive nociceptive primate reflexes, they hold promise for objective quantification of pain's behavioral correlates. A facial action coding system (FACS), developed by Ekman and Friesen [46], has been characterized with normal volunteers undergoing painful electric shock [47]. The original FACS requires that 44 separate action units be extracted from filmed behaviors observed frame by frame. Unsuitable for routine use, a practical alternative may prove to be the Global Rating Method developed by LeResche and Dworkin [48]. Such methods have not yet found their way into clinical pain research.

Pain assessment by monitoring medication requirement

The philosophical differences between *pain relief* and *analgesia* become critical when the medication requirement is used as an index of the underlying pain state. To recapitulate, pain relief is the diminution in perceived intensity of an endogenous pain state, whereas analgesia is the reduction in sensibility to an applied — external or incident — nociceptive stimulus. The measurement of analgesia *requires* the use of an applied nociceptive stimulus. The measurement of pain relief does not; one merely polls the opinion of perceived endogenous pain intensity. Medications can be pain relieving without being analgesic; aspirin in the treatment of inflammatory pain or anticonvulsant drugs used in treatment of the pain of tic douloureux and tabes dorsalis being examples, or tricyclic antidepressants in chronic pain [4,49]. Since the perception of pain is phenomenologically a psychic event, and since the biological substrate of this psychic event is, we believe, neurochemically mediated by endorphinergic and other neurochemical systems [50,51], the mechanism of pain relief engendered by analgesic opiate drugs is quite complex. Indeed, the opiate-abusing addict who is not a pain sufferer — the "street user" — experiences a painful hyperesthesia on drug withdrawal, accompanied by affective changes that can only be described as "psychic pain." Despite the widespread clinical belief that the same does not occur in pain patients, it is biologically impossible to separate the pain-relieving and affective actions of opiate analgesics using the pharmacological agents currently available. One can, however, measure the analgesic effect by means of a nociceptive stimulus and compare the results so obtained with the patient's subjective report of pain relief. In our own laboratory, we have used a radiant heat stimulus to measure the analgesic effect of standard doses of intravenous and intrathecal morphine on cutaneous pain tolerance in the pain patient [52]. We find major differences in the correlation between pain relief (assessed by VAS) and analgesia (assessed by elevated pain tolerance), depending upon the route of administration of the drug. Intrathecal administration engenders pain relief with, initially, no analgesia (no change in pain tolerance to the radiant heat-beam stimulus), and intravenous administration engenders both simultaneously.

Such measurement has unfortunately not yet become common practice in the clinic. Monitoring of the pain patient's demand for pain-relieving (and analgesic) medications is nevertheless common practice and is used as an index of the severity of the underlying pain state. Despite the limitations of this procedure — drug demand may outlast resolution of the organic basis of the pain and may reflect the avoidance of withdrawal hyperaesthesia — there is a certain usefulness in such measurement.

The advent of the patient-controlled "analgesia" (PCA) pump facilitates the collection of this data. The PCA pump is an automated intravenous infusion device capable of being programmed to deliver a limited quantity of drug (the prescribed maximum) per unit time. Individual doses are administered on a *pro re nata* basis by the patients themselves using a push-button control. There are various types of pumps available. Some emit a tone whenever the patient demands medication, whether or not medication is delivered, some emit a tone only when the delivery takes place. The time of each demand by the patient is recorded, and such records of demand, delivery rate, and cumulative dose form the overall estimate of the patient's perceived need for pain relief and — by reciprocal inference — of his or her underlying pain status.

Given the limitations of such data in the absence of an independent measure of analgesia, the PCA pump has restricted utility in pain research. Clinically it is, however, well tolerated by the patient and, needless to say, by the nursing staff. It is reported that patients using these pumps achieve better pain relief while requiring less pain medication than patients treated in the traditional p.r.n. fashion [53,54]. Clearly the placebo effect engendered by the greater sensation of self-control that is inherent in the use of these pumps is measurable thereby.

PSYCHOPHYSICAL AND PHYSIOLOGICAL METHODS OF ASSESSMENT

Psychophysical methods

As described earlier, and as recently phrased by Gracely [55], "due to an almost universal distrust of nonphysical — subjective — reports, the physical measures of behavior and physiology enjoy at least equality, if not presumed superiority, over verbal judgments . . . however . . . pain exists only in consciousness."

Psychophysical procedures attempt to establish the link between the external physical environment and its internal psychological representation. There are various depths to which the psychophysical researcher may delve in investigating this relationship. A simple stimulus-dependent psychophysical test, for example, forms the basis of the clinical audiometry examination. Sounds of various frequencies and amplitudes are directed to the human ear, and respondents indicate the range and acuity of their hearing by signalling their ability to detect these frequencies and amplitudes. The psychophysical relationship between stimulus intensity and perceptual quality is readily calculable. A portion of the audiometry examination entails a test of the subject's ability to understand spoken words against a background of various types and intensities of sound interference. The comprehension of such content comes also within the purpview of the audiometry test, even though the perception of content is a complex product of education and gestalt. The test does not purport to measure the cognitive psychological basis of the comprehension of speech and language, yet without such basis the test could not be conducted. Clearly more is involved than the sensitivity of the ear. The subject's comprehension is inherent to the test.

Psychophysical methods thus rely on the subjective report of the test subject, and they attempt to control for bias and sensitivity to stimulation by means of sophisticated experimental designs.

Psychophysical principles originated with the work of Fechner [56], who argued that sensation is proportional to the logarithm of stimulus intensity. More recently, Stephens [57] has introduced a simplified form of the relationship that has come to be called "Stephen's power law." It states:

Reported sensation intensity $= C \times S \times B$,

where C is a constant, S is the stimulus intensity, and B is the proportionality constant that maximizes the fit of reported sensation intensity to stimulus intensity.

Psychophysical methods have been used to investigate the phenomenon of pain sensibility in the experimental subject and, more recently, in the patient suffering endogenous pain.

Pain assessment in the experimental subject

Pain-free human volunteers are used for the most part in psychophysical procedures to investigate the relationship between the intensity of noxious stimulation and perceived pain intensity. Gracely [55] has elegantly reviewed and compared the psychophysical methods designed to assess this relationship and broadly divides them into two types: stimulus dependent and response dependent. In stimulus-dependent methods, the subject's predetermined responses constitute the fixed, independent variable and the intensity of stimulation required to evoke these responses is the dependent variable. Response-dependent methods present a series of fixed stimulus intensities to which the response judgement varies.

Stimulus-dependent methods have been used to investigate the features of the pain sensitivity range described by Stephen's psychophysical power law. A lower region of stimulus intensity, evoking a sensation termed *prepain*, has been recognized, particularly with electrical methods of stimulation [58]. The term *pain threshold* is used to describe the region of stimulus intensity where sensory judgement is "just noticeably" of pain, where prepain turns into pain. Suprathreshold stimuli, more intense than that required to elicit the pain threshold sensation, occupy what is commonly referred to as the *pain sensitivity range* or more properly, the *pain sensibility range*. At the upper limit of subjective pain sensation lies the *pain tolerance level*, defined as the stimulus intensity above which the volunteer is unwilling to endure — or incapable of enduring — further stimulation [59]. Scaling of subjective pain intensity along the pain sensitivity range is possible with both stimulus-dependent and response-dependent methods. The principal concern of the investigator engaged in such tasks is to measure and control response bias, and various test procedures have been designed to achieve this [55]. As with all psychophysical research, it is the judgement of the subject that forms the basis of the response. This judgement is subject to manipulation by various factors and thus may these factors be studied. Theoretically, the effect of an analgesic may be detected by its ability to modify the perceived intensity of any portion of the pain sensitivity range. In practice, most studies have been carried out on the boundary extremes — the threshold or tolerance levels.

Pain thresholds have been studied using a variety of noxious stimuli, including electrical stimulation [58], radiant heat [60], and pressure [61]. Pain tolerance levels are usually assessed by the use of a continuous, rather than a discrete, noxious stimulus. The elapsed time to the limit of endurance, or the total stimulus energy of this, is the measure of the pain tolerance level. The starting point of the measurement can be taken as the pain threshold or the start of the stimulus. Pain tolerance has been measured by a variety of means, including that of the "cold pressor test," in which the hand or limb is immersed in ice water until unendurable pain results [62], focal pressure [63], tourniquet ischemia [64], and radiant heat [65]. Of the types of noxious stimulation available, certain modalities have been criticized for their lack of "physiological" relevance. The sensation of electric shock, for instance, does not resemble any of the common clinical pain sensations. Electrical stimulation, moreover, indiscriminately engenders generalized neuronal barrages in both afferent and efferent circuits. The sensations of the tolerance level engendered by cold pressor, tourniquet ischemia, and radiant heat methods more closely resemble the clinical report of pain sensation in their quality. Tolerance methods using these techniques, unlike threshold methods, also evoke some not inconsiderable anxiety and apprehension on the part of the subject, which may loosely resemble the anxiety of the pain-suffering patient. Tolerance methods may possess a peculiar usefulness in that they are ideal for the detection of analgesic effects due to analgesic drugs [52,64].

Pain psychophysics in pain patients

For reasons that are not entirely clear, a schism has developed over the years between the work of those investigators who study pain sensory phenomena in normal volunteers and the work of those who seek to quantify pain in the clinical situation. In part this may represent ideological differences — turf battles — or, as suggested by Naliboff and Cohen [66] in their recent review, it may have arisen as a result of the finding by Beecher in 1959 [67] that pain *thresholds* to radiant heat are unaffected by various analgesics in doses known to relieve clinical pain in humans. This has led to a widely held view that clinical and experimental pain studies are inimicable. Recent evidence suggests that they are not.

Improvement in our understanding of pain has given new impetus to the reexamination of the use of laboratory methods to assess clinical pain in pain patients [66,68,69]. It is hypothesized that the state of suffering an endogenous pain influences the perceived intensity of an applied, experimental, pain; that is, the pain patients differ from pain-free normals in their judgment of the painfulness of a nociceptive stimulus.

The evidence to date is admittedly confusing at this early stage of the investigation. There are fundamentally two theories of how the clinical pain patient will judge the intensity of an incident — applied — pain. One theory, the *hypervigilance theory*, holds that the clinical pain patient will be more sensitive to an applied painful stimulus and will judge it to be more painful than would a pain-free individual. The second, opposing, *adaptation-level theory* holds that the pain patient judges the intensity of an applied pain stimulus in the context of his or her own pain and so will be less sensitive to an applied painful stimulus and will judge it to be less painful. Rollman's studies [68,70] in normal volunteers support the existence of an adaptation theory. Our own work, in chronic pain patients suffering from medical conditions permitting neurosurgical resolution, also supports the adaptation level theory. We have found that while these patients are in pain, before treatment, their pain tolerance to a radiant heat stimulus is elevated over that of normal pain-free volunteers. When their pain is relieved by surgical treatment of their patho-logical condition, their pain tolerance is reduced, and it is comparable to that of normal volunteers [65].

As reviewed by Naliboff [66], there is good evidence for the truth of both theories. How can this be? It is possible that both are indeed true; there may be two different *types* of chronic pain patients: those who are stoical and those who are hypervigilant. It is possible also that future studies may find that the pain sufferer is hypervigilant to certain types of stimulus and stoical to others. It is also important to realize that the studies conducted thus far are a mixed bag; some measure the pain threshold, others — like ours — the pain tolerance level. As stated by Rollman [70], "the method of pain induction is not an issue that can be examined in isolation . . . often the pain source is chosen on the basis of what apparatus is readily available rather than by an informed judgment regarding its capacity to mimic the sensory, affective or evaluative properties of particular clinical disorders". It is also possible that the normal psychophsical relationships of the pain sensitivity range are different in chronic pain patients, and indeed there is no certainty that they are comparable for the different modes of noxious stimulation, even in normal volunteers. The biological basis of different parts of the pain sensitivity range may not be the same. Thus morphine does not change the pain *threshold* to radiant heat [71], but it measurably increases the pain *tolerance* level [52]. This may indicate that endorphinergic processes are involved in the latter but not the former.

Studies that support the hypervigilance theory have largely used electrical stimulation or focal pressure to elicit the judgement of pain threshold. Even in trained normal subjects, the pain threshold, where prepain becomes just noticeably painful, is a composite of nuances and is difficult to judge. In the patient suffering excruciating endogenous clinical pain, the detection of such nuances may be overly difficult. Pain tolerance, in contrast, is a more easily recognized point. Defined as the limit of endurance, most subjects can readily identify this and reflexively signal when this level is reached.

It is to be hoped that future studies in algesiometry, as described above, will resolve the questions they have posed. It is possible, even probable, that the pain sufferer differs in reproducible and predictable ways from the individual not in pain, and thus may the pain state be measured. Since these studies are occurring in the arena of psychophysics, an arena well used to the experimental control of bias in subjective response, they hold out great hope for providing an "objective" method of pain "measurement" by using patients' own pain perceptive machinery to assess their pain status.

Physiological methods of assessment

The advantages of finding a physiological correlate of the "pain state" are manifold. To the clinician, it would represent an "objective" measure of this subjective condition. To the scientist, the pursuit of physiological correlates is doubly exciting, representing the search for the biological bases of pain perception and its physiological expression. In truth, the definition of pain is so inextricably bound up in the emotional context within which it is perceived that its biological separation from this context at the level of central neurochemical processing is probably neither desirable, possible, nor meaningful.

There are various levels at which physiological correlates are sought. On the efferent arm of the nervous system lies the autonomic response associated with pain. Measured at the central nervous system, we find the electrophysiological consequences of sensory detection and processing. These are both spinal and supraspinal. Within the neurochemistry of the brain reside the humoral mechanisms of synaptic action associated with neuronal function.

Autonomic correlates

Using galvanic skin response as a measure of autonomic sympathetic nervous system activation, Naifeh et al. [72] studied two patient groups. One group was surgically preoperative and was stressed, but not in pain. The other was surgically postoperative and considered to be in pain and stress. A group of normal volunteers acted as the control. All were subjected to a Valsalva maneuver and a mental arithmetic test. The pain patients gave smaller galvanic skin response changes to these tests, indicating decreased arousal of the sympathetic nervous system.

Nociceptive reflexes

Nociceptive reflexes occur in both nonverbal animals and humans, with the difference being that in humans a verbal report can be obtained on the perceived painfulness of the stimulus. In animal studies of analgesia, thermal or electrical stimuli [73,74], or other such methods, are used to evoke the nociceptive reflex that analgesics inhibit. Analgesia in humans is presumed to represent the antinociceptive effect in animal tests.

Electrical stimulation of the human sural nerve elicits such a reflex readily amenable to study [75,76]. Nociceptive rather than tactile stimulation of this nerve elicits a reflex withdrawal. Stimulated at the skin surface behind the external malleolar at the ankle, electromyelographic responses of the biceps femoris muscle are recorded at the posterior face of the thigh. Delivery of nociceptive stimuli of different intensities can be subjectively scaled over the pain sensitivity range by standard psychophysical techniques and can be related to reflex recruitment by the muscle. No muscle movement occurs until very near the maximum stimulus intensity. In reviewing this technique, De-Broucker, Willer, and Bergeret [77] have demonstrated, in normal volunteers, that the pain threshold (by self-report) covaries with the reflex threshold, and that the pain tolerance level covaries with the maximum recruitment reflex threshold. The effect of morphine administration is to shift the stimulus-response curve to the right, with a minimal effect on threshold and a maximum effect on tolerance. It is naloxone reversible. Supraspinal influences also modify the relationship [76]. The stimulus-reflex relationship holds true even in paraplegics, however, in contradistinction to radiant heat methods of pain tolerance assessment, which require intact pain perception. This leads one to conclude that the sural nerve reflex may be useful in studies of spinal nociception processes but not in studies of pain perception per se. Its value may lie in the elucidation of diffuse noxious inhibitory controls and in the assessment of supraspinal influences on these controls.

Electroencephalographic (EEG) methods

Insofar as cortical arousal is manifest by changes in the frequency domain of the EEG, modern computer methods of analysis of the EEG signal are capable of capturing this information. Typically the data are digitized as they are collected (in real time), or are stored as an analog magnetic tape signal for later (off-line) processing. Transposition of the original signal captured in the time domain into the frequency domain is usually accomplished by means of fast fourier transformation (FFT), and by this means the frequency spectrum may be numerically analyzed [78]. The transformed signal is then available in greatly simplified form and is amenable to statistical methods of computer analysis. Principal component analysis and discriminant function analysis, to name but two methods, have become quite common.

Curiously, the power of these computer methods to tell us which specific features of the EEG signal are associated with specific physiological states greatly exceeds our understanding of the physiological basis of the EEG itself. These techniques have nevertheless spawned the science of pharmaco-electroencephalography, a method and discipline that seeks to match the phenomenological features of the quantified EEG with the underlying psychic states associated with them, these latter engendered by psychoactive drugs of known action and mechanism [79]. Using principal component analysis, Bromm and Scharein [80] have derived a measure of arousal from the EEGs of volunteers undergoing evoked potential measurement. Similarly Bourne et al. [81] have used an expert system derived from discriminant function analysis features, which is sensitive to and correctly diagnoses the dementia of uremia in human subjects. Our own studies [82] have shown that these methods are applicable to the animal research laboratory.

Since the utility of the EEG is limited by our understanding of its physiological basis, and the linkage of this to cognitive and perceptual processes is poorly understood, researchers in the field do not hold out immediate hope that such methods will be successfully applied to pain measurement in the near future. The work is proceeding at a furious pace in both human and animal models, however, and may yet surprise us.

Evoked potential (EP) methods

Insofar as specific cortical arousal states may prove characteristic of the pain-perception process (as indexed by autonomic and electroencephalographic measures, see above), the evoked cortical potential arising from painful peripheral stimulation provides the most specific method for accessing brain signals associated with pain. Less general than EEG measurement, the EP signal is readily associated with the noxious signal evoking it. It provides a method, therefore, for examining psychophysical relationships at the level of their cortical processing.

Such psychophysical relationships have been examined in normal human volunteers using a variety of peripheral stimuli, including electrical tooth stimulation [83], ultrasonic stimulation of the joint [84], and laser stimulation [85]. As pointed out in recent reviews by Chapman and colleagues [23,49,83], waveform amplitude of the long-latency component measured from the vertex increases with the energy of peripheral stimulation. There is good correlation between such amplitudes and the subjective pain report. As with the EEG itself, EP signals are usually transposed into the frequency domain by fast fourier transformation or other methods. Using a further data reduction algorithm called the maximum entropy method, Bromm [49] has revealed that power in the delta range (between 1 and 4 Hz) is highly correlated with subjective pain rating where this is evoked by painful electrical stimulation.

EP studies show exceptional promise in the study of pain psychophysics in the normal volunteer. Furthermore, because the pain patient may process the perception of an applied pain in a different way from the pain-free individual (reviewed above), EP methods may provide the ideal means for quantifying this phenomenon at the level of the electrophysiological processing of pain. The work of Bromm and Scharein [80] suggests that this value lies latent.

Biochemical correlates of pain

The humoral basis of neuronal endocrine communication and intercommunication provides an observational window through which these processes may be observed.

At the level of the periphery, sampling from blood, the phenomenon of the pain state is associated with increased levels of circulating stress-related chemical mediators, including ACTH, cortisol, catecholamines, and the longer lived endorphins, including beta-endorphin and its precursor beta-lipotropin.

As recently reviewed by Noel and Nemeroff [50], beta-endorphin and several other endorphins are potent analgesic substances when centrally administered in animals. The finding that there is a proportional relationship between circulating levels of peripheral beta-endorphin and pain report, as has been described in burned children by Szyfelbein, Osgood, and Carr [86], thus implicates this moiety in the mediation of pain and the stress associated with pain. Since beta-endorphin is believed to act as a neuroendocrine mediator in the periphery, since the molecule is not known to penetrate the blood-brain barrier intact, and since it seems to act in an entirely different manner (as a neuromodulator) in the brain itself, it is unlikely that peripheral beta-endorphin is directly mediating the presumed autoanalgesic response of the "pain limb" of the pain-stress complex.

In apparent confirmation of the more general role of peripheral beta-endorphin in states not specifically painful, it has been found to increase in concentration during pregnancy and to undergo further increase during labor and parturition [87,88], with no specific correlation to the (self-reported) painfulness of these conditions [89].

We must look within the brain itself for the neurochemical correlates of pain perception, and at this level also beta-endorphin concentrations have not been found in proportional association with the pain state per se. However, lower levels of met-enkephalinlike immunoreactivity have been found in the ventricular fluid of chronic pain patients than in pain-free individuals [90].

The vast majority of CSF endorphins have not been characterized to identity, although their presence can be measured quantitatively in terms of their opiatelike effects [50,91]. It is amongst these uncharacterized endorphins that differences have been found between the pain patient and the pain-free individual. Terenius' group have found that a chromatographic region of the cerebrospinal fluid (CSF), which they term *fraction one* is present in lower concentration in the chronic pain patient with organic but not psychogenic pain [92,93]. In our own studies of this region of the chromatographically fractionated CSF, we have found that one of the components of fraction one, which we have termed *peak B* because it is the second of the many opioid fractions to elute from the system, is specifically associated with the chronic pain condition and the autoanalgesic processes of the placebo response. Peak B levels are reduced in chronic pain patients compared with normal volunteers. In those pain patients capable of engendering a placebo response, peak B levels are normalized after the patient has reported placebo-induced pain relief, but remain depressed in those patients that do not experience the autoanalgesic effect of the placebo [5]. Peak B is a potent analgesic in animals tests, and we have proposed, therefore, that it is the mediator of the autoanalgesic response engendered in the pain patient in response to the psychological cue of the placebo [94]. Peak B measurement may well prove to be useful in both clinical pain assessment and in furthering our understanding of the neurochemical processes of pain perception and its psychogenic control and modulation.

CONCLUSIONS

The aim of this review has been to bring together the established clinical methods used to assess both the self-report of pain and its externally observable signs. It has been attempted to illustrate the strengths and limitations of the methods historically used and the quite considerable advances that have been made at the cognitive-behavioral, psychophysical, physiological, and neurochemical frontiers on our understanding of these signs, and to explain how these relate to the elusive definition of "pain".

Pain research stands at a turning point in its development. Combined and concerted efforts of different scientific disciplines have been directed at the question of the biological basis of this perceptual phenomenon, and these efforts are beginning to bear fruit. Our future success in achieving a quantitative measure of the phenomenon of pain will be directly proportional to our understanding of its nature.

REFERENCES

1. Fordyce WE. 1974. Treating chronic pain by contingency management. In JJ Bonica (ed), Advances in Neurology, Vol. 4, International Symposium on Pain. New York, Raven Press, pp. 585–587.
2. Fordyce WE. 1976. Behavioral Methods for Chronic Pain and Illness. St Louis, C.V. Mosby.
3. Fordyce WE. 1979. Environmental factors in the genesis of low back pain and illness. In JJ Bonica, JE Liebskind, DG Albe-Fessard (eds), Advances in Pain Research and Therapy, Vol. 3.

4. Loeser JD. 1989. Pain relief and analgesia. In CR Chapman, Loeser JD (eds), Issues in Pain Measurement. New York, Raven Press.
5. Lipman JJ, Miller BE, Mays KS, Miller MN, North WC, Byrne WL 1990. Peak "B" endorphin concentration in cerebrospinal fluid: Reduced in chronic pain patients and increased during the placebo response. Psychopharmacology, in press.
6. Scott J, Huskisson EC. 1976. Graphic representation of pain. Pain 2(2):175–184.
7. Joyce CR, Zutish DW, Hrubes V, Mason RM. 1975. Comparison of fixed interval and visual analogue scales for rating chronic pain. Eur J Clin Pharmacol 8:415–420.
8. Downie WW, Leatham PA, Rhind VM, Wright V, Brancho JA, Anderson JA. 1978. Studies with pain rating scales. Ann Rheum Dis 37:378–381.
9. Nicholson AN. 1978. Visual analog scales and drug effects in man. Br J Pharmacol 6:3–4.
10. Stubbs DF. 1979. Visual analogue scales (letter). Br J Clin Pharmacol 7:124.
11. Melzack R, Torgerson WS. 1971. On the language of pain. Anesthesiology 34:50–59.
12. Wallenstein SL, Rogers A, Kaiko GH, Houde RW. 1980. Relative analgesic potency of oral zomepirac and intramuscular morphine in cancer patients with postoperative pain. J Clin Pharmacol 20(4 pt 2):250–258.
13. Frank AJM, Moll JMH, Hort JF. 1982. A comparison of three ways of measuring pain. Rheumatol Rehab 21:211–217.
14. Heft MW, Parker SR, 1984. An experimental basis for revising the graphic rating scale for pain. Pain. 19:153–161.
15. Chapman CR, Syrjala KL. 1989. Measurement of pain. In CR Chapman, JD Loeser (eds), Issues in Pain Measurement. New York, Raven Press. pp. 580–594.
16. Melzack R. 1975. The McGill pain questionnaire: Major properties and scoring methods. Pain 1(3):277–299.
17. Daut RL, Cleeland CS, Flannery, RC. 1983. Development of the Wisconsin Brief Pain Questionnaire to assess pain in cancer and other diseases. Pain 17:197–210.
18. Fishman B, Pasternak S, Wallenstein SL, Houde RW, Holland JC, Foley KM. 1986. The memorial pain assessment card: A valid instrument for evaluation of cancer pain (abstr). Am J Clin Oncol 5:239.
19. Reading AE. 1979. The internal structure of the McGill Pain Questionnaire in dysmenorrhea patients. Pain 7:353–358.
20. Byrne M, Troy A, Bradley LA, Marchisello PJ, Geisinger KF, Van Der Keide LH, Prieto EJ. 1982. Cross-validation of the factor structure of the McGill Pain Questionnaire. Pain 13: 193–201.
21. Reading AE, Everitt BS, Sledmere CM. 1982. The McGill pain questionnaire: A replication of its construction. Br J Clin Psychol 21:339–349.
22. Prieto EJ, Geisinger KF. 1983. Factor analytic studies of the McGill Pain Questionnaire. In R Melzack (ed), Pain Measurement and Assessment. New York, Raven Press, pp. 63–70.
23. Chapman CR, Casey KL, Dubner R, Foley KM, Gracely RH, Reading AE. 1985. Pain management: An overview. Pain 22:1–31.
24. Cleeland CS. 1985. Measurement and prevalence of pain in cancer. Semin Oncol Nurs 1: 87–92.
25. Cleeland CS, Shacham S, Dahl JL, Orrison W. 1984. CSF beta-endorphin and the severity of clinical pain. Neurology 34:378–380.
26. Cleeland CS. 1989. Measurement of pain by subjective report. In CR Chapman, JD Loeser (eds), Issues in Pain Measurement. New York, Raven Press, pp. 391–403.
27. Kerns RD, Turk DC, Rudy TE. 1985. The West Haven Yale Multidimensional Pain Inventory (WHYMPI). Pain 23:345–356.
28. Hunter M, Philips C, Rachman S. 1979. Memory for pain. Pain 6:35–46.
29. Kremer EF, Block AJ, Gaylor MS. 1980. Behavioral approaches to treatment of chronic pain: The innacuracy of patient self-report measures. Arch Phys Med Rehabil 62:188–191.
30. Sanders SH. 1983. Automated versus self-monitoring of "uptime" in chronic pain patients: A comparative study. Pain 15:399–406.
31. Budzynski TH, Stoyva JM, Adler CM, Mullaney DJ. 1973. EMG biofeedback and tension headache: A controlled outcome study. Psychosom Med 35:484–496.
32. Jensen MP, Karoly P, Braver S. 1986. The measurement of clinical pain intensity: A comparison of six methods. Pain 27:117–126.

33. Ready LB, Sarkis E, Turner JA. 1982. Self-reported vs actual use of medications in chronic pain. Pain 12:285–294.
34. Keefe FJ. 1989. Behavioral measurement of pain. In CR Chapman, JO Loeser (eds), Issues in Pain Measurement. New York, Raven Press, pp. 405–424.
35. Richards R, Nepomuceno C, Riles M, Sauer A. 1982. Assessing pain behavior: The UAB pain behavior scale. Pain 14:393–398.
36. Feuerstein M, Greenwald M, Gamache MP, Papciak AS, Cook EW. 1985. The pain behavior scale: Modification and validation for outpatient use. J Psychopathol Behav Assess 7(4): 301–315.
37. Keefe FJ, Block AR. 1982. Development of an observation method for assessing pain behavior in chronic low back pain patients. Behav Ther 13:363–375.
38. Follick MJ, Aher DK, Aberger EW. 1985. Development of an audiovisual taxonomy of pain behavior: Reliability and discriminant validity. Health Psychol 4:555–568.
39. Keefe FJ, Crisson JE, Trainor M. 1987. Observational methods for assessing pain: A practical guide. In JA Blumenthal, DC McKee (eds), Applications in Behavioral Medicine and Health Psychology. Sarasota, FL, Professional Resources Exchange, pp. 67–94.
40. Cinciripini PM, Floreen A. 1982. An evaluation of a behavioral program for chronic pain. J Behav Med 5:375–389.
41. Linton SJ. 1985. The relationship between activity and chronic pain. Pain 21:289–294.
42. Keefe FJ, Hill RW. 1985. An objective approach to qualifying pain behavior and gait patterns in low back patients. Pain 21:153–161.
43. Follick MJ, Ahern DK, Laser-Wolston N, Adams AA, Moloy AJ. 1985. Chronic pain: Electromechanical recording devices for measuring patients' activity patterns. Arch Phys Med Rehab 66:75–89.
44. Tryon WW. 1985. Measurement of human activity. In WW Tryon (ed), Behavioral Assessment in Behavioral Medicine. New York, Springer, pp. 200–256.
45. Morrell EM, Keefe FJ. 1988. The actometer: An evaluation of instrument applicability for chronic pain patients. Pain 52:265–270.
46. Ekman P, Frieson WV. 1978. Manual for the Facial Action Coding System. Palo Alto, CA, Consulting Psychologists Press.
47. Craig KD, Prkachim KM. 1983. Nonverbal measures of pain, In R Melzack (ed), Pain Measurement and Assessment. New York, Raven Press.
48. LeResch L, Dworkin SF. 1984. Facial expression accompanying pain. Soc Sci Med 19(12): 1325–1330.
49. Bromm B. 1989. Laboratory animal and human volunteer in the assessment of analgesic efficacy. In CR Chapman, JD Loeser (eds), Issues in Pain Measurement. New York, Raven Press, pp. 117–143.
50. Noel MA, Nemeroff CB. 1988. Endogenous opiates in chronic pain, In RD France, KR Krishnan (eds), Chronic Pain. Washington, D.C., A.P.A. Press, pp. 55–65.
51. Stimell B. 1983. Neuroregulators and pain. In Pain, Analgesia and Addiction — the Pharmacological Treatment of Pain. New York, Raven Press, pp. 18–38.
52. Lipman JJ, Blumenkopf B. 1990. Comparison of subjective and objective analgesic effects of intravenous and intrathecal morphine in chronic pain patients by heat beam dolorimetry. Pain 39(3):249–256.
53. Graves DA, Foster TS, Batenhorst RL, Bennett RL, Baumann TJ. 1983. Patient-controlled analgesia. Ann Intern Med 99:360–366.
54. White P. 1985. Patient controlled analgesia: A new approach to the management of post operative pain. Semin Anesthesia IV 3:255–266.
55. Gracely RH. 1989. Pain psychophysics. In CR Chapman, JD Loeser (eds), Issues in Pain Measurement. New York, Raven Press, pp. 211–229.
56. Fechner GT. 1860. Elemente der psychophysic. Reprinted In DH Howes, EC Boring (eds), HE Adler (translator), Elements of Psychophysics. Holt Rinehart and Winston.
57. Stephens SS. 1975. Psychophysics: Introduction to its Perceptual Neural and Social Prospects. New York, Wiley.
58. Brown AD, Beeler WJ, Kloka AC, Fields RW. 1985. Spatial summation of prepain and pain in human teeth. Pain 21:1–16.
59. Wolff BB. 1971. Factor analysis of human pain responses: Pain endurance as a specific pain factor. J Abnorm Psychol 78:292–298.

60. Hardy JD, Wolf HG, Goodell H. 1952. Pain sensations and reactions. Baltimore, Williams & Wilkins.
61. Mersky H, Evans PR. 1975. Variations in pain complaint threshold in psychiatric and neurological patients with pain. Pain 1:73–79.
62. Chery-Croze S. 1983. Relationship between noxious cold stimuli and the magnitude of pain sensation in man. Pain 15:265–269.
63. Malow RM, Olson RE. 1980. Changes in pain perception after treatment for chronic pain. Pain 11:65–72.
64. Smith GM, Egbert LD, Markowitz RA, Mosteller F, Beecher HK. 1966. An experimental pain method sensitive to morphine in man: The submaximum effort torniquet technique. J Pharmacol Exp Ther 154:324–332.
65. Lipman JJ, Blumenkopf B, Parris WCV. 1987. Chronic pain assessment using heat beam dolorimetry. Pain 31:59–67.
66. Naliboff BD, Cohen MJ. 1989. Psychophysical laboratory methods applied to clinical pain patients. In CR Chapman, JD Loeser (eds), Issues in Pain Measurement. New York, Raven Press, pp. 365–386.
67. Beecher HK. 1959. Measurement of subjective responses: Quantitative effects of drugs. New York, Oxford University Press.
68. Rollman GB. 1979. Signal detection theory pain measures: Empiricle validation studies and adaptation-level effects. Pain 6:9–12.
69. Chapman CR. 1983. On the relationship of human laboratory and clinical pain research. In R Melzack (ed), Pain Measurement and Assessment. New York, Raven Press, pp. 243–249.
70. Rollman GB. 1983. Measurement of experimental pain in chronic pain patients: Methodological and individual factors. In R Melzack (ed), Pain Measurement and Assessment. New York, Raven Press, pp. 251–257.
71. Chapman LF, Dingman HF, Ginzberg SP. 1965. Failure of systemic analgesics to alter the absolute sensory threshold for the simple detection of pain. Brain 88:1011–1022.
72. Naifeh KH, Heller PH, Perry F, Gordon NC, Levine JD. 1983. Electrodermal responsivity associated with clinical pain. Pain 16:277–283.
73. Lipman JJ, Spencer PSJ. 1980. A comparison of muscarinic cholinergic involvement in the antinociceptive effects of morphine and clonidine in the mouse. Eur J Pharmacol 64:249–258.
74. Paalzow G, Paalzow L. 1976. Clonidine antinociceptive activity: Effects of drugs influencing central monaminergic and cholinergic mechanisms in the rat. Naunyn Schmeidebergs. Arch Pharmacol 292:19–126.
75. Willer JC. 1977. Comparative study of percieved pain and nociceptive flexion reflex in man. Pain 3:69–80.
76. Willer JC. 1984. Nociceptive flexion reflex as a physiological correlate of pain sensation in humans. In B Bromm (ed), Pain Measurement in Man, Neurophysiological Correlates of Pain. Amsterdam, Elsevier, pp. 87–110.
77. DeBroucker T, Willer JC, Bergeret S. 1989. The nociceptive flexion reflex in humans: A specific and objective correlate of experimental pain. In CR Chapman, JD Loeser (eds), Issues in Pain Management. New York, Raven Press, pp. 337–352.
78. Lipman JJ. 1988. The electroencephalogram as a tool for assaying neurotoxicity. Meth Enzymol 165:270–277.
79. Herrmann WM. 1982. (ed). Electroencephalography in Drug Research. Stuttgart, Gustav Fischer.
80. Bromm B, Scharein E. 1982. Principal component analysis of pain related cerebral potentials to mechanical and electrical stimulation in man. Electroenceph Clin Neurophysiol 53:94–103.
81. Bourne JR, Hamel B, Giesg D, Woyce G, Lawrence PL, Ward JW, Teschan PE. 1980. The EEG analysis system of the national cooperative dialysis study. IEEE Trans Biomed Eng 27(11):656–664.
82. Lipman JJ, Lawrence PL, DeBoer D, Shoemaker MO, Sulser D, Tolchard S, Teschan PE. 1990. The role of dialysable solutes in the mediation of uremic encephalopathy in the rat. Kidney Int, in press.
83. Chapman Cr, Jacobson RC. 1984. Assessment of analgesic states: Can evoked potentials play a role? In B Bromm (ed), Pain Measurement in Man. Amsterdam, Elsevier, pp. 233–255.
84. Wright A, Davis II. 1989. A recording of brain evoked potentials resulting from intra articular

focussed ultrasonic stimulation: A new experimental model for investigating joint pain in humans. Neurosci Lett 97(1–2):145–150.

85. Kakigi R, Shibasaki H, Ikeda A. 1989. Pain related somatosensory evoked potentials following CO_2 laser stimulation in man. Electroencephalogr Clin Neurophysiol 74(2):139–146.
86. Szyfelbein SK, Osgood PF, Carr DB. 1985. The assessment of pain and plasma beta endorphin immunoreactivity in burned children. Pain 22(2):173–182.
87. Thomas TA, Fletcher JE, Hill RG. 1982. Influence of medication, pain and progress in labour on plasma beta-endorphin-like immunoreactivity. Br J Anaesthesiol 54:401–408.
88. Pilkington JW, Nemeroff CB, Mason GA, Prange AR Jr. 1983. Increase in plasma beta-endorphin-like immunoreactivity during parturition in normal women. Am J Obstet Gynecol 145:111–113.
89. Cahil CA, Akil H. 1982. Plasma beta endorphin-like immunoreactivity, self-reported pain perception and anxiety levels in women during pregnancy and labor. Life Sci 32:1879–1882.
90. Akil H, Watson SJ, Sullivan S, et al. 1978. Enkephalin-like material in normal human CSF: Measurement and levels. Life Sci 23:121–126.
91. Miller BE, Lipman JJ, Byrne WL. 1987. Partial characterization of a novel endogenous opioid in human cerebrospinal fluid. Life Sci 41:2535–2545.
92. Terenius L, Wahlstrom A. 1975. Morphine-like ligands for opiate receptors in human CSF. Life Sci 16:1759–1764.
93. Terenius L, Wahlstrom A, Johansson L. 1979. Endorphins in human cerebrospinal fluid and their measurement. In E Usidin, WE Bunney, N Kline (eds), Endorphins in Mental Health Research. New York, Oxford University Press.

10. SELECTIVE TISSUE CONDUCTANCE IN THE ASSESSMENT OF SYMPATHETICALLY MEDIATED PAIN

DAVID R. LONGMIRE AND WINSTON C.V. PARRIS

During the past decade there has been a significant renewal of interest in the role of the sympathetic nervous system as it relates to the mediation or modulation of pain [1–7]. Evidence to support this observation may be found in the increasing numbers of published reports and presentations to scientific societies regarding basic and clinical aspects of sympathetically maintained pain (SMP). The devastating features of SMP syndromes, including reflex sympathetic dystrophy (RSD), algodystrophy, allodynia, and other forms of the causalgia/hyperpathia complex, were described clinically in detail in the last century [8,9]. However, it is only recently that certain components of the complex pathophysiological process that creates SMP have been elaborated [10–13]. This apparent trend toward systematic, controlled research of the sympathetic nervous system and pain may represent, to the SMP sufferer, a future hope for relief from such debilitating symptoms.

Although the development of effective methods for treating SMP may be in progress, practicing physicians continue to be faced with the problem of differentiating this condition from other pain syndromes. Few test procedures by which the diagnosis of painful sympathetic dysfunction can be confirmed have ever existed, and many of these (e.g., Minor's test [14], starch-iodine application [15], or the quinizarin test [16]) are no longer used because of inconvenience or time requirements. Other, more modern tests, (e.g., infrared telethermography), although valuable, may not be readily available to many primary care physicians who treat SMP patients.

One alternative method for assessing sympathetic dysfunction in general, and SMP specifically, has been the electrophysiological evaluation of the post-ganglionic efferent nerve supply to the skin. The anatomical and physiological mechanisms by which regional changes in skin electrical activity occur in SMP are felt to be analogous to those that create local abnormalities in skin hidrosis, texture, color, hair loss, and temperature [17–19]. The neural events that may represent the common substrate for local skin conductance changes and the "vicious circle" of SMP [20] may include the following phenomena.

Local trauma or other inflammatory processes, however mild, may induce structural and chemical changes in neural tissue that affect the membrane integrity of sensory receptors and free nerve endings alike [21,22]. The hyper-excitability of nerve fibers thus created, and the resultant increase in afferent pathway activity [23,24], may indeed kindle secondary and tertiary neurons in the dorsal horn of the spinal cord grey matter. The substantia gelatinosa, from which any of several neural loops may be recruited, is particularly sensitive to this effect [25,26]. Regardless of how simple or complex such circuits may be, the pain-evoked firing patterns created therein eventually evoke post synaptic potential changes in preganglionic neurons within the spinal cord. These cells, located almost entirely in the intermediolateral fasciculus, have processes that exit the cord to terminate in the respective chain ganglion appropriate for each spinal level [27]. The terminal activity of the preganglionic fibers creates post-synaptic excitation or inhibition at the postganglionic cells, which, when activated, transmit impulses in an orderly, relatively limited fashion to sweat glands in a specific region of the skin [28]. Local changes in effector membrane function, regardless of the presence or absence of clinically detectable sweating [29], can then be detected as regional changes in skin electrical conductivity. Since skin conductance levels seem to be independent of cutaneous blood flow [30], the quantitative assessment of each component may provide compli-mentary data regarding separate disturbances of sudomotor and vasomotor sympathetic pathways, respectively, in different pain syndromes.

Various aspects of SMP have been studied for over 100 years, but only re-cently has the application of a new form of conductivity measurement to the study of pain been initiated. The following sections are presented as an intro-duction to the historical foundations, current research status, and future clini-cal potential of this interesting method, known as selective tissue conductance (STC) technology.

HISTORICAL PERSPECTIVES

Much of what is currently known about the physiological basis of pain has been founded on early studies of electrical currents produced by nervous tissue in response to noxious stimuli. This type of neurophysiological research was established during the middle decades of the 19th century only after the de-velopment of instruments that were sensitive enough to record the electrical activity of nerve and muscle tissues [31,32]. The excitement generated by these measurement methods was so great that by the 1860s a new field of investigation, electrophysiology, was formally established in Europe [33].

Unfortunately, the relatively rapid growth of this field had been based only on the study of so-called "active" components of electricity, i.e., voltage and current. For nearly a century, very little attention was paid to studies of any other electrical properties of tissue or membrane, such as resistance, impedance, or conductance, until electrophysiology was redefined to include such "passive" components [34]. The works of those investigators who chose to explore the neglected pathways of clinical neurophysiology by studying passive, rather than active, electrical phenomena have formed the basis of STC mapping.

Some of the earliest observations on the effects of electrical stimulation on central, peripheral, and sympathetic portions of the nervous system were made in the mid-1800s by Dunglison et al. [35]. These physicians applied Faradic, alternating currents (AC) or Galvanic, direct currents (DC) to many body parts in order to treat a wide range of painful disorders [36]. When reports of successful response to "electrization" treatments were disseminated, many physicians began to incorporate Galvanic or Faradic stimulation techniques in their clinical practices. As this form of therapy became more widespread, many clinicians began to report the results of their confirmatory research [37,38]. It was during this period that the resistance of the intact skin to electrical stimulation was described by Duchenne du Boulogne, who noted that various improvements in the clinical response to "electro-Galvanismus" could be obtained by inducing skin "blisters" at stimulation sites. This method of disrupting the epidermis lowered the skin resistance considerably, thereby increasing the amount of current available for use in the electrical treatment [39].

Although it was soon understood that the skin could oppose electrical current flow differently in various types of illness and death [40], it was not until 1879 that local changes in skin resistance were demonstrated in certain forms of peripheral nerve dysfunction. Credit for the first published report of this phenomenon belongs to Vigouroux, who noted regional increases in skin resistance in several patients with peripheral nerve lesions. He described such elevated values as occurring in the cutaneous territories of the affected nerves, but not over skin regions with normal innervation. However, Vigouroux confirmed that this effect had been recognized earlier by other researchers, whose unpublished observations he acknowledged in his own report [41].

One contemporary of Vigouroux was Féré, whose interest in relating mental disorders to nervous system dysfunction perhaps reflected more the wishes of his mentor, Charcot, than his own [42,43]. He discovered, by methods that remain unclear, that the resistance measurement techniques used clinically by Vigouroux could be applied to the study of patterns of sweating induced by emotional or sensory stimuli [44,45]. Féré's research soon received much attention and was subsequently supported by Tarchanoff's report of similar changes in the electrical skin potential [46]. Later, Veraguth [47] demonstrated that sensory and emotionally intense stimuli evoked, within a few seconds, a transient reduction in skin resistance *and* an increase in skin potential. It was he who first coined the phrase *psycho-Galvanic reflex* (PGR) and established a new focus of study in psychological research.

The need for an instrumental method to investigate the interactions of mind and brain soon appeared to be fulfilled by the PGR technique. Research activity in PGR grew rapidly, but without any attempts at standardization of instrumentation, terminology, technique, or interpretation. Eventually the term *psycho-Galvanic reflex* was replaced by the more general title of *Galvanic skin response* (GSR). This term is currently used to signify one or more of the following components of electrodermal activity that can be measured: 1) as a resting or basal value (skin resistance, conductance, or potential *level*) or 2) in response to sensory or emotional stimulation (skin resistance, conductance, or potential *response*). Although the term *GSR* is widely known, use of the appropriate name of the specific component being studied is encouraged [48,49]. Despite the individual differences in electrical characteristics measured for each component, all techniques involve the application of electrodes to the skin surface. These are used to detect changes in electrodermal activity through connections with specific instrumentation that can amplify, record, or display the results. Beyond these basic similarities, however, consistency of method was rare during the early development of GSR recording. In addition, studies of the underlying physiological mechanisms of GSR, or those relating GSR changes to neuropathological conditions, were nearly nonexistent before 1920. This situation soon changed as a result of the following clinical case report and the subsequent research interest that it evoked.

In 1924, Richter [50] reported on the effects of a structural lesion of the sympathetic chain on the evoked GSR. Remaining true to the classical "scientific method" of that era, Richter began his systematic study of these effects with the process of basic observation. He noted, in a single patient with a traumatic lesion of the cervical sympathetic chain, a marked difference in sweating between symptomatic and asymptomatic sides of the face, neck, upper chest, arms, and hands. With reference to the upper limbs of this patient, he attempted to obtain some objective measurement of this pathological state by using contemporary GSR methods and instrumentation. His detailed recordings of phasic resistance changes occurring at rest and after sensory stimulation revealed a loss of the expected GSR of the hand ipsilateral to the lesion. Responses recorded from the asymptomatic arm and hand remained consistent with those of normal controls [51]. These provocative findings soon led him to study other lesions, and shortly thereafter he abandoned the recording of evoked GSR to develop more clinically applicable techniques for measuring the passive, basal levels of skin resistance [52,53]. For more than 75 years, Richter applied this technique to hundreds of patients with pathological or surgical lesions of the sympathetic chain [54–56], peripheral nerves [57,58], and spinal cord [59]. Even today, this research remains the definitive work on the electrophysiological mapping of the sympathetic nervous control of the skin.

Richter's work always compared resistance levels before treatment (e.g., surgical sympathectomy) with those measured at several post-treatment intervals. Thus he was able to reveal the natural temporal course of the resistance effect associated with each treatment method. He also described pertinent symptoms and signs of sympathectomy patients and related regional skin resistance changes to the success of treatment. In several patients whose pretreatment symptoms included pain, Richter noted that the resistance of the skin was significantly decreased over the symptomatic regions [60,61]. Following surgical sympathectomy, however, the skin resistance in the territory of the sectioned ganglia or rami rose significantly. Nevertheless, certain patients whose original symptoms recurred weeks or months after the surgery were retested by Richter, who demonstrated that the resistance had returned to levels at, or less than, those measured preoperatively. A potential relationship between decreased skin resistance and the success or failure of surgical sympathectomy to provide long-term pain control was thus suggested, albeit indirectly, by Richter's early research.

It was not until 1949 that a clear-cut hypothesis relating regional skin electrical resistance to clinical pain was formulated by Van Metre [62], who found that the pain produced by marked sinusitis was accompanied by decreased resistance over symptomatic regions, but only rarely over asymptomatic sites. Several decades later, Riley and Richter [63] confirmed the existence of pain-related skin resistance changes by demonstrating that resistance levels were reduced over painful regions in patients with cervical musculoskeletal and nerve root injuries. In contrast, resistance levels were normal or increased over asymptomatic regions in the same patients.

Unfortunately the early instrumentation [64] and measurement methods [65,66] developed by Richter and his colleagues never gained widespread popularity, despite subsequent confirmation of his findings in peripheral nerve lesions [67,68]. Even after the U.S. War Department approved his design of the clinical dermohmeter for use in the diagnosis of peripheral and autonomic nerve injuries caused by missile wounds [69], use of the skin resistance method waned. However, the importance of his work did not go unnoticed by several renowned neuroscientists, including Jasper [70], Denny-Brown [71], and Gibbs [72], each of whom encouraged his students to consider research in the electrodermal evaluation of the sympathetic nervous system. Regardless of such support, the time and effort required to perform such testing, as well as the rapid growth of interest in other areas of neurophysiology, temporarily reduced both clinical and investigative use of this technique. Despite his advancing age and declining health, Richter continued to maintain a genuine interest in this aspect of his broad career in neurobiology [73], even until shortly before his death at the age of 94 [74].

Fortunately, a resurgence of interest in the measurement of pain–related electrodermal activity appears to have taken place early in the past decade. For example, in 1983 Naifeh et al. [75] attempted to determine possible relationships between abnormalities in electrodermal responses evoked in the distal extremities by sensory stimuli in subjects with clinical pain and in pain-free control subjects. Their equivocal results are perhaps explained on the grounds that those investigators made their electrodermal measurements over standard distal extremity sites, and not over the subjects' clinically painful regions. In 1984, Frexai-Baque et al. [76] reviewed the relationship between asymmetry of skin electrical changes and several conditions, including certain unilaterally painful syndromes. In the same year, Shahani et al. [77] developed a method for evoking the sympathetic skin response (SSR) in order to evaluate C-fiber conduction and dysfunction. Direct applications of the SSR to the study of clinical pain have not been widely published, but Green et al. [78] have related skin response abnormalities to those found on infrared thermography. Further, the use of a different electrodermal method to study pain reduction by sympatholytic blockade had been demonstrated successfully by Lofstrom et al. [79] in 1984. More recently, Katz et al. [80] have presented a case report in which they described significant correlation between stump skin conductance and paresthesias in a patient with unilateral lower extremity pain and phantom phenomena following amputation. With the introduction of the selective tissue conductance method, described in detail in the following section, it is hoped that many more reports of pain-related electrodermal phenomena will be forthcoming.

SELECTIVE TISSUE CONDUCTANCE MAPPING

The development of this new electrodermal technology was based on the historical reports described above, as well as on unpublished observations made by Longmire and Woodley. In 1962, Longmire, while attempting to record the clinical electroencephalogram (EEG) of a patient with unilateral hypesthesia, observed a significant increase in electrode/scalp resistance over the symptomatic hemicranium. In order to improve electrical contact with the skin, the scalp was abraded with a sterilized, blunted needle. This "skin drilling" technique, formerly developed by Shackel [81], was used on at least two occasions, with only a minimal decrease in the scalp resistance. This preliminary observations, regarding a potential relationship between increased skin resistance and reduced sensation, was consistent with those reports described in the preceding section. Subsequently, while collecting data for a technical study on EEG [82], Longmire observed an opposite effect in patients with unilateral migraine. During, or shortly after, migraine attacks the DC resistance of EEG electrodes applied to the scalp seemed to be less over the symptomatic hemicranium. This effect represented a contaminating factor for the specific purpose of that technical study, therefore any data obtained from migraine patients, although interesting, were excluded from the final published report.

Shortly thereafter, however, Longmire [83] undertook a study of the resistance of extracerebral tissues, which indicated the need for improved measurement methods. An extensive review of the literature on existing GSR methods indicated certain technical problems by which studies of pain-related skin resistance changes could be contaminated or otherwise made ineffective. The first problem was that resistance measurements provided an inversely, not directly, related method for monitoring the sympathetic efferent supply to the skin. The existing literature on GSR suggested that conductance, not resistance, represented a more physiological measurement of autonomic outflow functions [84,85]. The second problem involved the use of referential or "monopolar" methods on which most skin resistance testing had been based. This involved the application of a single electrode to a "neutral" site on the body, at some distance from the skin regions where the measurements would be made. A DC electrical source, varying in electromotive force from 9 to 22.5 V, would be wired in series with an ammeter of appropriate sensitivity, but the circuit would only be completed when a roving, or exploring, electrode was applied. This meant that the test current was permitted to flow between two separate sites on the body surface, by volume conduction, with the potential risk of excitation of electrically sensitive tissue, i.e., the conduction system of the heart. In addition, the placement of the exploring electrode at a distance from the neutral reference would result in a summation of the specific resistances of all body tissues interposed between the electrodes, producing false measurements.

The third problem, or source of error, suggested by earlier reports was related to the iontophoretic effect [86]. This phenomenon occurs when the application of a continuous DC current to living tissue results in progressive functional breakdown of the resting electrochemical gradient existing across cell membranes. Specifically, resistance to the current decreases over time. This membrane breakdown created by the iontophoretic effect has been applied successfully by forcing charged molecules of certain topical medications into the skin and subcutaneous tissue with external electrical currents [87]. However, the exponential increase in conductance caused by iontophoresis makes it undesirable in attempting to evaluate stable electrodermal levels.

With these three problems under consideration, Longmire and Woodley began a series of experiments, the primary goal of which was to create an electrophysiological technology that could be applied safely and without artifactual contamination, to the assessment of sympathetic outflow dysfunction and pain. By 1981 they had developed methods and instrumentation in a manner that avoided the technical problems described above, as follows: They bypassed the first problem by using only *conductance*, not resistance, levels. They then overcame the second problem, i.e., transcorporeal currents, by utilizing either of two types of bipolar, concentric surface electrodes, which limited the application of the test current to superficial skin (Figure 10-1).

The smooth surface of the type I electrode was found to be most appropriate

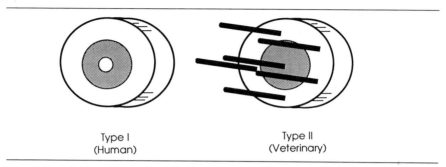

Type I
(Human)

Type II
(Veterinary)

Figure 10-1. STC electrode types.

for hairless skin, whereas the multipoint type II electrode allowed measurement of the conductance of hairy skin along insulated, small-diameter probes that passed between the individual hair shafts. Theif approach to the third problem, i.e., the iontophoretic effect, was to make brief measurements (<500 ms) only, and thereby avoid prolonged application of DC test currents. They also included numeric displays to permit quantification of each measurement. This new methodology was named *selective tissue conductance mapping* because of the ease with which the operator could make multiple measurements along different axes in order to "map" any field of interest. The electrophysiological changes thus measured, therefore, were operationally defined in 1987, as follows:

Selective Tissue Conductance (STC) is the relative ability of biological tissue to conduct a weak (DC) electrical signal which is applied, for a *selected* period of time to a *selected*, limited and restricted surface area of that tissue.[88]

INSTRUMENTATION AND TECHNIQUE

Selective tissue conductance devices currently in use in human and animal pain research consist of a battery-powered digital meter to which either a type I or type II concentric electrode is connected. Control switches are provided to select different sensitivity settings, which are used to compensate for interindividual or inter region variations in STC level. An audio circuit permits the presentation of each STC count as a clicking sound, and a liquid crystal numeric readout device displays the test result obtained for each measurement. Individual measurements are made by placing the concentric electrode against the skin until the result appears on the display. The values obtained may be recorded on a standardized form for statistical analysis, or on a body map in situations where the spatial distribution of the data is important.

For research purposes, measurements may be made at predetermined sites, preferably selected on the basis of anatomical landmarks. For clinical applications, more systematic examination guidelines must be followed to improve test–retest reliability. In current practice, STC assessment procedures may be performed using any of the following stages of complexity.

Stage I (linear gradient) STC tests consist of a sequence of several measurements, made along a predetermined parasagittal or transverse line connecting two anatomical landmarks (Figure 10-2). This method is particularly useful in detecting the presence of STC asymmetries or border zones of hyperhydrosis in reflex sympathetic dystrophy. When Stage I data are collected at several pretreatment or posttreatment intervals, the linear gradient plots may be stacked to allow visual analysis of spatial and temporal changes.

Stage II tests, also known as peak/perimeter determinations (PPD), incorporate the linear gradient technique, but do this relative to a zone of markedly decreased or increased STC counts. This method has been applied mostly to studies in which the borders of painful or hyperesthetic zones may need to be compared with the surrounding normal tissue.

Stage III, computer contour mapping (CCM), incorporates multidirectional LG data and provides a graphic display of overlapping (Stage II) polygons that represent the fields surrounding a focus of abnormal STC activity [89].

PRELIMINARY INVESTIGATIONS

STC measurements were first made on normal control volunteers by Longmire and Woodley in 1981. In those preliminary, unpublished studies, it became evident that certain somatic regions (e.g., palms, soles, axillae) were associated with elevated STC levels, corresponding to the expected zones of heightened activity or increased number of functional sweat glands [90,91]. However,

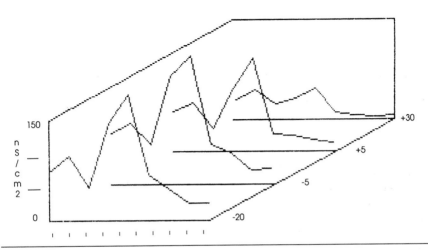

Figure 10-2. Linear gradient STC levels before (−20, −5 minutes) and after (+5, +30 minutes) stellate ganglion blockade.

almost all other areas of skin over the trunk or proximal limbs did not demonstrate an increased STC level. Exceptions to this observation included volunteers who had previously sustained painful but otherwise minor injuries that did not disrupt the epidermis. The values over asymptomatic sites varied between 1 and 3 nanoSiemens per square centimeter of skin surface (nS/cm²), as compared with the painful areas that were associated with levels between 17 and 129 nS/cm².

In 1982, the STC method was first applied investigatively to the assessment of sympathetically mediated pain. On that occasion, an adult male patient had been referred for evaluation of intractable thoracic pain that began shortly after undergoing neurolytic celiac plexus blockade with phenol for recurrent pancreatic pain. The new pain, which was severe and burning in character, occurred in a triangular distribution, the apex of which matched the injection site and the base of which was vertically aligned with and limited by the paravertebral fascia. In the region of intense superficial pain, STC values were in excess of 440 nS/cm². In regions of the original (preneurolytic) abdominal pain, levels between 38 and 46 nS/cm² were noted, whereas over asymptomatic zones all STC values were 5 nS/cm². The results of STC testing were found to be of value in establishing the etiology for the new pain as an early reflex sympathetic dystrophic effect, probably due to tracking of the phenol from the injection site along subcutaneous layers.

Following the HHS/FDA classification of the Epi-Scan STC meter as a regulatory Class II device, clinical studies were initiated in canine, equine, and human subjects. However, it was not until 1989 that the first blinded, controlled trials were performed by Parris et al. [92], who demonstrated significant changes in STC levels following unilateral stellate ganglion blockade. These authors observed that STC values were reduced unilaterally over the face, neck, chest, and hand on the side of successful blockade. They also noted a paradoxical increase in STC levels contralateral to the blocked side. Further studies of STC changes following stellate ganglion blockade using Stage I (linear gradient) and Stage III (computer contour mapping) methods by Longmire et al. [93] revealed the existence of STC dipole shifts. Those preliminary findings suggested that changes in stellate ganglion function in health and disease may be monitored using STC methods.

Subsequently, a case-control study was performed by Longmire and Woodley [94] on STC changes in patients with neck and shoulder pain and an equal group of age-and sex-matched asymptomatic control subjects. Their results indicated that STC levels are increased over painful regions, but not over pain-free sites. Only rarely were levels elevated in the asymptomatic control subjects. The data suggested that STC evaluation may also be helpful in delineating sympathetic abnormalities in clinical pain syndromes.

FUTURE APPLICATIONS TO CLINICAL PAIN RESEARCH

The preceding sections have demonstrated that an interest in the passive electrical characteristics (i.e., resistance or conductance) of tissue has existed for over a century. During the intervening years, and despite many technical difficulties, neurophysiologists have studied these electrodermal phenomena until finally their collective role as an electrophysiological expression of sympathetic nervous function is acceptable and reproducible. With the recent growth of research in sympathetically mediated pain, methods such as selective tissue conductance mapping may provide a quantifiable way by which to study SMP mechanisms, as well as many other clinical pain syndromes.

In animal research, the noninvasive nature of the veterinary STC technique may allay the fears of those who are concerned with the fair and humane treatment of nonhuman subjects. The application of STC testing of performance animals in the field is currently under study, with promising results in equine subjects. The clinical use of STC in veterinary medicine is undergoing rapid growth, but with better pathological correlation in canine patients than in felines.

In human subjects, the application of STC to monitoring the treatment outcome of neurolytic blockade has been described earlier in this chapter. Other forms of STC evaluation of medications using pre-treatment and post-treatment testing have been shown, in preliminary, unpublished studies, to be of potential clinical benefit. Similarly, comparison of STC levels before and after nonpharmacologic treatment, e.g., transcutaneous electrical nerve stimulation (TENS), may help to quantify treatment success.

The potential diagnostic value, once confirmed through appropriately blinded and controlled studies, may well be limited to detecting regional STC abnormalities with topographic distributions that suggest correlation with the patients' pain sites. If preliminary observations are substantiated scientifically, the potential benefit of correlating objective STC data to patients' subjective pain reports could be very useful in clinical pain assessment. However, if the future of STC mapping only provides the pain practitioner with a device that demonstrates results sufficient to suggest that an atypical pain complaint may deserve further investigation, then the application of this technology to pain medicine will have been worthwhile.

REFERENCES

1. Tasker RR, Organ LW, Hawrylyshin P. 1980. Deafferentation and causalgia. In JJ Bonica (ed), Pain. New York, Raven Press, pp. 305–329.
2. Kozin F, Ryan L, Carrera GF, 1981. The reflex sympathetic dystrophy syndrome (RSDS). Am J Med 70:23–30.
3. Payne R. 1986. Neuropathic pain syndromes, with special reference to causalgia and reflex sympathetic dystrophy. Clin J Pain 2:59–73.
4. Roberts WJ. 1986. A hypothesis on the physiological basis for causalgia and related pains. Pain 24:297–311.
5. Schwartzman RJ, McLellan TL. 1987. Reflex sympathetic dystrophy: A review. Arch Neurol 44:555–561.
6. Procacci P, Maresca M. 1987. Reflex sympathetic dystrophies and algodystrophies: Historical and pathogenic considerations. Pain 31:137–146.
7. Hendler N. 1989. Reflex sympathetic dystrophy and causalgia. In CD Tollison (ed), Handbook of Chronic Pain Management. Baltimore, Williams & Wilkins.

8. Mitchell SW, Morehouse GR, Keen WW. 1864. Gunshot wounds and other injuries of nerves. New York, J.B. Lippincott.
9. Mitchell SW. 1872. Injuries to Nerves and their Consequences. Philadelphia, J.B. Lippincott.
10. Emmers R. 1980. Pain: A spike-interval coded message in the brain. New York, Raven Press.
11. Devor M. 1983. Nerve pathophysiology and mechanisms of pain in causalgia. J Auton Nerv Syst 7:371–384.
12. Roberts WJ, Fogelsong ME. 1988. Spinal recordings suggest that wide-dynamic-range neurons mediate sympathetically maintained pain. Pain 34:289–304.
13. Roberts WJ, Fogelsong ME. 1988. Identification of afferents contributing to sympathetically evoked activity in wide-dynamic range neurons. Pain 34:305–314.
14. Minor L. 1923. Uber erhoten elektrischen hautwiderstand bei traumatischen affektionen des hals sympathias. Z ges Neurol Psychiat 85:482–507.
15. Wada M, Arai T, Takagaki T, Nakagawa T. 1952. Axon reflex mechanism in sweat response to nicotine, acetylcholine and sodium chloride. J Appl Physiol 4:745.
16. Guttmann L. 1941. A demonstration of the study of sweat secretion by the quinizarin method. Proc R Soc Med 35:77–78.
17. De Takats G. 1937. Reflex dystrophy of the extremities. Arch Surg 35:939–956.
18. Livingston WK. 1938. Post-traumatic pain syndromes. West J Surg Obstet Gynecol 46: 426–434.
19. Lewis T. 1942. Pain. New York, Macmillan.
20. Livingston WK. 1943. Pain Mechanisms. New York, Macmillan.
21. Tower SS. 1943. Pain: Definition and properties of the unit for sensory reception. In HG Wolff (ed), Pain: Proc ARNMD. Baltimore, Williams & Wilkins, pp. 16–43.
22. Seyffarth H. 1969. Tissue injury and local anesthetic. In S, Locke Modern Neurology. Boston, Little Brown, pp. 599–605.
23. Gasser HS. 1943. Pain-producing impulses in peripheral nerves. In HG Wolff (ed), Pain: Proc. ARNMD. Baltimore, Williams & Wilkins, pp. 44–62.
24. Perl ER. 1968. Myelinated afferent fibers innervating the primate skin and their response to noxious stimuli. J Physiol (London) 197:593–615.
25. Devor M, Wall PD. 1978. Reorganization of spinal cord sensory map after peripheral nerve injury. Nature 275:75–76.
26. Wall PD, Devor M. 1981. The effect of peripheral nerve injury on dorsal root potentials and on transmission of afferent signals into the spinal cord. Brain Res 209:95–111.
27. Brodal A. 1981. Neurological Anatomy in Relation to Clinical Medicine, 3rd ed. New York, Oxford University Press.
28. Crosby EC, Humphrey T, Lauer E. 1962. Correlative Anatomy of the Nervous System. New York, Macmillan.
29. Thomas PE, Korr IM. 1957. Relationship between sweat gland activity and electrical resistance of the skin. J Appl Physiol 10:505–510.
30. Prout BJ. 1967. Independence of the galvanic skin reflex from the vasoconstrictor reflex in man. J Neurol Neurosurg Psychiat 30:319.
31. Biedermann W. 1898. Electro-Physiology. London, Macmillan.
32. Brazier MAB. 1951. The Electrical Activity of the Nervous System. London, Pitman.
33. DuBois-Reymond EH. 1848–1849. Untersuchungen uber Tierische Elektricitat. Berlin, Reimer. 2 vol.
34. Walter WG. 1950. Introduction. In D Hill, G Parr, Electroencephalography: A Symposium on its Various Aspects. London, Macdonald, pp. 10–24.
35. Dunglison R. 1851. New Remedies with Formulae for their Administration. Philadelphia, Blanchard and Lea, pp. 392–399.
36. Beard GM, Rockwell AD. 1871. A practical treatise on the medical and surgical uses of electricity including localized and general electrization. New York, William Wood & Co.
37. Matteucci M. 1845. [Electro-Magnetismus]. Med Chirurg Rev.
38. Pereira S. 1842. Elements of Materia Medica. London, p. 42.
39. Duchenne du Boulogne M. 1850. Mémoire sur la galvanisation localisée. Arch Gen de Medecine pp. 257, 420.
40. Beard GM, Rockwell AD. 1867. The medical use of electricity. Trans NY State Med Soc.
41. Vigouroux R. 1879. Sur le role de la résistance électrique des tissus dans l'électrodiagnostic. C R Séance Soc Biol 31:336–339.

42. Goetz C. 1987. Charcot the clinician: The Tuesday lessons. New York, Raven Press.
43. Goetz C. 1988. Personal communication.
44. Fere C. 1888. Note sur les modifications de la résistance électrique sous l'influence des excitations sensorielles et des émotions. C R Séance Soc Biol 40:217–219.
45. Neumann E, Blanton R. 1970. The early history of electrodermal research. Psychophysiology 6:453–475.
46. Tarchanoff J. 1889. Décharges électriques dans la peau de l'homme sous l'excitation des organes des sens et d'activité psychiques. C R Séance Soc Biol 41:447–451.
47. Veraguth P. 1906. Die Verlegung diaskleral in das menschliche auge einfallender lichtreize in den raum. Z Psychol 42:162–174.
48. Brown CC. 1967. Methods in Psychophysiology. Baltimore, Williams & Wilkins.
49. Martin I, Venables PH. 1980. Techniques in Psychophysiology. New York, John Wiley & Sons, pp, 4–67.
50. Richter CP. 1927. A study of the electrical skin resistance and the psychogalvanic reflex in a case of unilateral sweating. Brain 50:216–235.
51. Richter CP. 1924. The sweat glands studied by the electrical resistance method. Am J Physiol 68:147.
52. Richter CP. 1929. Physiological factors involved in the electrical resistance of the skin. Am J Physiol 88:596.
53. Richter CP. 1929. Nervous control of electrical resistance of the skin. Bull Johns Hopkins Hosp 45:56–74.
54. Tower SS, Richter CP. 1931. Injury and repair within the sympathetic nervous system. I. The preganglionic neurons. Arch Neurol Psychiat Chicago 26:485–495.
55. Tower SS, Richter CP. 1932. Injury and repair within the sympathetic nervous system. II. The postganlionic neurons. Arch Neurol Psychiat Chicago 28:1139–1148.
56. Tower SS, Richter CP. 1932. Injury and repair within the sympathetic nervous system. III. Arch Neurol Psychiat Chicago 28:1149–1152.
57. Richter CP, Katz DT. 1943. Peripheral nerve injuries determined by the electrical skin resistance method. I. Ulnar nerve. JAMA 122:648.
58. Richter CP, Malone PD. 1945. Peripheral nerve lesion charts. J Neurosurg 2:550–552.
59. Richter CP, Shaw MB. 1930. Complete transections of the spinal cord at different levels. Their effect on sweating. Arch Neurol Psychiat Chicago 24:1107–1116.
60. Richter CP, Levine M. 1937. Sympathectomy in man. Its effect on the electrical resistance of the skin. Arch Neurol Psychiat Chicago 38:756–760.
61. Richter CP, Otenasek FJ. 1946. Thoracolumbar sympathectomies examined with the electrical skin resistance method. J Neurosurg 3:120–134.
62. Van Metre TH Jr. 1949. Electrical skin resistance studies of the region of pain in painful acute sinusitis. Bull Johns Hopkins Hosp 85:409.
63. Riley LH, Richter CP. 1975. Uses of the electrical skin resistance method in patients with neck and upper extremity pain. Johns Hopkins Med J 137:69–74.
64. Richter CP. 1946. Instructions for using the cutaneous resistance recorder or "Dermometer." J Neurosurg 3:181–191.
65. Richter CP, Woodruff BG. 1942. Facial patterns of electrical skin resistance. Bull Johns Hopkins 70:402–455.
66. Whelan FG, Richter CP. Electrical skin resistance technique used to map areas of skin affected by sympathectomy. Arch Neurol Psychiat Chicago 49:454–456.
67. Jasper HH, Robb JP. 1945. Studies of electrical skin resistance in peripheral nerve lesions. J Neurosurg 2:261–268.
68. Egyed B, Eory A, Veres T, Manninger J. 1980. Measurement of electrical resistance after nerve injuries of the hand. The Hand 12(3):275–281.
69. U.S. War Department. 1944. Technical Bulletin (TB Med 76), Neurological Diagnostic Techniques. Washington DC, U.S. Govt Printing Office.
70. Jasper HH. 1945. An improved clinical dermohmmeter. J Neurosurg 2:257–260.
71. Denny-Brown D. 1957. Handbook of Neurological Examination and Case Recording. Cambridge Press, 175 pp.
72. Gibbs FA. 1989. Personal communication.
73. Richter CP. 1987. Personal communication.
74. McHugh PR. 1989. Obituary of Curt Paul Richter. JAMA 261(21):3174.

75. Naifeh KH, Heller PH, Perry F, Gordon NC, Levine JD. 1983. Altered electrodermal responsivity associated with clinical pain. Pain 16:277–283.
76. Frexai-Baque E, Catteau E, Miossec Y, Roy JC. 1984. Asymmetry of electrodermal activity: A review. Biol Psychol 18:219–239.
77. Shahani BT, Halperin JJ, Boulu P, Cohen J. Sympathetic skin response — A method of assessing unmyelinated axon dysfunction in peripheral neuropathies. J Neurol Neurosurg Psychiat 47(5):536–542.
78. Green J, Reilly A, Hazelwood C, Becker C. 1987. Sympathetic skin response abnormalities correlated with abnormal infrared thermogram in patients with low back pain and radiculopathy. Mod Med (Suppl):89–92.
79. Lofstrom JB, Malmquist LA, Bengtsson M. 1984. Can the sympathogalvanic reflex be used to evaluate the extent of sympathetic block in spinal analgesia? Acta Anaesthesiol Scand 28:578–582.
80. Katz J, France C, Melzack R. 1989. An association between phantom limb sensations and stump skin conductance during transcutaneous electrical nerve stimulation (TENS) applied to the contralateral leg. Pain 36:367–377.
81. Shackel B. 1959. Skin-drilling: A method of diminishing galvanic skin potentials. Am J Psychol 72:114–121.
82. Longmire DR. 1963. Some considerations on bipolar and monopolar recording. Spike & Wave (J CAET) 12:23–33.
83. Longmire DR. 1965. Some effects of extra-cerebral resistance on the electroencephalogram. Spike & Wave (J CAET) 14:21–40.
84. Brown CC. 1967. A proposed standard nomenclature for psychophysiological measures. Psychophysiology 4:260–264.
85. Boucsein W, Hoffman G. 1979. A direct comparison of skin conductance and skin resistance methods. Psychophysiology 16:66–70.
86. Fricke H. 1932. The theory of electrolytic polarization. Phil Mag 14:310–318.
87. Glass JM, Stephen RL, Jacobson SC. 1980. The quantity and distribution of radiolabelled dexamethasone delivered to tissue by iontophoresis. Int J Dermatol 19:519–525.
88. Longmire DR, Woodley WE. 1988. Selective Tissue Conductance Meter, K874850A, Office of Device Evaluation, Food and Drug Administration, U.S. Dept of Health & Human Services.
89. Longmire DR. 1989. Selective tissue conductance mapping: Application to aerospace research. TABES, NASA/Ames Conf. Huntsville.
90. Kuno Y. 1956. Human Perspiration. Springfield, IL, Charles C. Thomas.
91. Richter CP, Woodruff BG, Eaton BC. 1943. Hand and foot patterns of low electrical skin resistance; their anatomical and neurological significance. J Neurophysiol 6:417–442.
92. Parris WCV, Longmire DR, Lindsey K, Harrison MD, Woodley WE. 1989. Changes in selective tissue conductance levels following stellate ganglion blockade. APS.
93. Longmire DR, Parris WCV, Woodley WE, Moore C. 1990. Computerized contour mapping of selective tissue conductance in sympathetically mediated pain. Pain Suppl 5:S423.
94. Longmire DR, Woodley WE. 1989. Selective tissue conductance levels in neck and shoulder pain. APS, Phoenix AZ, in press.

11. VISCERAL AND REFERRED PAIN

PAOLO PROCACCI AND MARCO MARESCA

In classical textbooks, pain is categorized as cutaneous, deep somatic or musculoskeletal, and visceral pain. In the clinic situation, this division into categories is not always so clear. There are, however, some characteristics peculiar to the sensations aroused from the viscera. These characteristics are varied and not as well defined as somatic sensations. Typical examples are the feeling in the stomach known as "appetite" and also the sensation in the rectum and the bladder giving a "sense of fullness." These sensations are generally known as "common sensations" or "coenaesthesia" (from the Greek *koine* = common and *aisthesis* = sensation).

A common sensation can become clearly unpleasant yet not painful, as in the case of motion sickness or in the sensation of "air hunger." We must note that in viscera (much more than in somatic tissues) transitory and unpleasant feelings are often felt. When they rise to a certain level of intensity, they become painful. Keele [1], in his studies on sensations induced by chemicals on cantharidin blister in the skin, used the term *metaesthesia* to indicate these feelings. The term seems very appropriate for many visceral sensations that are unpleasant but below the level of pain, such as a feeling of disagreeable fullness or acidity of the stomach, a sensation of light cramp in the abdomen, or the desire to micturate when it is not possible. These "metaesthesic sensations" can arise from every viscus, but more often from the hollow viscera, i.e., from the gastrointestinal and urogenital tracts. Even though they can remain under the level of pain for a long time, these sensations can nevertheless cause a strong sense of malaise and anxiety. They can disappear, but they can also precede the onset of visceral pain, such as a typical attack of angina pectoris, a renal or biliary colic, or a strong gastric pain.

The metaesthesic sensations are not generally considered in modern textbooks of pain, but we observed that they are extremely important.

Not infrequently a myocardial infarction is described as painless, but a careful clinical history shows that the patient felt a sense of gastric fullness or "indigestion" prior to the attack. These sensations are also important as possible signals of other diseases, such as gastritis or irritable colon.

Visceral pain can arise from a common visceral sensation. Sensations from the bladder are typical examples. One common sensation is the feeling of fullness, accompanied by the desire to micturate. If it is inconvenient to micturate, the desire to do so becomes stronger and even unpleasant, but it is still not painful. In urinary retention, as occurs in acute urinary bladder obstruction, this unpleasant feeling becomes severe and increasingly painful.

VISCERAL RECEPTORS AND AFFERENT FIBERS

The origin of metaesthesic and painful visceral sensations has been discussed in the past and also in the present; however, the discussion is still open. High-threshold receptors, considered as true nociceptors by some researchers, have been identified in the skin [2–4]. With respect to visceral organs, there is some experimental evidence of the existence of a separate category of high-threshold receptors in some organs, such as the heart, lungs, gallbladder and biliary ducts, testes, and perhaps the uterus [5–9]. On the other hand, Iggo [10], Wall [11], and Malliani and his coworkers [12] have observed that painful stimuli can induce an increased activity of receptors, which at a low level of activity are involved in regulating reflexes. They have suggested that such receptors at a high level of activity break through to give the conscious perception of pain, and consequently, they refute the existence of true nociceptors, at least in the viscera. This is the old problem of specificity of sensory receptors, which has been widely debated in the past and in recent times. There are still two main schools of thought: one assumes that receptors are specific for each type of sensation, and the other considers the specificity of sensation as due to a different pattern or processing of information. Procacci and Maresca have reviewed the subject extensively [13].

It is well known that most internal organs have a dual afferent innervation. Some afferent fibers are joined to sympathetic nerves, while other afferent fibers are connected to the parasympathetic nerves. Visceral pain has been considered only as the result of impulses transmitted by afferent fibers running in sympathetic nerves; however, afferent fibers running in parasympathetic nerves can also play a role in visceral pain, at least for some particular pain radiations (a typical example is cardiac pain radiating to the neck and to the jaws).

Visceral afferent fibers are few in number in comparison to somatic afferent fibers (about 10% of the total amount of spinal afferent fibers in the cat) [14,15]. But the relatively small number of visceral afferent fibers innervate an area equivalent to at least a quarter of the body surface, with extensive ramifications of fibers and a great overlap between the fields of adjacent dorsal roots (even up to 100%) [14]. As a consequence, afferent impulses from a given visceral area enter the central nervous system via many dorsal roots. This "multiple entry" may ensure widespread evocation of reflexes and spatial summation in the central nervous system of impulses evoking pain.

VISCERAL ALGOGENIC CONDITIONS

The stimuli apt to induce pain in viscera are different from those that induce pain in somatic structures. This explains why in the past the viscera were thought to be insensitive to pain. In fact, it was observed that viscera could be exposed to such stimuli as burning or cutting without evoking pain. This apparent insensitivity of viscera was due to failure to apply adequate stimuli.

The main factors capable of inducing pain in visceral structures are the following [16,17]:

1. Abnormal distension and contraction of the hollow viscera muscle walls
2. Rapid stretching of the capsule of such solid visceral organs as the liver, spleen, and pancreas
3. Abrupt anoxemia of visceral muscles
4. Formation and accumulation of pain-producing substances
5. Direct action of chemical stimuli, especially important in the esophagus and stomach
6. Traction or compression of ligaments and vessels
7. Inflammatory states
8. Necrosis of some structures (myocardium, pancreas)

Some of these factors may be concomitant and interact in many clinical conditions.

With respect to the contraction of the hollow viscera wall, it must be noted that a strong contraction in isometric conditions provokes a more severe pain than in isotonic conditions. This may explain the strong pain of some diseases, as in acute mechanical intestinal obstruction and the biliary or ureteral colics.

The different visceral structures show different pain sensitivity. Serous membranes have the lowest pain threshold and are followed, in order of ascending threshold, by the hollow viscera wall and by parenchymatous organs.

Experimental investigations have been carried out in humans on algogenic visceral conditions. Esophageal pain has been induced by many authors, using mechanical, electrical, and chemical stimuli. Gastric algogenic conditions were studied by Wolf and Wolff [18] on a patient with a large gastric stoma.

Different kinds of stimuli were applied. No pain could be induced when healthy mucosa of the fundus of the stomach was squeezed between the blades of a forceps. Electrical stimuli, intense enough to cause pain in the tongue, and chemical stimuli, such as 50% or 90% alcohol, 1.0 N HCl, 0.1 N NaOH, and 1:30 suspension of mustard, were also ineffective in evoking pain when applied to healthy gastric mucosa. However, if the mucosa was inflamed, all the above-mentioned procedures induced a strong pain. Kinsella [19] observed that squeezing the inflamed appendix provoked pain.

The sensibility of pleura has been investigated by means of electrical, thermal, and mechanical stimuli during a Jacobaeus operation (section of pleural synechiae) [20]. Pain was induced by stimulation of areas of normal and inflamed pleura. When the stimuli were applied to the inflamed serosa, pain was more intense, sharp, and localized than when the stimuli were applied to the normal pleura. Similar phenomena were observed in all cases of electrical, mechanical, and chemical endobronchial stimulation.

All these findings suggest that inflammation plays an important role in the genesis of pain in many viscera, inducing a sensitization to normally nonpainful stimuli. Many pain-producing substances have been identified, such as kinins, 5-hydroxytryptamine, histamine, prostaglandins, and potassium ions, which could be active in visceral painful diseases. The algogenic activity of some substances has been demonstrated in experiments in which the substances were introduced in the arteries or in the peritoneum [21,22]. However, it must be noted that when an algogenic substance is released in pathological conditions, many factors are present. These factors include activating or inhibiting agents, and changes of pH and of capillary permeability, and may modify the effect of the algogenic substance. This complex biochemical and biophysical situation cannot be reproduced in experiments.

TRUE VISCERAL PAIN AND REFERRED PAIN
Visceral pain has different characteristics in different patients or in the same patient at different times. Two main types of visceral pain are distinguished: true visceral pain and referred pain. True visceral pain is deep, dull, not well-defined, and is described in a unique way by the patients. It is difficult to locate this type of pain, which tends to radiate and frequently reaches parts of the body that are far from the affected organ. It is often accompanied by a sense of malaise. It induces strong autonomic reflex phenomena, including diffuse sweating, vasomotor responses, changes of arterial pressure and heart rate, and an intense psychic alarm reaction.

When an algogenic process affecting a viscus recurs frequently or becomes more intense and prolonged, the location becomes more exact and the painful sensation is progressively felt in more superficial structures, sometimes far from the site of origin. This phenomenon is usually called *referred pain*. This type of pain may be accompanied by allodynia, cutaneous, and muscular hyperalgesia.

MECHANISMS OF REFERRED PAIN

A classical interpretation of the phenomenon of referred pain was proposed by Henry Head [23], on the basis of previous observations of Sturge [24] and Ross [25]. Head wrote that

a painful stimulus to an internal organ is conducted to that segment of the cord from which its sensory nerves are given off. There it comes into close connection with the fibres for painful sensation from the surface of the body which also arose from the same segment . . . the localising power of the surface of the body is enormously in excess of that of the viscera, and thus by . . . a psychical error of judgment . . . the pain is referred on to the surface of the body instead of on to the organ actually affected [23].

Head's concepts were further developed by MacKenzie [26]. According to MacKenzie, the convergence of impulses from viscera and from the skin in the central nervous system plays a fundamental role in the genesis of referred pain. Sensory impulses from the viscera create an "irritable focus" in the segment at which they enter into the spinal cord. Afferent impulses from the skin are thereby facilitated, giving rise to true cutaneous pain. This interpretation is called the *convergence-facilitation theory*.

The importance of convergence in the genesis of referred pain has also been stressed by Sinclair, Weddell, and Feindel [27], and by Ruch [28]. In the interpretation proposed by Ruch, some visceral afferents subserving pain sensation converge with cutaneous afferents to end on the same neuron at some point in the sensory pathway. The resulting impulses, on reaching the brain, are interpreted as having come from the skin, an interpretation that has been learned from previous experiences in which the same tract fiber was stimulated by cutaneous afferents. This interpretation is called the *convergence-projection theory*. Many experimental findings support the above theories by showing that nociceptive impulses from visceral and cutaneous areas converge in the central nervous system [29–31].

MacKenzie [26] furthermore suggested that 1) visceral afferent impulses activate anterior horn motor cells to produce rigidity of the muscles; 2) a similar activation of anterolateral autonomic cells induces piloerection, vaso-constriction, and other sympathetic phenomena. He called these motor re-actions the *viscero-motor reflexes*. This mechanism, that in modern terms can be defined as a positive sympathetic and motor feedback loop, is to be considered as fundamental in referred pain. A classic experiment in humans was performed by MacLellan and Goodell [32], who observed that following a faradic stimulation of the ureter or of the pelvis of the kidney, the muscles of the abdominal wall on the stimulated side remained contracted and, after about half an hour, this side began to ache. The ache became quite severe and lasted for 6 hours, with the side still tender the following day. Therefore, it is clear that painful stimulation of visceral structures evokes a visceromuscular reflex, so that some muscles contract and become a new source of pain.

In respect to the activation of the autonomic system, it has been demonstrated that algogenic conditions in the skin and some related phenomena are induced through a reflex arc, the efferent limb of which is sympathetic. In fact, it has been observed that the local anesthetic block of the sympathetic ganglia led to the disappearance, or at least to a marked decrease, of referred pain, allodynia, hyperalgesia, and alteration of dermographia and of skin electrical impedance [33,34].

Thus, referred pain is caused by two phenomena: 1) central convergence of visceral and cutaneous impulses; 2) visceromuscular and viscerocutaneous reflexes that give rise to algogenic conditions in the periphery. The two phenomena are always linked, because when the strong afferent barrage arrives at the posterior horn, a strong efferent discharge is induced both in the anterior and anterolateral horn, i.e., in motor and sympathetic efferent fibers.

The importance of an antidromic activation of afferent fibers, with release in peripheral tissues of substance P and other active substances, is still a matter of conjecture. It is interesting to note that the axon reflexes, hypothesized by Lewis [35], Sinclair, Weddell, and Feindel [27], and other authors more than 40 years ago, are now again considered very important [36,37].

In some conditions, referred pain is long lasting, increases progressively, and is accompanied by dystrophy of somatic structures, as in the shoulder-hand syndrome that may follow a myocardial infarction. This is probably due to the onset of a self-maintaining "vicious circle" of impulses "periphery — afferent fibers — central nervous system — somatic and sympathetic efferent fibers — periphery," as suggested by Livingston [38] and Bonica [39] for causalgia and other reflex dystrophies.

INTRICATE CONDITIONS

As we have stated in the beginning of this chapter, in clinical practice the distinction among true visceral pain, referred pain, and somatic pain is often difficult: these are the so-called intricate conditions. This concept was firstly proposed by Froment and Gonin [40], who observed that angina pectoris can be related to cervical osteoarthritis, esophageal hernia, or cholecystitis. A very important clinical problem often arises as to whether such a syndrome can be defined; according to Heberden's difinition, "angina pectoris" is due in different patients to diseases of the esophagus, to ischemia of the heart, to fibrositis of the chest muscles, or to many of these factors. We have observed all these possibilities, i.e., that a single algogenic factor gives origin to the pain or that many factors intermingle.

It is difficult to ascertain whether the "intricate conditions" are due to a simple addition of impulses from different sources in the central nervous system or to viscerosomatic and somatovisceral reflex mechanisms, which may induce a typical "vicious circle" between different structures.

MNEMONIC TRACES

Mnemonic traces may play an important role in visceral pain. It has been demonstrated that the mnemonic process is facilitated if the experience to be retained is repeated many times or is accompanied by pleasant or, above all unpleasant, emotions [41]. Pain experience develops not only in learning avoidance reflexes but also as memory [42]. Nathan [43] observed that in some subjects different kinds of stimuli could call to mind forgotten painful experiences. Nathan concluded that traces had been laid down in the central nervous system, which were subliminal as far as consciousness was concerned, but could be reactivated and reinforced in later episodes.

We carried out a series of investigations on patients with previous myocardial infarction and on patients with angina pectoris, who appeared normal at a complete exam of sensibility [44,45]. In these patients, we provoked a sensory stimulation in the same metameres of the heart by inducing ischemia of the upper limbs, with the limbs at rest. In normal subjects, ischemia of the limbs at rest induces paresthesic sensations but never pain. In many patients with previous myocardial infarction, ischemia of the upper limbs provoked the onset of pain with characteristics similar to those of the pain felt during the infarction. In many patients with angina pectoris, ischemia of the upper limbs provoked the onset of pain with characteristics similar to those of anginal pain. These phenomena are probably due to the activation of mnemonic traces. The formation of mnemonic traces is facilitated in myocardial infarction by the strong emotions that accompany pain, and in angina pectoris by the repetition of attacks.

Similar mechanisms may also be active in painful diseases of the abdominal organs. We have observed that, during the first biliary or renal colic, referred pain followed true visceral pain after a variable interval. In subsequent episodes, referred pain developed promptly and was not preceded by true visceral pain. These phenomena may be considered as arising from the activation of mnemonic traces.

CONCLUDING REMARKS

We have seen how the problem of visceral pain is difficult and far from the schematizations found in many textbooks. As a final clinical comment, we must remember that visceral pain is extremely significant for a correct diagnosis and for appropriate medical or surgical therapy. In this aspect, visceral pain is somewhat different from deep somatic and cutaneous pain. In general, pain in these conditions can be long lasting, but without reflecting an immediate danger for the patient.

REFERENCES

1. Keele CA. 1962. Sensations aroused by chemical stimulation of the skin. In CA Keele and R Smith (eds), The Assessment of Pain in Man and Animals. Edinburgh, Livingstone, pp. 28–31.

2. Burgess PR, Perl ER. 1967. Myelinated afferent fibers responding specifically to noxious stimulation of the skin, J Physiol (London), 190, 541–562.
3. Bessou P, Perl ER. 1969. Response of cutaneous sensory units with unmyelinated fibers to noxious stimuli. J Neurophysiol 32:1025–1043.
4. Perl ER. 1985. Unraveling the story of pain. In HL Fields, R Dubner, F Cervero (eds), Advances in Pain Research and Therapy, Vol. 9. New York, Raven Press, pp. 1–29.
5. Widdicombe JG. 1974. Enteroceptors. In JI Hubbard (ed), The Peripheral Nervous System. New York, Plenum Press, pp. 455–485.
6. Baker DG, Coleridge HM, Coleridge JCG, Nerdrum T. 1980. Search for a cardiac nociceptor: Stimulation by bradykinin of sympathetic afferent nerve endings in the heart of the cat. J Physiol (London) 306:519–536.
7. Cervero F. 1982. Afferent activity evoked by natural stimulation of the biliary system in the ferret. Pain 13:137–151.
8. Kumazawa T. 1986. Sensory innervation of reproductive organs. In Cervero F, Morrison JFB (eds), Visceral Sensation. Amsterdam, Elsevier, pp. 115–131.
9. Robbins A, Sato Y, Hotta H, Berkley KJ. 1987. Response of uterine afferent fibers in the rat to sodium ajamide and CO_2. Pain Suppl. 4: S20.
10. Iggo A. 1974. Pain receptors. In JJ Bonica, P Procacci, CA Pagni (eds), Recent Advances on Pain. Springfield, IL, Charles C. Thomas, pp. 3–35.
11. Wall PD. 1988. Stability and instability of central pain mechanisms. In R Dubner, GF Gebhart, MR Bond (eds), Proceedings of the Vth World Congress on Pain. Amsterdam, Elsevier, pp. 13–24.
12. Malliani A, Pagani M, Lombardi F. 1989. Visceral versus somatic mechanisms. In PD Wall, R Melzack (eds), Textbook of Pain. Edinburgh, Churchill Livingstone, pp. 128–140.
13. Procacci P, Maresca M. 1984. Pain concept in Western civilization: A historical review. In C Benedetti, CR Chapman, G Moricca (eds), Advances in Pain Research and Therapy, Vol. 7. New York, Raven Press, pp. 1–11.
14. Downman CBB, 1965. Viscerotomes and dermatomes: Some comparison of the innter and outer surfaces of the body. In DR Curtis, AK McIntyre (eds), Studies in Physiology. Berlin, Springer, pp. 47–51.
15. Cervero F, Connell LA, Lawson SN. 1984. Somatic and visceral primary afferents in the lower thoracic dorsal root ganglia of the cat. J Comp Neurol 228:422–431.
16. Ayala M. 1937. Douleur sympathique et douleur viscerale. Rev Neurol 68:222–242.
17. Procacci P, Zoppi M, Maresca M. 1986. Clinical approach to visceral sensation. In F Cervero, JFB Morrison (eds), Visceral Sensation. Amsterdam, Elsevier, pp. 21–28.
18. Wolf S, Wolff HG. 1947. Human Gastric Function. An Experimental Study of a Man and his Stomach. New York, Oxford University Press.
19. Kinsella VJ. 1948. The Mechanism of abdominal Pain. Sydney, Australasian Medical Publishing Company.
20. Teodori U, Galletti R. 1962. Il Dolore Nelle Affezioni Degli Organi Interni del Torace. Roma, Pozzi.
21. Lim RKS. 1966. A revised concept of the mechanism of analgesia and pain. In RS Knighton, PR Dumke (eds), Pain. London, Churchill, pp. 117–154.
22. Lim RKS. 1967. Pharmacologic viewpoint of pain and analgesia. In EL Way (ed), New Concepts in Pain and its Clinical Management. Philadelphia, Davis, pp. 33–47.
23. Head H. 1893. On disturbances of sensation with especial reference to the pain of visceral disease. Brain 16:1–132.
24. Sturge WA. 1883. The phenomena of angina pectoris, and their bearing upon the theory of counter-irritation. Brain 5:492–510.
25. Ross J. 1888. On the segmental distribution of sensory disorders. Brain 10:333–361.
26. MacKenzie J. 1909. Symptoms and their Interpretation. London, Shaw and Sons.
27. Sinclair DC, Weddell G, Feindel WH. 1948. Referred pain and associated phenomena. Brain 71:184–211.
28. Ruch TC. 1960. Pathophysiology of pain. In TC Ruch, JF Fulton (eds), Medical Physiology and Biophysics. Philadelphia, W.B. Saunders, pp. 350–368.
29. Hugon M. 1971. Transfer of somatosensory information in the spinal cord. In WA Cobb (ed), Handbook of Electroencephalography and Clinical Neurophysiology, Vol. 9. Somatic Sensation. Amsterdam, Elsevier, pp. 33–44.

30. Wall PD. 1974. Physiological mechanisms involved in the production of pain. In JJ Bonica, P Procacci, CA Pagni (eds), Recent Advances on Pain. Springfield, IL, Charles C. Thomas, pp. 36–63.
31. Cervero F. 1988. Visceral pain. In R Dubner, GF Gebhart, MR Bond (eds), Proceedings of the Vth World Congress on Pain. Amsterdam, Elsevier, pp. 216–226.
32. MacLellan AM, Goodell H. 1943. Pain from the bladder, ureter and kidney pelvis. Proc Assoc Res Nerv Ment Dis 23:252–262.
33. Galletti R, Procacci P. 1966. The role of the sympathetic system in the control of somatic pain and of some associated phenomena. Acta Neuroveg 28:495–500.
34. Procacci P. 1960. A survey of modern concepts of pain. In PJ Vinken, GW Bruyn (eds), Handbook of Clinical Neurology, Vol. 1. Amsterdam, North-Holland Publishing Company, pp. 114–146.
35. Lewis T. 1942. Pain. New York, Macmillan.
36. Wall PD, Devor M. 1983. Sensory afferent impulses originate from dorsal root ganglia as well as from the periphery in normal and nerve injured rats. Pain 17:321–339.
37. Devor M. 1984. The pathophysiology and anatomy of damaged nerve. In PD Wall, R Melzack (eds), Textbook of Pain. Edinburgh, Churchill Livingstone, pp. 49–64.
38. Livingston WK. 1943. Pain Mechanisms. New York, Macmillan.
39. Bonica JJ. 1953. The Management of Pain. Philadelphia, Lea & Febiger.
40. Froment R, Gonin A. 1956. Les Angors Coronariens Intriques. Paris, Expansion Scientifique Francaise.
41. Benedetti G. 1969. Neuropsicologia. Nilano, Feltrinelli.
42. Melzack R. 1973. The Puzzle of Pain. Harmondsworth, Penguin Books.
43. Nathan PW. 1962. Pain traces left in the central nervous system. In CA Keele, R Smith (eds), The Assessment of Pain in Man and Animals. Edinburgh, Livingstone, pp. 129–134.
44. Procacci P, Buzzelli G, Voegelin MR, Bozza G. 1968. Esplorazione della funzione sensitiva degli arti superiori in soggetti con pregresso infarto miocardico. Rass Neurol Veg 22:403–418.
45. Procacci P, Passeri I, Zoppi M, Burzagli L, Voegelin MR, Maresca M. 1972. Esplorazione della funzione sensitiva degli arti superiori in soggetti con angina pectoris. Giorn Ital Cardiol 2:978–984.

12. NERVE BLOCK THERAPY IN CHRONIC PAIN MANAGEMENT

WINSTON C.V. PARRIS

Chronic pain management continues to be a major challenge for the medical profession, and whereas about two decades ago the problem was not adequately addressed, it is gratifying to note that this challenge and its implications is increasingly recognized by almost all segments of the health delivery team. This fact is borne out by the large number of pain centers and pain clinics that have developed nationwide, and this number continues to increase yearly [1]. Unfortunately, the increase in the number of pain facilities has not corresponded with the increase in the quality of chronic pain management. Moreover, the "conquest" of pain is elusive and is still very far from satisfactory resolution. The good news is that tremendous direct and indirect progress is being made at several levels during the process of solving this major scourge of humankind. Testimony of this progress is borne out by the impressive list of pain-oriented scientific papers that continue to be delivered at international, national, and local pain meetings, and also at several medical specialty meetings (notably anesthesiology, neurosurgery, rehabilitation medicine, orthopedic surgery, psychology, and neurology). Nerve blocks have always formed an important part of perioperative pain management and are also a major modality in chronic pain management. At the recently concluded 6th World Congress of Pain held in Adelaide, Australia, an entire plenary session was allocated to postoperative pain. The work of Woolf [2], Kehlet [3], and Handwerker [4] suggest that hyperexcitability of the spinal cord interneurons was the end result of a series of events that resulted from injury (including surgery), pain, and inflammation. This concept was supported by Cousins [5] et al. and Kehlet [6], who presented data to show that preoperative nerve blocks or nerve blocks immediately postinjury diminish the intensity and severity of subsequent pain. The purpose of this chapter is, therefore, to review some of the more commonly administered nerve blocks and to discuss their relevant application to the management of chronic pain patients.

Before discussing specific nerve blocks and their relevance to pain management, it may be appropriate to review some general considerations that may be helpful in the overall evaluation of nerve blocks as effective modalities in pain management. These considerations include history of nerve blocks; prerequisites for nerve block administration; resuscitation, drugs, and equipment personnel for nerve blocks; the pharmacology of agents used in the performance of nerve blocks; accessories for nerve block therapy; complications of nerve blocks; and mechanism of actions of local anesthetics in nerve block therapy.

GENERAL CONSIDERATIONS

History of nerve blocks

A possible place for nerve blocks in the archives of pain management was assured as early as 1826 by Mueller [7], who proposed "the doctrine of specific energies of the senses." This concept stimulated contemporary thought that resulted in the "specificity hypothesis" of pain, as formulated by Schiff [8] in 1858. In 1845, Rynd [9] described the infiltration of morphine in a peripheral nerve for neuralgic pain using a hypodermic needle — this may have been the first documentation of a nerve block. The discovery of the syringe by Pravaz [10] in 1853 contributed to a variety of "neural procedures" by notable researchers, including Wood and Hunter.

Koller, in 1884, first used cocaine topically for eye surgery, and in 1885 Corning described the epidural anesthetic. Reclus proposed infiltration anesthesia in 1890, and Quincke described the lumbar puncture technique in 1891; these advances led the way for the introduction of spinal anesthesia, which was first described by Bier [11] in 1898. A flurry of important events, including the development of local anesthetics, the use of epinephrine for augmenting conduction anesthesia, the development of regional anesthesia, and the formation of national and international pain societies (see Chapter 1) have led to the establishment of an important role of nerve blocks in anesthesia in general and in pain management in particular.

Prerequisites for nerve blocks

Nerve blocks may produce significant systemic as well as local effects on the body. For anesthetic purposes, there was an initial misconception that vigilance, which was a monitoring hallmark of general anesthesia, could be relaxed or eliminated when nerve blocks and regional anesthesia were administered. This assumption is (and was) a total fallacy. The effects of some nerve blocks, notably spinal and epidural blocks, on the cardio-respiratory, circulatory, and central nervous systems may be profound enough to be life threatening if adequate prophylactic measures and thorough monitoring techniques are not implemented. In the presence of these measures, however, nerve blocks are relatively safe and complication-free.

It is important, at this juncture, to deal with a major controversy that exists in the anesthesia community regarding nerve blocks and monitoring. This controversy centers around the issue of the amount of monitoring (EKG, blood pressure monitoring, pulse oximetry, etc.) that is required for nerve block performance in pain clinics and the need for preblock establishment of intravenous access in pain clinics. As in most controversies, the issues are not clear cut. In the operating room setting where nerve blocks (regional anesthesia) are performed, the concentration and volume of local anesthetic administered are usually high (in contrast to the pain clinic setting) in order to provide optimum surgical conditions for analgesia and muscle relaxation. To provide these optimal surgical conditions, profound analgesia and muscle relaxation are the desired endpoint, and major hemodynamic and cardiorespiratory changes may occur. It is therefore necessary to monitor this perioperative period very closely and frequently so as to manage effectively those physiological changes as soon as they occur.

The management of the hemodynamic effects of regional anesthesia is facilitated by the presence of a reliable intravenous access to administer fluids rapidly and also to administer appropriate supportive medications. In the setting of the pain clinic, profound analgesia and muscle relaxation are not desirable physiological or therapeutic endpoints. Here, sympathetic and mild sensory blockade are ideal. The concentration and volume of local anesthetic used to achieve these goals are lower than that necessary to achieve satisfactory regional anesthesia and do not usually produce the hemodynamic and cardiorespiratory changes that may be seen in the operating room setting if the nerve blocks are performed competently. Since mishaps may occur from time to time, even under the most ideal circumstances, it becomes mandatory to conduct nerve blocks in a pain clinic setting where resuscitation drugs and equipment are always available to be administered by skilled individuals trained and certified in Advanced Cardiac Life Support (ACLS) [12]. Under the normal circumstances, this is usually an anesthesiologist. However, a medical specialist with the appropriate training, experience, and expertise may function in that capacity, although the medicolegal implications of any subsequent misadventure may be complicated to defend.

There is another reason to support the practice of minimal monitoring, i.e., pre- and post-nerve block pulse, respiration, and blood pressure in the *healthy* chronic pain patient, and also to refrain from having intravenous access in those patients. The reason evolves around the unique clinical characteristics of the chronic pain patient. The patient is usually depressed, angry, frustrated, tense, fed up with the conventional medical system, and usually dependent on drugs and the medical infrastructure. The establishment of intravenous lines (unless indicated by the patient's medical condition, e.g., dehydration, vaso-vagal phenomena, preblock hypotension, etc.) and a plethora of monitoring paraphernalia may enhance dependency on the "medical system" when clearly one of the most important strategies in chronic pain management is the promotion of wellness behavior and self-coping techniques. However, it must be emphasized that each case must be individualized and evaluated by the medical pain specialist and that the patient's clinical condition supercedes any behavioral factors that may otherwise be extremely important for pain management.

Resuscitation: Drugs, personnel and equipment for nerve blocks

As previously mentioned, nerve blocks should only be performed in locations where resuscitation drugs and equipment are easily accessible. The drugs available should not only include the essential resuscitation drugs (sodium bicarbonate, epinephrine, calcium chloride, lidocaine, etc.) and intravenous fluids, but also drugs used to treat grand mal seizures secondary to inadvertent intravenous injections (sodium thiopental, diazepam). Resuscitation equipment should include endotracheal tubes, laryngoscopes, oropharyngeal airways and suction devices. As important as the drugs and equipment required to resuscitate appropriate patients is the need for a physician skilled and credentialed in the art of cardio-pulmonary resusitation.

Pharmacology of drugs used in nerve block therapy

The following drug groups are commonly used in nerve block therapy:

1. Local anesthetics
2. Steroids
3. Neurolytic agents
4. Miscellaneous agents

Local anesthetics are the main drugs used in the performance of nerve blocks. To facilitate sympathetic and sensory blockade without undesirable motor blockade, a lower concentration (than that used for surgical conditions) of local anesthetic is usually employed in most nerve blocks. A variety of local anesthetics are used, and the choice depends on the individual physician. However, adequate knowledge of the structural-activity relationships [13] of the various local anesthetics (molecular structure, pKA or dissociation constant, protein binding properties, lipid solubility) allows one to make a more informed choice of the various local anesthetics.

The author's preference for the performance of most nerve blocks is 0.25% bupivacaine (Marcaine®, Sensocaine®). That concentration appears to fulfill most of the above-mentioned conditions for nerve block administration in the pain clinic setting. However, a variety of other drugs could be used. Knowledge of the potential side effects of the various local anesthetics and of their toxic dosages should be ascertained. It is important to emphasize a few known complications of local anesthetics: 0.75% bupivacaine may cause sudden and progressive cardiac arrest [14], which is usually difficult to treat successfully; 2-chloroprocaine, if inadvertently introduced intrathecally, may produce severe and irreversible neurological complications [15]; and prilocaine may cause methemoglobinemia [16] if administered in doses in excess of 500 mg.

Steroids are used extensively in the management of cervical, thoracic, lumbar, and sacrococcygeal back pain [17]. When slow-releasing or depotsteroids are used judiciously, the customary biochemical complications of steroids (e.g., suppression of the adrenal axis, Cushing's syndrome, osteoporosis) are not observed. Methylprednisolone diacetate (Depomedrol®) and triamcinolone (Aristocort®) are the commonly used agents. The author's preference of a depot-steroid is methylprednisolone. A dose of 2 or 3 ml of 4% methylprednisolone with 7 or 8 ml of 0.25% bupivacaine is routinely used for the healthy adult patient (18–55 years) having a lumbar epidural steroid injection. The local anesthetic may provide almost immediate relief following administration, while the methylprednisolone may provide later-onset pain relief approximately 1–2 weeks later. The mechanism of action of steroids in pain control is not precisely known; however, several mechanisms have been postulated. These include 1) an antiinflammatory effect [18], 2) perispinal and intraspinal steroid receptors [19], and 3) increased phospholipase A_2 activity induced by steroids [20]. More work needs to be done to elucidate the precise mechanism of action of steroids in pain management. It is important to stress at this point that the depot steroids are not recommended for intrathecal use. The presence of preservatives in these drugs may produce arachnoiditis and other serious neurological sequelae, which may produce unacceptable morbidity for the patient and uncomfortable medicolegal difficulties for the physician [21].

Neurolytic agents are used to manage chronic intractable pain in patients with terminal neoplastic disease, and more recently in patients with terminal HIV disease. There are a few situations in which neurolytic nerve blocks may be used to treat patients with chronic benign pain; these patients usually have well-demarcated peripheral lesions that respond to a peripheral nerve block (e.g., suprascapular nerve block or ulnar nerve block) and in whom the resultant sensory and motor blockade are acceptable to the patient. Naturally, informed consent from the patient and thorough discussion with the family have to be obtained prior to the performance of the neurolytic block, as indeed for all nerve blocks. However, the "permanent" implications of neurolytic blocks make this prerequisite even more mandatory.

Neurolysis of nerves may be attained with a number of agents. Absolute alcohol [22] and 6% phenol [23] with glycerine are the more frequently used drugs. The author's preference is 6% phenol in glycerine, because absolute alcohol produces alcohol neuritis, which is associated with intense burning pain after injection, and also because the regeneration of nerves following alcohol injection is very slow or nonexistent. Phenol, on the other hand, does not produce pain following injection, and nerve regeneration may occur 3–6 months after injection. Systemic toxic effects could be limited if overdoses of phenol are avoided. These toxic effects include convulsions, central nervous system depression, and cardiovascular collapse. Less serious complications of phenol toxicity including gastrointestinal symptoms, skin eruptions, and renal dysfunction. Before neurolytic blocks are performed, it is clinically expedient to have demonstrated satisfactory pain relief after "temporary" or diagnostic nerve block with local anesthetic. Further, the precise placement of a needle should be ascertained and verified by means of radiological and fluoroscopic control. A radiograph (P.A. and lateral views) of that needle placement makes good medicolegal sense, even though it can be generalized that chronic pain patients as a group, and more especially chronic pain patients with neoplasms, are not usually litigious.

Other clinically used neurolytic agents include glycerol, ammonium sulfate, chlorocresol, and cold saline. Glycerol is gaining popularity in the treatment of trigeminal ganglion block for tic douloureux. Neurolysis of nerves may be accomplished by radiofrequency lesioning or thermocoagulation, cryotherapy (thermal neurolysis), and possibly laser techniques. All these techniques require the same precautions as neurolytic blocks with conventional neurolytic agents. It is hoped that as newer techniques and newer drugs are developed, they may be associated with less morbidity than the older drugs and techniques.

There is a varied group of drugs used to supplement and potentiate local anesthetics for nerve block therapy in chronic pain management. Sometimes these drugs may be used instead of local anesthetics. These drugs may come from diverse pharmacological groups and exert their effects in different ways. The alpha-adrenergic antagonists may be used to treat resistant reflex sympathetic dystrophy (RSD) by intravenous administration using the "Bier" or intravenous regional sympathetic block [24]. Guanethidine, reserpine, and clonidine have been used in these cases. The combined alpha- and beta-adrenergic antagonist, labetalol, has been used to treat resistant RSD. Verapamil [25] has been used in in-vitro animal studies to potentiate the neural conduction blockade of bupivacaine. However, similar experiments using in-vivo animal models have not been successful in duplicating these results [Parris and Nyhuis, unpublished data; 26].

Narcotic analgesics (morphine) have been injected intrathetically since the work of Wang [27] in 1979. Initial reports of unacceptable complications have decreased as newer narcotic analgesics with different pharmacological characteristics (e.g., lipid solubility) have been utilized. Further, these analgesics are now mixed with local anesthetics and cumulatively their analgetic effects are potentiated while the undesirable side effects are minimized. Currently, epidural opioids and epidural opioid/local anesthetic mixtures are used increasingly for pain management, particularly for acute pain management and for cancer pain management. There are, in addition, a number of synthetic compounds that are currently being investigated, and these drugs may have an important place in nerve block therapy for pain management. These drugs include substance P antagonists, synthetic endorphins and enkephalins, parenteral nonsteroidal antiinflammatory drugs (e.g., Ketorolac®), somatostatin, and calcitonin. As the complex mechanisms of pain are unraveled, more therapeutic options may become available, and consequently more drugs may become available for nerve block therapy.

Accessories for nerve block therapy

As previously mentioned, nerve blocks should be administered under optimal conditions, in ideal locations with reliable equipment, and by competent well-trained personnel. This statement may be considered ultra-idealistic, and the author offers no apology for these recommendations. A nerve block tray of some kind is desirable, because all the component parts are to be consistently found in a sterile location and standardization of equipment is usually assured. The composition of a typical nerve block tray is shown in Figure 12-1. This tray consists of a prep section with a receptacle for the cleansing antiseptic (usually betadine) and a compartment with sponge-tipped cleaning applicators: This compartment is considered "nonsterile." The other section of the tray is considered to be sterile. This section contains a compartment where the local

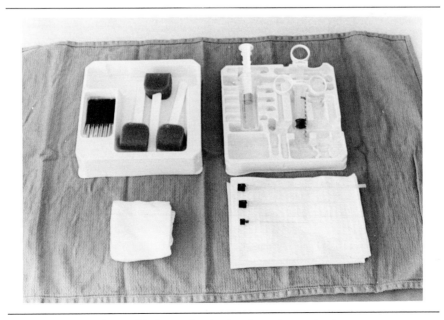

Figure 12-1. Typical nerve block tray showing luer-loc syringe and pulsator.

anesthetic is kept prior to injection. There is a second drug compartment for use of a second drug if necessary. The other compartment of the tray contains three 22-gauge needles (2.5, 4.5, and 5.5 inches long), 6-gauge sponges, a pulsator syringe, and a 10-ml luer-lok syringe. The pulsator syringe facilitates the determination of the "loss-of-resistance" technique, as used for epidural blocks and paravertebral lumbar sympathetic block. The luer-lok syringe adds a safety feature to nerve block administration by allowing the drug (local anesthetic) to be administered in small doses of 1–2 ml at a time while allowing for immediate postinjection aspiration. This technique, which is made possible and simple with this syringe, minimizes inadvertent intra-vascular injection, with all its potential morbidity and mortality. It is important to have the antiseptic agent kept in separate compartments from the local anesthetic so as to eliminate major neurological complications that may occur if neurotoxic components of the antiseptic cleansing agent were to be inad-vertently injected intrathecally or epidurally. It is this very unfortunate com-plication in the United Kingdom (Wooley and Roe) [78] that adversely affected the development of regional anesthesia in that country for several decades.

Mechanism of action of local anesthetics in nerve block therapy

Since local anesthetics are the drugs commonly used in the performance of nerve blocks, it is appropriate to consider, at this juncture, their mechanism of action. Under normal conditions, various stimuli may exceed a given minimum potential (known as the resting potential) and initiate the develop-ment of an action potential that travels orthodromically along the axonal fiber of a sensory or afferent nerve. At the end of the nerve, a synapse with another nerve or with a muscle (neuromuscular junction) occurs. To facilitate con-tinued activation and response to the original stimulus, a neurotransmitter is released. This is usually acetylcholine and it may act on the motor end plate or on the dendrites of another nerve. It is very likely that a number of other neuropeptides and vasoactive substances (secondary messengers) may inhibit or potentiate this basic action. Nevertheless, the primary effect of local anesthetics is to inhibit the generation of an action potential, thereby pro-ducing conduction blockade. The conduction blockade not only affects sensory nerves, but also motor and sympathetic nerves. The schema (Table 12-1) pro-posed by Covino [28] is a logical approach to consider the sequence of events in local anesthetic-induced conduction blockade:

SEQUENCES OF EVENTS OF LOCAL ANESTHETIC BLOCK

To accomplish these physiological events, local anesthetics block impulses by interfering with the function of sodium channels and consequently nerve depolarization and conduction blockade. In effect, local anesthetics convert these critical sodium channels from a preblock active state into an inactivated state during which the conduction of normal action potential ceases. From a molecular standpoint, the mechanism of action of local anesthetics is much

Table 12-1. Sequence of events in local anesthetic-induced conduction blockade.

BINDING OF LOCAL ANESTHETIC MOLECULES TO RECEPTOR SITES IN
THE NERVE MEMBRANE
↓
REDUCTION IN SODIUM PERMEABILITY
↓
DECREASE IN THE RATE OF DEPOLARIZATION
↓
FAILURE TO ACHIEVE THRESHOLD POTENTIAL LEVEL
↓
LACK OF DEVELOPMENT OF A PROPAGATED ACTION POTENTIAL
↓
CONDUCTION BLOCKADE

more complex than outlined above. However, for purposes of this chapter, this simple outline would suffice. The various local anesthetics have different effects in blocking the transmission of nociceptive stimuli, depending on their individual pharmacological characteristics. The pharmacological characteristics that may influence the activity of local anesthetics include molecular structure, pKA or dissociation constant, lipid solubility, protein binding, intrinsic vasodilation activity, tissue diffusibility, and rate of drug biodegradation. Other factors that may also affect the quality and duration of a nerve block may be the site of nerve block, the concentration and total mass of drug used, and the presence or absence of a vasoconstrictor or other adjuvant.

In the operating room setting where nerve blocks are administered for regional anesthesia, the course and duration of a nerve block is more predictable. This predictability may be altered by hepatic disease, cardiac disease, renal disease, and also by drug interactions in patients taking diverse medications. In the setting of the pain clinic, where local anesthetics are used in nerve block administration to treat chronic pain patients, the duration of analgesia is even more unpredictable. There are many explanations for the phenomenon. The inherent neurophysiological properties of nervous tissue and the pathophysiological effects induced by chronic and sustained nociceptive stimuli on these tissues may produce biochemical changes that ultimately affect the "normal" action of local anesthetics. In these patients, behavioral implications of chronic pain may produce psychogenic effects that alter the perception of and reaction to pain. These events serve to emphasize the concept that the psychological (as well as medical) evaluation of the chronic pain patient is necessary in order to attempt to determine all aspects of the pain process.

Complications of nerve block therapy

When properly conducted under ideal conditions, nerve blocks are relatively safe and complication-free. At the outset, it is important to differentiate between side effects of a properly conducted nerve block and complications of a nerve block. This difference becomes important in obtaining informed consent prior to performing a nerve block and has important medicolegal significance. For example, the droopy eyelid, red eye, hoarseness, nasal stuffiness, and warm face following a stellate ganglion block may be occasionally unpleasant but are anticipated side effects of this block, while convulsions and hypotension are complications of a stellate ganglion block. Side effects are normal and expected, whereas complications are abnormal and undesirable. However, these may occur following nerve blocks by the most experienced personnel and should be explained with compassion to the patient as part of the process of informed consent.

Prior to the performance of a nerve block, information should be obtained to determine the presence of bleeding diatheses. In the presence of any doubt or if the patient had been taking anticoagulants in the recent past, appropriate coagulation studies should be performed. Some diseases, e.g., porphyria, hemophilia, Christmas disease, pyoderma gangrenosum, etc., may preclude the administration of nerve blocks. Major neurological complications may occur in these patient groups secondary to the effects of accumulating hematoma following nerve blocks.

The more common complications of nerve blocks include the following:

A. Central nervous system effects
    1. Tinnitus, circumoral numbness, dizziness, visual disturbances, numbness of tongue with metallic taste
    2. Loss of consciousness
    3. Convulsion
    4. Coma
    5. Respiratory arrest
B. Cardiovascular system effects [29]
    1. Hypotension
    2. Bradycardia
    3. Arrhythmias
    4. Cardiac muscle toxicity
    5. Peripheral vascular collapse
    6. Cardiac arrest
C. Allergic effects [30]
    1. Anaphylactic reactions
    2. True allergic reactions
    3. Hypersensitivity reactions
    4. Idiosyncratic reactions
    5. Vasovagal reactions
D. Local tissue effects
    1. Prolonged paresthesia and other sensory and motor deficits (especially following 2-chloroprocaine)
    2. Muscle atrophy (following bupivacaine) [31]
    3. Methemoglobinemia (following prilocaine)
    4. Infection (following poor sterile technique)

All these complications can be usually prevented by meticulous attention to technical details. Further, most of these complications are completely reversible if diagnosed early, treated promptly, and managed with professional competence.

SPECIFIC NERVE BLOCKS

This section of the chapter deals with specific nerve blocks; their applications, indications, and unique characteristics; and potential complications. The application of these nerve blocks in the setting of a multidisciplinary pain clinic is proposed as a supplement to the many modalities that may be used to manage chronic pain. There are some conditions for which a particular nerve block is specifically indicated, e.g., suprascapular nerve block for the patient with the "frozen shoulder" or adhesive capsulitis, while in other situations nerve blocks may represent a component of a group of modalities to treat a given pain syndrome, e.g., chronic low back pain. Nerve blocks are expected to assume an expanded role in the prevention of chronic pain. The works of Woolf [32], Wall [33], Kehlet [34], and Cousins [35] demonstrate that preoperative nerve blocks and immediate postinjury nerve blocks play a significant role in preventing the development of chronic pain. These studies and others would enhance the role of nerve blocks in the algologist's armamentarium for the prophylactic management of chronic pain.

Sympathetic nerve blocks

The significance of the autonomic nervous system, and in particular the sympathetic nervous system, in pain mechanisms is indisputable. The manipulation of that system is utilized directly and indirectly by sympathetic nerve blocks in an attempt to inhibit or control nociception. The specific mechanisms of action of these nerve blocks are not clearly understood. Several theories have been proposed [36,37]. Recent studies propose that pain is mediated through the sympathetic nervous system [38]. It has been demonstrated that some pain originating from the upper abdominal viscera and the gastrointestinal tract as far as the descending colon can be relieved by celiac plexus block. Sympathetic efferent and afferent nerves both play roles in mediating pain in different viscera. Further, sympathetic nerve endings may release a variety of neurotransmitters, including vasoactive compounds, e.g., bradykinin, vasoactive intestinal peptide, tachykinins, etc., as a response to tissue inflammation, injury, and pain. These compounds, through a variety of diverse mechanisms, increase the sensitivity of peripheral nociceptors. They may also produce profound microcirculatory changes that may disrupt the biochemical environment and enhance nociceptor activity [39]. Consequently, it is reasonable and feasible to propose that sympathetic blocks may reverse the deleterious effects induced by autonomic dysfunction, and ultimately decrease pain. It is important to stress that there are several factors that partially or totally contradict the validity of that premise.

Sympathetic blocks [40] may be administered at three levels and may influence the following organs:

1. Stellate ganglion block or cervico-thoracic ganglion block:
   This block may affect sympathetic distribution to the brain, eye, ear salivary glands, heart, lungs, neck, and upper extremity.
2. Paravertebral lumbar sympathetic block:
   This block interferes with the sympathetic innervation to the urogenital organs, gastrointestinal tract from the transverse colon to the rectum, skin, and vessels of the lower extremities.
3. Celiac plexus block:
   This block impacts upon the sympathetic innervation to the gastrointestinal as far distal as the transverse colon, pancreas, liver, spleen, and major abdominal vessels.

Stellate ganglion block

The stellate ganglion is formed by the union (partial or complete) of the inferior cervical ganglion and the first thoracic ganglion, and is most frequently located in the proximity of the anterior tubercle of the transverse process of the seventh cervical vertebra. The sympathetic nerve supply to the head, neck, and upper extremities exit the spinal cord via the ventral roots from the first through sixth thoracic segments. Their cell bodies originate in the intermediolateral columns of the spinal cord and run separately as white rami communicantes towards the cervical sympathetic chain. The cervical sympathetic chain consists of a superior cervical ganglion, a middle cervical ganglion, an intermediate cervical ganglion, and an inferior cervical ganglion. The efferent preganglionic sympathetic fibers converge on the stellate ganglion, but several fibers bypass it, seeking other cervical sympathetic ganglia. This anomalous situation probably accounts for failure to demonstrate signs of a successful block despite apparent accurate anatomical placement of the needle.

The commonly accepted technique for stellate ganglion block is the anterior paratracheal technique [41]. This technique involves the placement of the needle just lateral to the trachea at the cricoid cartilage or sixth cervical vertebra level. This placement should bring the needle in contact with the anterior tubercle of the transverse process of the sixth cervical vertebra. (Chassaignac's tubercle). Prior to the performance of this block, the carotid artery is indentified and retracted laterally along with the anterior border of the sternocleido-mastoid muscle. The two fingers used to retract the carotid artery laterally serve to stretch the tissues in the neck so that only fat and subcutaneous tissue remain present between the skin and Chassaignac's tubercle. Consequently, the insertion of the needle should not exceed 1 cm after puncturing the skin in average-sized patients. A clean puncture with a perpendicularly placed needle minimizes trauma to the periosteum of the transverse process and decreases the incidence of transverse process osteitis.

Positioning of the patient becomes very important, especially in patients with short, muscular necks. A rolled sheet placed between the scapulae provides extension of the neck and facilitates accurate needle placement. The vertebral artery is in close proximity to the stellate ganglion, thus puncture of the vertebral artery is always possible during the performance of a stellate ganglion block. Less than 1 ml of local anesthetic injected into the vertebral artery (which goes directly to the posterior fossa of the brain) may produce a rapid onset of grand mal convulsions, which could evolve into cardiovascular collapse. Therefore, the injection of the local anesthetic should not be a bolus-type injection but a process of 1 ml injection followed by careful sequential aspiration of the luer-lok syringe containing the local anesthetic. At the earliest observation of blood in the syringe, the injection is discontinued, the needle removed, and the patient is meticulously observed for central nervous system (seizures) and cardiovascular system (hypotension and cardiac arrest) complications associated with injection of the vertebral artery. As a prophylactic measure, at our institution the patient is asked to count during the injection and to inform the physician of any subjective perception of tinnitus, dizziness, vertigo, or metallic taste. These prodromal signs (especially tinnitus) usually herald the onset of seizures. The treatment of these complications is intravenous thiopental or diazepam, along with thorough cardiorespiratory monitoring.

Although the stellate ganglion is located at the C7 level, the ganglion is blocked by introducing the needle at the C6 level. This maneuver eliminates pneumothorax as a complication, since the stellate ganglion is close to the apex of the lung, especially on the right side. A volume of 10–15 ml of 0.25% bupivacaine is the author's preference to block the stellate ganglion; the local anesthetic spreads inferiorly beneath the prevertebral fascia to eventually block the stellate ganglion. Thus, the term *cervico-thoracic sympathetic block* is more appropriate than stellate ganglion block. The signs of a successful stellate ganglion block include Horner's syndrome (meiosis, enophthalmos, and ptosis), unilateral nasal congestion, conjunctival engorgement, anhydrosis, and ipsilateral plethora of the face, neck, and upper extremity. In our institution, stellate ganglion blocks are used frequently for treating reflex sympathetic dystrophy [42], herpes zoster [43], postherpetic neuralgia, Raynaud's disease and Raynaud's phenomenon, vascular insufficiency states, phantom limb, diabetic neuropathy, causalgia, unilateral headache [44], and Pancoast tumor with upper extremity pain. In pediatric patients, stellate ganglion blocks may be performed for treatment of the Romano-Ward (prolonged Q-T) syndrome [45] and for arteriovenous malformations of the subclavian system [46]. In these patients, some intravenous sedation may be desirable and the dose of the local anesthetic is decreased according to the infant's body weight.

Stellate ganglion blocks are associated with the following complications: grand mal seizures following intravascular injection; hypotension, cardiorespiratory arrest following intrathecal injection; cardiovascular collapse following intravenous injection; transverse process osteitis, protracted hoarseness, pneumothorax, hematoma of the neck, brachial plexus block, and phrenic nerve block.

Paravertebral lumbar sympathetic block

Lumbar sympathetic blocks are performed for the same clinical indications as stellate ganglion blocks when these lesions are in the lower abdomen and in the lower extremities. There are several techniques described for blocking the lumbar sympathetic chain. This block was first described by Mandl in 1926 and involved a two-needle technique. This technique is almost obsolete nowadays, since it has been demonstrated that if one needle is introduced in the correct fascial plane, a satisfactory block of the lumbar sympathetic ganglia may be obtained. The author prefers the paravertebral technique using a single needle at the L2 level. This level is indentified by finding the intercristal (Tuffier's) line, i.e., L4 neural spine or the L4–5 interspace and counting upwards to L2, or more reliably, by drawing a perpendicular line from the distal end of the 12th rib to the midline spinous process. This latter technique of locating L2 is more reliable in patients with six lumbar vertebrae. Figure 12-2 shows the location of the lumbar sympathetic chain in relation to the vertebral body, aorta, inferior vena cava, and the psoas major muscle.

The needle is inserted at the L2 level approximately 3–4 cm from the midline. If the needle comes into contact with the transverse process, this is an indication that the needle is approximately at the halfway mark. The needle is then partially withdrawn and redirected cephalad or caudad while remaining as

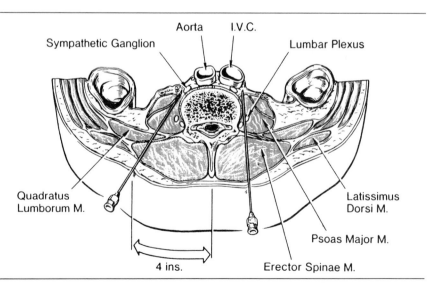

Figure 12-2. Cross-section of posterior back region showing sympathetic ganglia in relation to the major vessels, the psoas major muscle, and the vertebral body. (Reprinted with permission).

close as possible to the vertebral body. In that direction, the needle (a 6-inch, 22-gauge needle with a serrated hub) traverses the psoas major muscle to enter the potential space beyond the prevertebral fascia containing the sympathetic ganglia and the great vessels. This potential space is identified by a "give" that is felt during the advance of the needle. This sensation is facilitated by the serrated hub of the needle and the position is confirmed by a loss of resistance technique. The sympathetic ganglia are blocked with 20 ml of 0.25% bupivacaine. As in the stellate ganglion block, the injection of the local anesthetic is not a bolus injection but a technique of 2-ml aliquot injections followed by sequential aspirations. This technique is necessary since the needle position may be altered during the course of the injection. Of course, prior to the initial injection, careful needle aspiration is carried out to ensure that the needle tip is not inadvertently located in a vessel or viscus.

The traditional indications for lumbar sympathetic block include reflex sympathetic dystrophy, causalgia, lower extremity herpes zoster and postherpetic neuralgia, vascular insufficiency of the lower extremity, low back pain radiating to a lower extremity, diabetic neuropathy affecting the lower extremities, phantom limb pain, stump pain, frostbite, brown recluse spider bite, ulcers, and acrocyanosis.

The complications of lumbar sympathetic blocks include inadvertent intravascular injection associated with seizures, hypotension, and circulatory collapse; renal trauma (especially in patients with undiagnosed horseshoe kidney or polycystic kidney); subarachnoid or epidural injection with cardiorespiratory arrest; lumbar somatic nerve block with temporary (4–6 hours) paresis of the leg; neuralgia of the somatic nerve, especially the genitofemoral nerve; perforation of the intervertebral disc; and, very rarely, infection. This latter complication may occur following use of a continuous catheter technique for prolonged lumbar sympathetic block.

Celiac plexus block

Celiac plexus block is commonly used initially as a diagnostic and prognostic block in patients with carcinoma of the pancreas [47]. If the block with local anesthetic produces adequate pain relief in patients with terminal pancreatic carcinoma, then a neurolytic (therapeutic) celiac plexus block is administered. Unfortunately, this block is not as effective in patients with chronic pancreatitis, although there have been reports of efficacy of celiac plexus block when depot steroids were mixed with local anesthetics in that patient group.

The technique for celiac plexus block is almost the same as for lumbar sympathetic, except for four important differences [48]: First, the block is performed at the T12–L1 level; second, if the transverse process is encountered during the performance of the block, the needle is withdrawn and redirected caudad (never cephalad) to avoid pneumothorax by perforating the crus of the diaphragm; third, a volume of 30 ml of local anesthetic is used; and fourth, the injection site is slightly closer to the midline (approximately

2–3 cm) than in paravertebral lumbar sympathetic block. The author's preference of local anesthetic is 0.25% bupivacaine, since that concentration provides optimal sympathetic block with minimal sensory and motor blockade. There is considerable controversy regarding needle placement or even the number of needles to be used. Moore [49] advocates a three-needle technique. This technique, however, has been demonstrated to be unnecessary, since accurate placement in the correct fascial plane results in adequate caudad and cephalad distribution of the local anesthetic. This phenomenon has been adequately demonstrated by several investigators using contrast media studies. Other clinicians have proposed a more lateral placement (greater than 12 cm) of the needle to block the celiac plexus. This approach, however, is unfortunately associated with a high incidence of renal trauma.

There are other indications for celiac plexus block. These include chronic pain secondary to colon, liver, and spleen, and stomach pathology. It has been reported to be effective in controlled liver carcinoma pain. Complications of celiac plexus block may resemble those complications of lumbar sympathetic block, but the former may be more severe, because a larger volume of drug is used and because the celiac plexus lies in close proximity to the diaphragm and the aorta. The specific complications include intravascular injection with hypotension and cardiovascular collapse; subarachnoid, epidural, and intramuscular (intrapsoas) injections; retroperitoneal hematoma; renal damage; pneumothorax; temporary paresis of the lower extremities; sexual dysfunction (rare); and infection (very rare).

Epidural steroid injection

In the average multidisciplinary pain clinic, back pain accounts for approximately 40–60% of all patients seeking treatment. Back pain may be classified anatomically according to the corresponding vertebrae (or more precisely, spinal segments) where the pain originates. Thus, back pain may be cervical, thoracic, lumbar, or sacrococcygeal. After comprehensive medical evaluation and psychological assessment of the chronic back pain patient, a plan of management is usually outlined. One of the modalities frequently prescribed in appropriate patients includes the epidural steroid injection. The more common indications for epidural steroid use include cervical and lumbosacral radiculopathy; nonspecific trauma degenerative and inflammatory lesions of the ligaments, muscles, tendons, and joints of the vertebral column; and in particular, discogenic disease.

Lievre [50] first introduced hydrocortisone into the epidural space in 1957, and since that time the practice has proliferated. It is almost accepted as standard practice in medicine today. Unfortunately, many of the earlier discoveries were not exposed to the rigorous standards enforced by contemporary scientific methods. Fortunately, this deficiency is being corrected and many studies are currently underway (or have recently been concluded) to investigate the efficacy and mechanisms of epidural steroids in back pain. The initial speculations were that epidural steroids were effective because of an antiinflammatory effect resulting in decreased pressure of the protruding discs on the spinal nerves. This concept was partially dispelled by Wilson [51], who found that 37% of patients with myelographic evidence of disc protrusion did not have any pain. Other investigators [52] showed that the disc narrowing, spur formation, and facet joint sclerosis were not necessarily good predictors of back pain. However, the antiinflammatory concept still persists, and the membrane-stabilizing effects of steroids are espoused as promoting edema reduction of inflamed tissues and resolution of chronic back pain.

The various degenerative phenomena of the vertebral column include disc protrusion producing inflammation and irritation of the nerve roots with resulting hyperemia, swelling, and secretion of a variety of nociceptive substances. These nociceptive substances produce pain via a number of neuro-humoral mechanisms. Steroids may directly inhibit this process through a possible mechanism of increasing phospholipase A2 activity, which enhances the fatty acid substrate that is necessary for the production of arachidonic acid and its subsequent cascade. Dirksen et al. [53] recently proposed the presence of "steroid receptors" in the spinal cord and that steroids may have a direct analgesic effect at the spinal level. Notwithstanding, none of these theories has been fully tested, and much more work needs to be done to explore and validate these concepts.

The injection of steroids into the epidural space may facilitate pain relief in a variety of chronic back pain syndromes, including nerve root entrapment, discogenic disease, spondylolisthesis, degenerative arthritis, and a variety of trauma and sports-related injuries to the vertebral column. As in other chronic pain syndromes, comprehensive medical psychological evaluation should be carried out and appropriate modalities instituted to meet the needs of a particular patient. In patients with chronic benign back pain, physical therapy, stress control, narcotic detoxification, occupational therapy, biofeedback, and patient education are usually always necessary. Epidural steroids should be injected as close as possible to the site of the nerve root lesion, and this may be in the 1) cervical region, 2) thoracic region, 3) lumbar region, and 4) sacrococcygeal region. Three milliliters of 4% methylprednisolone (depot-medrol) suspended in 7 ml of 0.25% bupivacaine may be injected in any region of the epidural space. In older patients (older than 60 years) or immunocompromised patients, the dose of methylprednisolone should be decreased. Great care should be employed to make sure that the subarachnoid-dural membrane is not inadvertently punctured. The steroids contain certain preservatives [54] (polyethylene glycol and myristyl-gamma-picolinium chloride) that may produce irreversible neurotoxic changes in the spinal cord and its associated neural structures. Thus, intrathecal steroid injections are to be avoided at all costs. Another steroid that may be used for epidural injection with local anesthetic is triamcinolone diacetate (Aristocort®). There are a variety of protocols for epidural steroid injections utilized with diverse outcomes. The author's preference is based on a consideration of the potential complications that may occur. After the first epidural injection, the patient is cautioned that the pain may worsen when the local anesthetic effect wears off. Approximately 2 weeks later, the "steroid effect" may become manifest and pain relief may occur. Nevertheless, the patient is evaluated about 3–4 weeks after the first injection. If there has been no pain relief, an alternative modality is implemented. If there is some pain relief but still unacceptable residual pain, the epidural steroid injection is repeated. In general, if repeat injections may become necessary because of recurrence of pain, attempts are made to restrict epidural injections to three or fewer per year.

Complications of epidural steroid injections [55] include inadvertent intrathecal injection with consequent meningeal irritation and arachnoiditis, transient bladder paralysis, cauda equina syndrome, steroid psychosis, suppression of adrenal function, and conus medulla syndrome. Meticulous attention to proper technique almost always eliminates these potential complications.

Intrathecal and epidural opiates

Intrathecal and epidural opiate injections are used perioperatively for intraoperative and postoperative analgesia. Intrathecal opiate analgesia was first described by Wang [27] in 1979, and soon afterwards reports of complications were frequently described. These complications included early-, and more ominously, late-onset respiratory arrest, nausea, vomiting, pruritus, and urinary retention. Pharmacological developments of new narcotic analgesic drugs and greater understanding of the lipophilicity of these drugs has to a more effective utilization for both intraoperative and postoperative applications. Recently, a mixture of a lowered concentration of narcotic analgesic and lowered concentration of local anesthetic has been safely and effectively administered via both the epidural and the intrathecal routes. Nevertheless, careful monitoring is still necessary, although the reported incidence of undesirable side effects is markedly reduced. This application is somewhat limited for chronic pain management. However, as catheter technology, delivery systems, and pump devices are improved, the role of intrathecal and epidural opiates with or without supplemental drugs could expand in chronic pain management, especially in cancer pain management.

It is appropriate to discuss at this point the differential spinal block and its place (or the lack of it) in chronic pain management. The differential spinal block [56] has possible diagnostic applications in the evaluation of some chronic pain syndromes. This proposal is based on the work of Gasser and Erlanger [79], who showed that nerve fibers of different sizes are blocked by different concentrations of local anesthetics. In support of their findings, they used the cathode ray oscilloscope to demonstrate that individual nerve fibers in a peripheral nerve had different conduction velocities and that these properties were directly related to the individual fiber size. The implications of these findings were that different fibers had specific functions and that these fibers may be blocked by different local anesthetic concentrations. Thus, the classification of the individual components of a peripheral nerve into the following fibers: A-alpha, A-beta, A-gamma, A-delta, and B- and C-fibers made more anatomical and physiological sense.

The fundamental premise of the differential spinal block is that different concentrations of local anesthetic may selectively block specific nerves. In theory, the premise is sound; in practice, it is cumbersome, time consuming, and subject to manipulation by the patient and the physician. Thus, the modified differential spinal block has been proposed and may have a place in the anesthesiologist/algologist's armamentarium for the evaluation of selected pain syndromes, including pelvic pain, perineal pain, and sacrococcygeal pain. The author has used the modified differential spinal block to investigate and subsequently treat psychogenic pain in a young soldier who developed hysterical conversion reactions following an emotional crisis. Two milliliters of normal saline produced a dramatic decrease in back and leg pain, and increased motor function in a man who had suddenly developed unexplained back and lower extremity associated with motor dysfunction. Further, there are some patients who continue to have pain in spite of complete motor and sensory block with 1.0% procaine. It is proposed that this phenomenon is due to a "central" mechanism called encephalization, occasionally seen in phantom limb pain and various forms of neuropathic pain.

Intravenous regional sympathetic block

The First and Second World Wars produced a series of traumatic injuries in some wounded soldiers who developed chronic pain syndromes. These syndromes posed major clinical problems for the physicians who attempted to treat those veterans. It was in these patients that John Bonica [58] saw that conventional medicine was ineffective in treating the pain, and he accordingly proposed the concept of the multidisciplinary pain clinic. Further, he advocated sympathetic blocks to treat these patients with sympathetically mediated pain, e.g., reflex sympathetic dystrophy, causalgia, etc. The intravenous regional sympathetic block is a form of sympathetic block that is localized to a particular extremity.

Intravenous regional anesthesia was first described by August Bier in 1908 and was used as anesthesia for surgery of the hand. In 1974, Hannington-Kiff [59] used guanethidine to perform localized sympathetic blocks of the upper and lower extremities. The block is performed by exsanguinating the extremity after inserting a needle or catheter into the dorsum of the hand (or foot). The exsanguination process is accomplished by elevating the extremity and using an esmarch bandage distally and moving proximally. A pneumatic cuff is used proximally to maintain a pressure of 100 torr above the preblock systolic pressure. Guanethidine is injected intravenously and produces a sympathetic block by depleting norepinephrine in the peripheral nerve endings of the affected extremity. Guanethidine is not yet available in the United States (but is widely used in Europe). Thus, alternative agents must be used to produce sympathetic blocks in this technique. Reserpine [60] has been used previously, but the parenteral form is not currently manufactured in the United States. Clonidine [61], prazocin [62], bretylium [63], and labetalol [64] have been used by different investigators with varying success. The author's preference for intravenous regional sympathetic block (Bier block) of the upper extremity is labetalol 10 mg, 0.125% bupivacaine 25 ml, heparin 500 IU, and hydrocortisone 100 mg. The dose is doubled for the lower extremity. The pneumatic cuff is maintained inflated for 15–20 minutes after injection. The results obtained with labetalol in patients with reflex sympathetic dystrophy are satisfactory.

Intravenous regional sympathetic block is best utilized for the early management of sympathetically mediated pain, especially when prior stellate ganglion blocks have been ineffective. It is also used in patients who develop "postsurgical sympathectomy escape," in patients who refuse stellate ganglion blocks, in patients on anticoagulant medication, and in situations when stellate ganglion blocks are contraindicated.

Neurolytic blocks

Neurolysis [65] is a technique that ultimately produces destruction of nerve fibers and specific histological alteration of neuronal tissues. These histological changes include Wallerian degeneration, alteration of endoneurial blood supply, increasing endoneurial fluid pressure, changes in endoneurial electrolyte concentration, and increasing perineurial edema. The net effect of all these pathophysiological changes is disruption of normal and abnormal (or in the case of chronic pain patients) sensory or motor function. One of the major advantages of neurolysis over surgical transection of nerves is that in neurolysis the basal lamina around the Schwann cell tube, i.e., the bands of Büngner, remain intact, allowing for the normal and unimpaired regeneration of nerve fibers. In surgical nerve transection, these bands of Büngner are absent and the formation of uncontrolled neuromas occur, this phenomenon results in unacceptable postsurgical, neuroma-induced pain.

There are a variety of neurolytic agents and neurolytic techniques that produce the same basic effect via variations of the same basic mechanism. The ultimate result is alteration of sensory or motor dysfunction that produces pain relief. The neurolytic agents most commonly used in pain management are 6% phenol in glycerine or absolute alcohol. Other neurolytic agents include 50% glycerol, ammonium salts (sulfate, chloride, or hydroxide), chlorocresol, benzyl alcohol, bromsalizol, hypertonic solutions (saline), and hypotonic solutions. Neurolytic techniques include the use of the cryoprobe to "freeze" that portion of the nerve in contact with the probe, hyperthermic techniques, pressure application, and laser irradiation. There may be specific indications that may be appropriate for a particular technique. However, a general principle is that neurolysis may be associated with permanent and occasionally unacceptable motor, sensory, and visceral dysfunction, and the patient and his/her family should be aware of these potential complications. Thus, informed consent must always be obtained and properly documented prior to the neurolytic procedure. Neurolysis is, therefore, usually reserved for patients with terminal carcinoma.

In the author's practice, there are two neurolytic procedures that are frequently performed with satisfying results, both to the patient and the physician. These procedures include a neurolytic celiac plexus block for terminal carcinoma of the pancreas, and to a lesser extent, neurolytic caudal epidural block for some cases of terminal carcinoma of rectum, prostate, ovary, cervix, and uterus. The celiac plexus block is first performed with local anesthetics (30 ml of 0.25% bupivacaine), and if adequate analgesia is obtained consistently after two or three nerve blocks, then a neurolytic celiac plexus block using radiological control is performed. In our practice 20–30 ml of 6% phenol in 10% glycerine is used for neurolysis of the celiac plexus. Other clinicians used 50–90% alcohol with great success. However, absolute alcohol may cause an excruciating burning sensation on rejection, and this is due to alcoholic neuritis.

Patients with terminal carcinoma of the prostate, ovary, uterus, cervix, and rectum may develop severe lumbar-sacral pain due to metastatic bony involvement or to direct tumor invasion. A caudal epidural block with 15–20 ml of 0.25% bupivacaine may provide adequate pain relief to approximately 30–40% of these patients. If this pain control can be consistently reproduced, then a neurolytic caudal epidural block with 6% phenol in 10% glycerine is performed. An alternative procedure to the neurolytic caudal epidural block is the neurolytic transacral block. This procedure is particularly useful for patients with terminal carcinoma of the rectum.

Trans-sphenoidal chemical hypophysectomy [66] is performed with increasing frequency for patients with intractable pain in several locations produced by disseminated metastatic carcinoma, usually of the breast, thyroid, bronchus, and prostate. Hypophysectomy may be accomplished by open transcranial surgical technique, open microsurgical technique, transnasal cryoprobe, or transnasal alcohol injection. The technique employed does not affect the quality of the analgesia obtained. Therefore, the least invasive technique, i.e. transnasal or trans-sphenoidal hypophysectomy, is most desirable. For neurolysis, 0.4–2.0 ml of absolute alcohol is usually administered. For this technique, light general anesthetic with endotracheal intubation is used, and the procedure is done using a Todd-Wells stereotaxic head holder with the patient in the supine position. The mechanism of action of transsphenoidal chemical hypophysectomy is unclear. Clinical observations support the hypothesis that the resulting pain relief may be due to a stimulation of a hypothalamic pain-suppressing response, while other theories postulate the involvement of the endogenous opioid system. The complications of this procedure may be serious but, fortunately, they are usually transient (2–5 days) when present. These include epistaxia, pupillary dilation, drowsiness, neuritis, rhinorrhea, headache, blurred vision, and focal sensory or motor deficit. Diabetes insipidus does occur, but not with the anticipated frequency one might expect given the nature of the procedure.

Other neurolytic blocks have been used to manage intractable pain, but the complications of these procedures are high and generally unacceptable, even in the patient with terminal carcinoma. As other modalities, techniques, and drugs are developed and successfully used in pain management, less reliance on neurolytic blocks would occur. For example, the development of long-acting morphine (M.S. Contin®) enables a patient to take one tablet for approximately 12 hours of pain relief. This is made possible by the development of M.S. Contin in strengths of 15, 30, 60, and 100 mg. The development of substance P antagonists [67] and a newer generation of parenteral nonsteroidal antiinflammatory drugs may revolutionize neurolytic procedures and render some of the more invasive ones obsolete. The subarachnoid and epidural neurolytic blocks, along with cranial nerve blocks, may possibly become procedures of historical interest rather than practical use.

Nerve blocks of the chest wall

Chest pain is fairly common in patients coming to pain clinics. The etiology may include postherpetic neuralgia, post-thoracotomy, or poststernotomy syndromes; chest pain associated with bronchogenic carcinoma (Pancoast's tumor); and, more recently, chest pain associated with HIV-induced pneumonia. As with any other chronic pain syndrome, a complete medical evaluation and psychological evaluation, along with appropriate use of biofeedback, relaxation therapy, group therapy, patient counseling, and education, in addition to selective nerve blocks, are administered to the patient based on diagnostic considerations and personal needs.

Various nerve blocks may be used for the patient with chronic chest pain. For the patient with herpes zoster, postherpetic neuralgia, and sympathetically mediated chest pain cephalad to T4, a stellate ganglion block series may be necessary. For the patient with thoracic back pain, a thoracic epidural steroid injection is a useful modality to use when appropriate. For the patient with chronic chest pain secondary to post-thoracotomy syndrome, a series of intercostal nerve blocks may be effective in controlling the pain. Finally, for the patient with chronic chest pain secondary to poststernotomy syndrome, costochondritis, and HIV-induced pneumonia, interpleural analgesia [68] appears to have some efficacy in controlling the pain. This technique holds great promise for the management of chest pain and some forms of abdominal pain. It is important to stress that interpleural analgesia differs from intercostal nerve blocks in several respects. First, the mechanism of action is different in that splanchnic nerves may be involved in interpleural analgesia. Intercostal blocks provide the highest blood level of local anesthetics in the blood stream and is associated with a relatively high incidence of convulsive activity,

especially when several intercostal nerves are blocked. Moreover, the incidence of pneumothorax is higher in intercostal nerve blocks than in interpleural
analgesia.

Nerve blocks of the upper extremity

The brachial plexus provides almost total innervation to the upper extremity.
The nerve roots contributing to the form the brachial plexus include C5, C6,
C7, C8, and T1. Insignificant contributions do come from C4 and T2, the
latter innervating the axillary floor of the upper extremity. The brachial plexus
can be blocked at four levels: 1) axillary, 2) interscalene, 3) supraclavicular, and
4) infraclavicular [69]. Whereas these techniques are usually applied intraoperatively for surgery on the upper extremity, there are situations involving
patients with severe, unrelenting, chronic pain of the upper extremity when
brachial plexus blocks are used to interrupt the pain cycle and occasionally to
control successfully the pain long after the local anesthetic effect has ceased.
Special mention must be made of the infraclavicular approach to the brachial
plexus, since the technique is very useful when a continuous infusion of the
brachial plexus is indicated. The infraclavicular approach to the brachial plexus
is attained by inserting the needle at a point 1 inch below the midpoint of the
clavicle and directing it laterally towards the brachial artery with the patient
lying supine and the arm abducted to 90°. Paresthesiae indicate successful
placement of the needle, but a neurostimulator may be used in the localization
of this plexus.

Patients with rotator cuff lesions, osteoarthritis of the shoulder, adhesive
capsulitis, and "frozen shoulder" may present with chronic pain of the affected
shoulder area. These lesions may follow trauma or be the result of degenerative disorders of the musculoskeletal tissue in the shoulder region. Pain control
in these patients is best managed with progressive physical therapy preceded
by suprascapular nerve blocks with 4% methylprednisolone (1 ml) and 0.25%
bupivacaine (9 ml). The block is performed with the patient in the sitting
position. A 22-gauge needle is inserted on finger's breath superior to the
midpoint of the spine of the scapula, and the needle is advanced towards the
suprascapular notch until a paresthesia is elicited in the affected shoulder. One
of the complications of this procedure is pneumothorax, which may occur by
inadvertent puncture of the posterior chest wall between the ribs. Parris [70]
has described a technique of blocking the suprascapular nerve while minimiz-
ing or eliminating the incidence of pneumothorax. This technique involves the
placement of the hand on the side being blocked on the opposite shoulder after
the needle has been advanced 3–4 mm in the correct location. After the hand
placement, the needle advancement is continued until shoulder paresthesia is
elicited. This movement of the hand unto the opposite shoulder raises the
scapula from the posterior chest wall, thus increasing the distance from the
suprascapular notch to the chest; this effectively eliminates or decreases the
incidence of pneumothorax (Figures 12-3 and 12-4). The median, ulnar, and

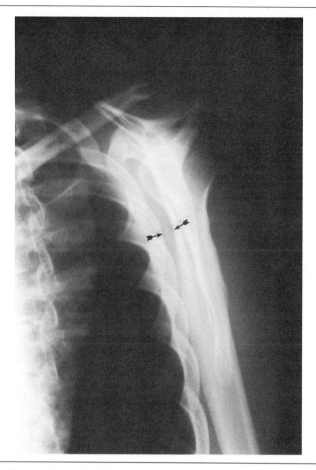

Figure 12-3. Chest radiograph: oblique view (with arm in the anatomical position), showing distance between chest wall and scapula. (Reprinted with permission).

radial nerves can be blocked, usually at the elbow, but occasionally at the wrist for a variety of pain syndromes. Those syndromes usually include postsurgical incisional pain, various peripheral neuropathic states, and neuropraxia. Further, these nerve blocks are useful in "salvaging" regional anesthetic procedures intraoperatively.

Nerve blocks of the lower extremity

The nerve supply to the lower extremity emanates from the anterior primary rami of L4, L5, S1, S2, and S3. The nerve roots form the lumbar-sacral plexus and the major nerves of that plexus: The sciatic, femoral, obturator, and lateral cutaneous nerve of the thigh can be blocked for specific dermatomal pain. These blocks, as in the nerve blocks of the upper extremity, may be used to

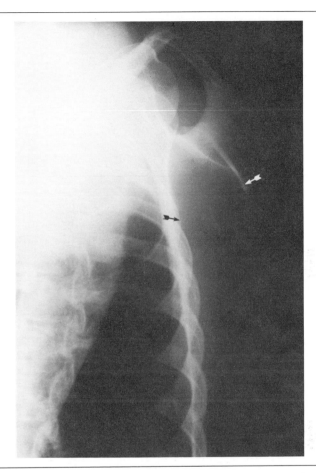

Figure 12-4. Chest radiograph: oblique view (with arm flexed at elbow and placed on opposite shoulder) showing distance between chest wall and scapula. (Reprinted with permission).

interrupt the cycle of pain and to control chronic pain in a region of the lower extremity. Sacral nerves can be accessed by identifying the sacral foramina and injecting local anesthetic (with or without steroids) into these foramina. These blocks are effective in sacral back pain, and neurolytic sacral nerve blocks are used as described above. Genitofemoral and ilioinguinal nerve blocks are used to manage pain following inguinal hernia repairs. Though not always success-ful in managing these pain syndromes, their use is still advocated, since they are relatively noninvasive.

Nerve blocks of the head and neck

Headaches represent approximately 20–25% of the patients seen in an average pain clinic. To reiterate a concept previously mentioned in this chapter (but that cannot be overemphasized), it is important to implement a multidisciplinary approach to the evaluation of the headache patient and to administer the appropriate modalities [71] that may be assessed as necessary for a given patient. Thus, the use of nerve blocks is only one of a group of therapeutic modalities that may be utilized for a given patient. It is not the author's intention to suggest that a given nerve block per se would be the "cure" of a particular headache, although every pain clinician has multiple anecdotal reports of success in treating selective pain syndromes with a particular nerve block.

The complexity of the pathogenesis of most headaches, and the fact that more than one mechanism may be contributing to the headache, makes headache management less than straightforward to implement. There are clinical situations when nerve blocks may be used to effectively control headaches that follow a particular anatomical distribution. These nerve blocks include supraorbital nerve blocks, occipital nerve blocks, and infraorbital nerve blocks. These nerves are superficial in location and usually lie in close proximity to a bony structure, making the block relatively easy to administer. In appropriate cases, thermal neurolysis (cryotherapy) is not difficult to apply. Sphenopalatine block [72] may be administered for sinus headache or other kinds of headache, and is accomplished by instilling pledgets soaked in local anesthetics into the nostrils parallel to the line of the external nose until contact with the superior region of the nasal cavity is made. A second local anesthetic-soaked pledget is inserted horizontally along the floor of the nose until contact with the sphenopalatine fossa is made. Together, these two pledgets can provide excellent block of the sphenopalatine ganglion, possibly producing adequate control of some headaches.

Tic douloureux can be treated in some cases by trigeminal nerve block. If this procedure gives temporary pain relief, then a neurolytic block with glyercol or radiofrequency lesioning of the trigeminal ganglion may be instituted. Some patients with unilateral headache may be treated with a series of stellate ganglion blocks [44] on the same side. The mechanism of action of these blocks on migraine headache is unclear, although an adrenergic mechanism has been postulated [73]. Other nerve blocks of the head and neck region that may have a place in chronic pain management include cervical plexus block, glossopharyngeal nerve block (for pain associated with lesions of the posterior tongue area and for headache secondary to trauma to the styloid process or Eagle's syndrome), and accessory nerve block. This latter block may be used to manage intractable hiccups and torticollis.

MISCELLANEOUS BLOCKS

There are several other nerve blocks that may have a place in the management of chronic pain. As a general rule, nerve blocks are relatively noninvasive and reversible as far as their sensory and motor side effects are concerned. The fascinating and intriguing aspect of nerve blocks is their capacity to produce prolonged pain relief in certain pain syndromes. Thus, nerve blocks will continue to be exploited for this capability, especially as new drugs or new applications of old drugs become available. In the group of miscellaneous nerve blocks, there should be some discussion of epidural blood patch and trigger point injections.

Epidural blood patch

During the performance of an epidural nerve block, following a myelogram and postoperatively after subarachnoid analgesia, patients may experience an acute severe, throbbing headache, occipital or frontal in location, which is aggravated by ambulation and relieved by recumbency; this is the classic post-dural puncture headache. In the first 48 hours of this headache, conservative measures consisting of supine bed rest, oral, or parenteral narcotic analgesics, excessive oral or intravenous fluid administration, and the use of abdominal binders may be applied. If these conservative measures fail, an epidural blood patch [74] is then the standard treatment of choice.

The pathogenesis of post-dural puncture headache is due to loss of cerebrospinal fluid via a hole in the dura and the consequent decrease in the volume and pressure of cerebrospinal fluid. This phenomenon produces sagging of the cerebral tissue with stretching of the meninges and the falx cerebri; these effects produce the post-dural puncture headache. DiGiovanni [75] first demonstrated that the injection of 10–15 ml of aseptically collected autologous blood into the epidural space at or close to the level of the dural "hole" produces almost immediate and sustained cessation of the headache. This is the epidural blood patch. This procedure has a success rate of 90–99%. The mechanism of action of epidural blood patch is not clearly elucidated. Several theories have been postulated. The author's preference is towards some biochemical mechanism given the immediacy of the pain relief. There are a select group of patients who present with headaches similar to those caused by dural puncture but in whom no nerve block or procedure has been performed in or close to the epidural or subarachnoid space. Some of these patients have been successfully treated with the epidural blood patch [76]. The mechanism of action of headache in these patients is also unclear. It is postulated that they have developed low-CSF pressure syndromes secondary to trauma or congenital anomalies of the dural sleeves or extensions along the intervertebral foramina. Thus, epidural blood patch is a reasonable consideration in that difficult headache patient group after other medical, psychogenic, and behavioral factors have been excluded.

Trigger point injection

Chronic pain consists in a large part of musculoskeletal dysfunction, which has been described as myofascial pain syndrome by Travell et al. [77]. Thorough musculoskeletal examination reveals the presence of discreet tender areas that produce pain and discomfort in contiguous (trigger points) or distant areas (target areas). Trigger points are characterized by specific clinical features consisting of palpable nodules, skin-fold hyperesthesia, positive "jump" sign, and increased hyperemia following palpation. These trigger points respond to a variety of biostimulation techniques, including nerve blocks or trigger point injections with local anesthetics with or without steroids. The fact that pain control can be achieved by "dry needling" suggests that the local anesthetic is not a *sine qua non* for adequate pain relief. Thus, other mechanisms (though not clearly understood) are involved. This is further borne out by the fact the acupuncture, acupressure, low-power laser modulation, iontophoresis, transcutaneous electrical nerve stimulation (TENS), and more recently magnetic field therapy have been all successfully used to treat trigger points or myofascial pain syndrome.

In conclusion, chronic pain is a multifaceted syndrome that requires a multimodal strategy to effectively manage these unique patients. Although specific nerve blocks may have a place in treating individual chronic pain syndromes, effective pain relief is never assured. To assist in the management of residual pain or to deal with intractable chronic pain, other modalities may need to be utilized singly or jointly to decrease or eliminate pain, to advance coping skills, to alleviate dependence on the medical system, and to promote the wellness concept. Thus, nerve blocks represent one of several therapeutic modalities that may be used to manage chronic pain. It is hoped that as research and development in pain medicine continue to expand, new techniques, including nerve blocks, will become available to solve the pain puzzle and ultimately to make our patients more pain-free and more comfortable.

REFERENCES

1. Brena SF, Chapman SL (eds). 1985. Chronic Pain: Management Principles. Clinics in Anaesthesiology. Philadelphia, W.B. Saunders, pp. 1–16.
2. Woolf CJ. 1983. Evidence for a central component of post-injury pain hypersensitivity. Nature 306:686–688.
3. Kehlet H. 1989. Surgical stress: The role of pain and analgesia. Br J Anaesth 63:189–195.
4. Handwerker HO. 1990. Pain and inflammation. Pain 5:S217.
5. Cousins MJ, Mather LE (editorial). 1989. Relief of postoperative pain: Advances awaiting application. Med J Aust 150:354–355.
6. Kehlet H. 1988. The stress response to surgery: Release mechanisms and the modifying effect of pain relief. Acta Chir Scand Suppl 550:22–28.
7. Riese W, Arrington GE Jr. 1963. The history of Johannes Müller's doctrine of the specific energies of the senses: Original and later versions. Bull Hist Med 37:179–183.
8. Dallenbach KM. 1939. Pain: History and present status. Am J Psychol 52:331.
9. Rynd F. 1845. Introduction of fluid to the nerve. Dublin Med Press 13:167.
10. Pravaz CG. 1853. Sur un nouveau moyen d'opérer la coagulation du sang dans les artères, applicable à la guérison des anéurismes. CR Acad Sci (Paris) 36:88.
11. Bier A. 1899. Versuche über cocainisirung des rückenmarkes. Dtsch Z Chir 51:361.
12. Standards for cardiopulmonary resusitation (CPR) and emergency cardiac care (ECC) JAMA 227 (Suppl.):883.
13. Ritchie JM, Ritchie B, Greengard P. 1965. The active structure of local anesthetics. J Pharmacol Exp Ther 150:152.
14. Albright GA. 1979. Cardiac arrest following regional anesthesia with etidocaine or bupivacaine. Anesthesiology 51:285.

15. Ravindran RS, Bond VK, Tasch MD, Gupta CD, et al. 1980. Prolonged neural blockade following regional analgesia with 2-chloroprocaine. Anesth Analg 58:447.

16. Lund PC, Cwik JC. 1965. Propitocaine (Citanest) and methemoglobinemia. Anesthesiology, 26:569–571.

17. Brown FW. 1977. Management of diskogenic pain using epidural and intrathecal steroids. Clin Orthop 129:72.

18. Burn JMB, Langdon L. 1970. Lumbar epidural injection for the treatment of chronic sciatica. Rheumatol Phys Med 10:368.

19. Duncan GE, Strumpf WE. 1984. Target neurons for ^{3}H-corticosterone in the rat spinal cord. Brain Res 307:321–326.

20. Green LN. 1975. Dexamethasone in the management of symptoms due to herniated lumbar disc. J Neurol Neurosurg Psychiatry 38:1211.

21. Wilson F. 1981. Neurolytic and other locally acting drugs in the management of pain. Pharmacol Ther 12:599.

22. Woolsey RM, Taylor JJ, Nagel HH. 1972. Acute effects of topical ethyl alcohol on the sciatic nerve of the mouse. Arch Phys Med Rehabil 53:410.

23. Wood KM. 1978. The use of phenol as a neurolytic agent: A review. Pain 5:205.

24. Bengon HT, Chomka CM, Brenner EA. 1980. Treatment of reflex sympathetic dystrophy with regional intravenous reserpine. Anesth Analg 59:500–502.

25. Parris WCV, Misculis KE, Kambam JR, Franks JJ, Dettbarn WD. 1987. Verapamil potentiates bupivacaine-induced neural conduction blockade. Anesth 67(3A):A252.

26. Parris WCV, Nyhuis G, Dirksen R. Unpublished data.

27. Wang JK, Nauss LA, Thomas JE. 1979. Pain relief by intrathecally applied morphine in man. Anesthesiology 50:149–151.

28. Covino BG, Bush DF. 1975. Clinical evaluation of local anesthetic agents. Br J Anaesth 47:289.

29. Blair MR. 1975. Cardiovascular pharmacology of local anaesthetics. Br J Anaesth 47:247.

30. Aldrete JA, Johnson DA. 1970. Evaluation of intracutaneous testing for investigation of allergy to local anesthetic agents. Anesth Analg 49:173.

31. Parris WCV, Dettbarn WD. 1988. Muscle atrophy following bupivacaine trigger point injection. Anesthesiol Rev 16(3):50–53.

32. Woolf CJ. 1983. Evidence for central component of postinjury pain hypersensitivity. Nature 306:686–688.

33. Wall PD. 1988. The prevention of postoperative pain. Pain 33:289–290.

34. Kehlet H. 1984. The stress response to anaesthesia and surgery: Release mechanisms and modifying factors. Clin Anaesth 2:315.

35. Cousins MJ. 1989. Acute and postoperative pain. In PD Wall, R Melzack (eds), Textbook of Pain, 2nd ed. Churchill Livingstone, New York, pp. 284–305.

36. Bryce-Smith R. 1951. Injection of the lumbar sympathetic chain. Anaesthesia 6:150.

37. Bonica JJ. 1953. The Management of Pain. Philadelphia, Lea & Febiger.

38. Levine J, Baubaum A. 1987. The peripheral nervous system and the inflamatory process. Pain Suppl 4:S109.

39. Zimmerman M. 1979. Neurophysiology of nociception. Pain and pain therapy. In JJ Bonica, V Ventafridda (eds), Advances in Pain Research and Therapy. New York, Raven Press.

40. Boas RA. 1978. Sympathetic block in clinical practice. Int Anesthesiol Clin 16(4).

41. Bonica JJ. 1959. Clinical Applications of Diagnostic and Therapeutic Nerve Blocks. Springfield, IL, Charles C. Thomas.

42. Linson MA, Leffert R, Todd DP. 1983. The treatment of upper extremity reflex sympathetic dystrophy with prolonged continuous stellate ganglion blockade. J Hand Surg 8:153.

43. Mayne GE, Brown M, Arnold P, Moya F. 1986. Pain of herpes zoster and postherpetic neuralgia. In PP Raj (ed), Practical Management of Pain, Chicago, Year Book Medical Publishers, pp. 345–361.

44. Parris WCV, Jamison RN, Lin S, Kambam JR. 1988. The use of stellate ganglion blocks in treating unilateral migraine headaches. Regional Anesth 13(1S):78.

45. Yanagida H, Kemi C, Suwa K. 1976. The effects of stellate ganglion block on idiopathic prolongation of the Q-T internal with cardiac arrhythmia (the Romano-Ward syndrome). Anesth Analg 55:782–787.

46. Parris WCV, Reddy B, White H. 1991. Stellate ganglion block in pediatric patients. Anesth Analg 67:993–995.

47. Kune GA, Cole R, Bell S. 1975. Observations on the relief of pancreatic pain. Med J Aust 2:789.
48. Parris WCV. 1985. Nerve block therapy. In SF Brena, SL Chapman (eds), Chronic Pain: Management Principles. Clinics in Anaesthesiology. Philadelphia, W.B. Saunders, pp. 93–109.
49. Moore DC. 1971. Regional Block, 9th ed. Springfield, IL, Charles C. Thomas.
50. Lievre JA, Bloch-Michel H, Attali P. 1957. L'injection trans-sacree: Etude clinique et radiologique. Bull Mem Soc Med Hôp Paris 73:1110–1118.
51. Wilson CB, Hoff JR. 1984. Clinical features and surgical treatment of cervical discogenic radiculopathy and myelopathy. In HK Genant (ed), Spine Update 1984. San Francisco, Radiology Research and Education Foundation, pp. 273–279.
52. Swerdlow M, Sayle-Creer W. 1970. The use of extradural injections in the relief of lumbosciatic pain. Anaesthesia 25:128.
53. Dirksen R, Rutgers MJ, Coolen JM. 1987. Cervical epidural steroids can reflect sympathetic dystrophy. Anesthiology 66:71–73.
54. Delaney TJ, Rowlingson JC, Carron H, et al. 1980. The effects of steroids on nerves and meninges. Anesth Analg 59:610–614.
55. Knight CL, Burnell JC. 1980. Systemic side-effects of extradural steroids. Anaesthesia 35:593.
56. Raymond SA, Gissen AJ. 1986. Differential nerve block. In GR Strichartz (ed), Handbook of Experimental Pharmacology, Vol. 81, Local Anesthetics. New York, Springer-Verlag.
57. Gasser HS, Erlanger J. 1929. Role of fiber size in establishment of nerve block by pressure or cocaine. Am J Physiol 88:581–591.
58. Bonica JJ. 1953. The Management of Pain. Philadelphia, Lea & Febiger.
59. Hannington-Kiff JG. 1970. Intravenous regional sympathetic block with guanethidine. Lancet 1:1019–1020.
60. Bengon HT, Chomka CM, Brenner EA. 1980. Treatment of reflex sympathetic dystrophy with regional intravenous reserpine. Anesth Analg 59:500–502.
61. Yaksh TL, Reddy SVR. 1981. Studies in the primate on the analgetic effects associated with intrathecal actions of opiates, alpha-adrenergic agonists and baclofen. Anesthiology 54: 451–461.
62. Fleetwood-Walker S, Mitchell R, Hope PJ, et al. 1985. An alpha$_2$ receptor mediates the selective inhibition by noradrenaline of nociceptive responses of identified dorsal horn neurones. Brain Res 334:243–254.
63. Ford SR, Forrest WH, Eltherington L. 1988. The treatment of reflex sympathetic dystrophy with intravenous regional bretylium. Anesthesiology 68:137–140.
64. Parris WCV, Harris R, Lindsey K. 1987. Use of intravenous regional labetalol in treating resistant reflex sympathetic dystrophy. Pain 4(Suppl.):S206.
65. Arner S. 1982. The role of nerve blocks in the treatment of cancer pain. Acta Anaesthesiol Scand 74(Suppl.):104.
66. Levin AB, Katz J, Benson RC, Jones AG. 1980. Treatment of pain of diffuse metastatic cancer by stereotactic chemical hypophysectomy: Long term results and observations on mechanism of action. Neurosurgery 6:258.
67. Hanley MR. 1985. Substance P antagonists. In D Bousfield (ed), Neurotransmitters in Action. Elsevier, Amsterdam, pp. 170–172.
68. Kambam JR, Hammon JW, Parris WCV, Lupinetti MD. 1989. Intrapleural analgesia for post-thoracotomy pain and blood levels of bupivacaine following intrapleural injection. Can J Anaesth 36(2):106–109.
69. Raj PP, Montgomery SJ, Nettles D, et al. 1973. Infraclavicular brachial plexus block: A new approach. Anesth Analg 52:897–904.
70. Parris WCV. 1990. Suprascapular nerve block: A safer technique. Anesthesiology 72:580–581.
71. Brena SF. 1985. Pain control facilities: Pattern of operation and problems of organization in the USA. In SF Brena, SL Chapman (eds), Chronic Pain: Management Principles. Clinics in Anaesthesiology. Philadelphia, W.B. Saunders, pp. 183–195.
72. Eagle WW. 1942. Sphenopalatine ganglion neuralgia. Arch Otolaryngol 35:66–70.
73. Moskowitz MA. 1984. The neurobiology of vascular head pain. Ann Neurol 16:157–168.
74. Gormley JB. 1960. Treatment of post spinal headaches. Anesthesiology 21:565–566.
75. Di Giovanni AJ, Galbert MW, Wahle WM. 1972. Epidural injection of autologous blood for post lumbar headache. II. Additional clinical experiences and laboratory investigations. Anesth Analg 51:226–232.

76. Parris WCV. 1987. The use of epidural blood patch in treating chronic headache: Report of six cases. Can J Anaesth 34(4):403–406.
77. Travell J. 1976. Myofascial trigger points: Clinical view. In JJ Bonica, DJ Albe-Fessard, (eds), Advances in Pain Research and Therapy, New York, Raven Press, pp. 919–926.
78. Cope RW. 1954. The Wooley and Roe case. Wooley and Roe vs. the ministry of health and others. Anaesthesia 9:249–270.
79. Gasser HS, Erlanger J. 1929. Role of fiber size in establishment of nerve blocks by pressure or cocaine. AMJ Physiol 88:581–592.

13. MANAGEMENT OF HEADACHE

HOWARD S. KIRSHNER

When you're lying awake with a dismal headache,
and repose is taboo'd by anxiety,
I conceive you may use any language you choose
to indulge in, without impropriety.
                        Gilbert & Sullivan, Iolanthe

Headache is arguably the most common pain syndrome afflicting humankind.
It is estimated that 15–29% of normal people suffer from migraines at some
time during life [1,2], and the stresses of modern life make "tension" or muscle
contraction headaches nearly a universal part of the human condition. Perhaps
for this reason, many headache patients seek to distinguish their headaches
from the "normal headaches" that they or their friends have experienced.
Headaches are caused by a variety of mechanisms, and proper classification
and diagnosis of headache syndromes is essential to proper management. This
chapter will discuss mechanisms of headache pain, differential diagnosis of
headache syndromes, and treatment of the common headache types: migraine
and muscle contraction headaches.

MECHANISMS OF HEADACHE

Any discussion of headache mechanisms must begin with the pain-sensitive,
structures of the head [3,4]. First, the brain parenchyma itself is not pain sensitive, as any neurosurgeon who operates on the awake brain can attest. The

meninges and vessels on the surface of the brain, however, carry nerve endings that are sensitive to pressure, distention, and inflammation. Traction on the dura and distention of venous sinuses or arteries are therefore involved in the pathogenesis of many causes of headache pain. Migraine and related vascular headaches may result from vasospasm and subsequent distention of these vessels, though recent research suggests that the vascular changes may be secondary to changes in neuronal activity within the brain itself. The headaches associated with vasculitis, brain tumors, subdural hematomas, brain abscesses, and meningitis all relate to stimulation of nerve endings within the vascular structures of the meninges. Other pain-sensitive structures in the head include the linings of the nasal sinuses, the teeth and nerve endings of the trigeminal nerve, the temporomandibular joints, and the paraspinal muscles of the neck. The eyes may also be a source of headaches. An ocular source of headaches is clearest in syndromes of increased intraocular pressure, such as glaucoma. "Eyestrain" related to muscle contraction of the extraocular muscles, as in prolonged reading, is debated as a cause of headache. Sustained muscle contraction of the cervical paraspinal muscles, and the frontalis, temporalis, and other muscles of the cranium, may lead to aching, dull pain.

DIFFERENTIAL DIAGNOSIS OF HEADACHE

Acute headaches are often the harbingers of serious neurological disease. The most abrupt of all headaches are those caused by subarachnoid hemorrhage. The classic history involves the sudden onset of the most severe headache of the individual's life. Many of these patients have no history of preexisting headaches, or at least no more than an "ordinary" headache history, but a few have had premonitory, severe headaches. These "sentinel" headaches may reflect minor leaks from an aneurysm, before the main vascular rupture [5,6]. The headache itself is split-second in onset, sometimes accompanied by a brief loss of consciousness, and followed by persistent headache and stiff neck. Focal neurological signs are usually absent, though some patients become stuporous or comatose from the onset. The most common cause of subarachnoid hemorrhage is a ruptured aneurysm. Saccular or "berry" aneurysms are dilatations of cerebral arteries, occurring at sites of bifurcation, almost always in arteries close to the circle of Willis. The most common sites are the internal carotid at the origin of the posterior communicating artery, the anterior cerebral at the origin of the anterior communicating artery, and the middle cerebral artery. The "posterior communicating artery aneurysm," as it is called, often announces its presence by the development of a painful third cranial nerve palsy, usually involving the pupil, even before the aneurysm ruptures. Prompt diagnosis may permit curative surgery before a hemorrhage occurs. Anterior communicating artery aneurysms have a tendency to rupture into the brain parenchyma of the frontal lobe, producing drowsiness, increased intracranial pressure, and sometimes focal signs. The remaining aneurysms can occur at multiple other sites, including the basilar artery. About 20% of cases have multiple aneurysms.

Once a subarachnoid hemorrhage is suspected, the diagnosis is usually confirmed by CT scan. If the CT scan fails to demonstrate blood in the subarachnoid space, a lumbar puncture is indicated [7]. Confirmation of the presence and location of an aneurysm requires cerebral arteriography. The treatment of a patient with aneurysmal subarachnoid hemorrhage involves intensive medical supportive care, followed by surgical clipping of the aneurysm. Medical management includes regulation of blood pressure and fluids, prophylactic antiepileptic therapy, prevention of vasospasm with the calcium-channel blocker nimodipine [8], and sometimes reduction of rebleeding via plasminogen inhibitors such as epsilon-amino-caproic acid [9]. The timing of surgery is controversial [10,11]. Delayed headache and drowsiness in patients with subarachnoid hemorrhage may be secondary to hydrocephalus, which may require shunting [12].

Arteriovenous malformation (AVM) is the second most common cause of subarachnoid hemorrhage. Because of their varied presentations [13,14], these lesions are challenging to the physician. AVMs can bleed, either purely into the subarachnoid space, or into the brain parenchyma, in which case focal neurological signs are the rule. They can present as slowly enlarging mass lesions, mimicking tumors, or they can cause focal or generalized seizures. AVMs as a cause of headache alone are controversial. Many patients with AVMs describe migrainelike headache, but migraines are so much more common than AVMs that a search for AVM is unlikely to be successful in the average migraine patient. Even consistently unilateral migraines only occasionally lead to the diagnosis of an otherwise unsuspected AVM. Diagnosis is aided by listening for ocular or cranial bruits, but brain imaging or angiography is often necessary.

Subarachnoid hemorrhage can also be seen with minor head injuries, blood dyscrasias, anticoagulation, and occasionally cerebral vasculitis. Occasionally, a patient with a spontaneous subarachnoid hemorrhage will have no source of bleeding discovered, despite CT or MRI scanning, cerebral arteriography, and immunological and clotting studies. Such patients usually have a benign course, with a low incidence of rebleeding or vasospasm. An occult AVM or small aneurysm is often assumed to be the cause.

Infections represent another relatively acute and serious cause of headache. Fever and stiff neck, often with severe headache and delirium, are the hallmarks of infectious meningitis. In the case of bacterial meningitis, prompt diagnosis by lumbar puncture and institution of antibiotics is lifesaving. If the patient is drowsy or has focal signs, the concern is often raised that a CT scan should be done before the lumbar puncture, to exclude a brain abscess. In such cases, the antibiotics should be begun before the CT scan, with the spinal tap performed immediately thereafter, to avoid delay in treatment. Viral meningitis often produces similar clinical signs, except that the sensorium and mental status are usually normal. The CSF formula is also different from that of bacterial meningitis, featuring a predominance of mononuclear cells, usually a normal glucose, and a lower level of protein, usually but not always below 100 mg/100 cc [15]. Fungal, tuberculous, or parasitic infections usually have a more subacute course, but otherwise the symptoms and signs are similar. Rickettsial infections, such as Rocky Mountain spotted fever, may present relatively acutely with headache, fever, and stiff neck, but here the skin rash is the clue to the specific etiology. Brain abscess is frequently difficult to diagnose, in that up to 50% of patients have no history of fever, though more complain of headache [16]. These lesions may present in the manner of tumors, with gradual development of focal neurological symptoms and signs, or with seizures. Viral encephalitis usually presents with headache, drowsiness, stupor, and coma. Herpes simplex encephalitis may be associated with focal, temporal lobe symptoms, such as aphasia, partial complex seizures, and personality change. In the late 1980s, AIDS emerged as a frequent cause of central nervous system infections. AIDS patients have a high frequency of secondary CNS infections, most commonly toxoplasmosis [17]. In addition, the HIV virus itself causes a low-grade encephalitis, characterized by headache, confusion, and dementia [18].

Sinusitis is a frequent but often improperly diagnosed cause of headache. Headache, usually associated with tenderness over the nasal sinuses, nasal congestion, and discharge are the common symptoms. Infection of the sphenoid sinuses is commonly associated with headache, often at the vertex, and the other signs may be absent [19]. The frontal and maxillary sinuses do not drain well in the supine position, and infection of these sinuses generally causes headache on awakening, with improvement after the upright posture is assumed. If sinusitis is suspected, transillumination of the sinuses, sinus X-rays, or a CT or MRI scan with attention to the nasal sinuses are helpful in diagnosis. Failure to treat acute sinusitis can lead to bacterial meningitis, venous sinus thrombosis, or subdural or epidural empyema. Treatment involves a combination of antibiotics, decongestants, and antihistamines, with surgical drainage for refractory cases [20]. In many cases, however, patients attribute to sinus congestion headache syndromes that are more likely related to migraine or tension mechanisms.

Vasculitis is another, relatively uncommon but serious cause of headache. Temporal or giant cell arteritis is a major cause of headache in elderly persons. Common symptoms, in addition to headache, are jaw claudication or pain on chewing, loss of vision in one eye, and the polymyalgia rheumatica syndrome of diffuse joint and muscle aches, low grade fever, and anemia [21]. The laboratory clue to temporal arteritis is a markedly elevated erythrocyte sedimentation rate (ESR). Rare cases of temporal arteritis in younger patients and in patients with normal ESR have been documented [22]. If the disease is suspected, temporal artery biopsy is indicated, and steroid treatment may be dramatically effective in relieving the headaches. Other types of cerebral vasculitis, including isolated CNS angiitis or granulomatous arteritis, polyarteritis nodosa, and even cocaine-induced vasculitis, cause prominent complaints of headache, as well as multifocal neurological symptoms and signs [23–25].

Stroke syndromes, both ischemic and hemorrhagic, may be associated with headache, usually on the basis of brain swelling and pressure on the meningovascular structures. The abrupt onset of focal neurological signs usually gives away the diagnosis of stroke. In the Harvard Stroke Registry, only 9% of thrombotic strokes, 8% of embolic strokes, and 36% of intracerebral hemorrhages had prominent complaints of headache at onset [26]. Gorelick and colleagues [27] also found headaches more common in subarachnoid (100%) and intraparenchymal (55%) hemorrhage than in ischemic stroke (17%). Cerebellar hemorrhages cause headache, dizziness, nausea, and vomiting. The supine neurological examination may be surprisingly normal, but the patient usually cannot walk. If cerebellar hemorrhage is suspected, prompt diagnosis by CT scan and consideration of surgical drainage are mandatory [28]. Another vascular cause of headache is hypertension. The syndrome of hypertensive encephalopathy includes headache, confusion, focal neurological signs, and obtundation or seizures. Papilledema and renal failure are frequent accompaniments. The syndrome occurs only in the setting of malignant hypertension, however, with diastolic blood pressures in excess of 120 mmHg. The pathology involves focal areas of ischemia, edema, and petechial hemorrhage [29]. Hypertension of milder degree can cause headaches in some patients, but headache is not generally a reliable indicator of hypertension.

Brain tumors and other mass lesions cause headache by increased pressure and traction on the dura. Morning headaches, often relatively mild in severity, are frequently associated with brain tumors. Most patients with tumors present with focal symptoms and signs or seizures, in addition to or instead of headaches, and only rarely does a patient whose sole complaint is of headache prove to have a brain tumor. The exceptions include mass lesions of the deep midline structures, such as craniopharyngiomas, third ventricular cysts, or posterior fossa tumors, often associated with hydrocephalus. These patients are the bane of headache clinics, in that the presence of a tumor may be diagnosable only by a brain imaging study. For this reason, patients whose headaches are atypical or fail to respond appropriately to therapy should receive a CT or MRI scan of the brain, though not all headache patients warrant routine brain imaging [30].

Benign intracranial hypertension, or "pseudotumor cerebri," is a syndrome of headaches, papilledema, and elevated CSF pressure, without focal signs except for the occasional presence of a sixth cranial nerve palsy [31]. The syndrome is most common in young, overweight females but is also associated with anemia and with a number of drugs. The diagnosis in confirmed by elevated CSF pressure, normal CSF chemistries and cell count, and normal brain imaging studies. Treatment includes serial lumbar punctures, diuretics, or acetazolamide to reduce CSF formation, and surgery for unusually refractory cases. Surgical approaches include shunting, usually from the lumbar peritoneal space into the peritoneum, or decompression of the optic sheath. The principal danger of the condition, if untreated, is loss of vision secondary to prolonged papilledema [32].

Subdural hematoma represents another mass lesion that can present with headache. Patients with subdural hematoma may not recall any episode of head trauma. Subacute symptoms of headache, drowsiness, confusion, and sometimes focal neurological symptoms then ensue. The neurological examination may reveal only subtle focal neurological signs [33]. As in brain tumor, an imaging study is necessary for diagnosis.

Head injuries, including mild trauma such as concussion, are often followed by headache. The "postconcussive syndrome" involves severe headaches, irritability, poor concentration, and insomnia [34,35]. Brain imaging is necessary to exclude such structural causes of headache as subdural hematoma or hydrocephalus. Other post-traumatic headache syndromes include vascular headaches similar to migraine [36] and muscle strain syndromes resembling tension headache. These are treated with the same symptomatic approaches used in non-traumatic headaches.

Headaches of cervical spine origin are very common, especially in the elderly. The upper cervical nerve root dermatomes extend up the back of the head, and referred head pain in this region is frequently related to cervical spondylosis. The mechanism is thought to be irritation of nerves, secondary muscle spasm, and then aching pain secondary to overcontraction of the paraspinal muscles and trapezii [37]. The headache of cervical spondylosis is thus an example of muscle contraction headache. A similar syndrome of "cervicogenic headache" has been described in young persons with headache beginning in the neck on one side, usually unassociated with demonstrable spine pathology [38]. The syndrome of "occipital neuralgia" is closely related [39]. Localized posterior headaches, in the manner of other musculoskeletal pain syndromes, are sometimes treated by injections of local anesthetic agents and corticosteroids over the local "trigger points" on the occipital scalp or neck.

Temporomandibular joint (TMJ) headache is another musculoskeletal headache syndrome. The typical "TMJ headache" is unilateral, located in the frontotemporal region just above the TMJ, worsened by chewing, and generally present after meals. Patients with nocturnal bruxism may have morning headaches. Improvement with bite blocks or with surgical procedures to the TMJ confirm this diagnosis. Many patients with definite TMJ pathology do not complain of headaches, however, and caution should be exercised in attributing headaches to TMJ dysfunction. One study of 100 prospective headache patients found that 11% had probable or definite TMJ dysfunction syndrome as a cause [40].

A number of other, miscellaneous headache syndromes will not be discussed here. These include ice cream headache; headaches related to withdrawal from caffeine, alcohol, cocaine, and other drugs; and lumbar puncture or "low pressure" headache. Lumbar puncture headaches are treated with supine bed rest, fluids, and occasionally epidural patch techniques for resistant cases. The treatment of all headaches involves removal of the underlying cause, if possible, and then symptomatic treatment of the headache pain. The remainder of the chapter will be devoted to the three common headache syndromes: muscle contraction, migraine, and cluster.

TENSION (MUSCLE CONTRACTION) HEADACHE

In theory, any sustained contraction of a muscle group in proximity to the pain-sensitive structures of the head and neck may cause headache. Cervical spondylosis and TMJ dysfunction syndrome are thus examples of muscle contraction headache. More commonly, however, individuals without obvious pathology experience dull, aching, bandlike, bilateral headaches, usually gradual in onset or present from awakening [41]. Such headaches may occur daily, throughout the day, and last for weeks; in fact, headaches of such long duration usually are related to muscle contraction. Nausea, vomiting, and photophobia occur only when the headache is at its most severe, generally after a long period of buildup. These vascular features, however, do cast some doubt as to whether there is a firm separation, or rather a spectrum, between muscle contraction and vascular or migraine headaches. Many headache patients seem to suffer from both vascular and muscle contraction headaches ("mixed headache") [42]. In terms of mechanism, patients who are tense or anxious may unconsciously contract muscles of the scalp, such as the frontalis, and the muscles of the neck, leading to the gradual onset of headache. Depressed patients often complain of similar headaches, though the mechanism may not be as simple. For all of these reasons, the 1988 International Headache Classification [43] has dropped the term *muscle contraction headache* in favor of the older term, *tension headache*. The diagnosis of tension headache is usually obvious, and diagnostic studies are not necessary unless the clinical features are atypical or the patient fails to respond to treatment.

The treatment of tension or muscle contraction headaches is multifaceted. Reassurance is often sufficient; once patients no longer fear that they are harboring brain tumors or other serious illness, they may be able to cope with the headaches on their own. Relaxation techniques and biofeedback training have had considerable success [44]. Drug therapy should be considered as an adjunct in tension headaches, especially since their frequent or chronic occurrence makes drug dependency a considerable risk. Mild muscle-relaxant, tranquilizing drugs, such as lorazepam and nonsteroidal antiinflammatory agents, may provide short-term, symptomatic relief. Tricyclic antidepressant drugs may prove more helpful in chronic therapy. Doses are usually begun low, for example, with 10–25 mg nightly of amitriptyline, doxepin, or nortriptyline, to avoid undesirable side effects, including sedation. Episodic headache relief may also be gained by analgesics or by one of the commonly prescribed combinations of butalbital, caffeine, and acetaminophen or aspirin (Fiorinal®, Esgic®, Phrenilin®). These drugs have considerable dependency potential, and their indiscriminate use has been implicated in the development of interstitial nephritis and renal failure. Analgesic treatment of tension headaches should be carefully monitored and combined with nonpharmacological treatments to alter the long-term headache pattern.

MIGRAINE

Migraine is a varied syndrome of "vascular" headaches, having at its core the common features of throbbing head pain, nausea, photophobia, and prostration [45]. An "aura," or prodrome, frequently heralds the onset of headache. The aura usually involves visual disturbances, such as positive scintillations or fortification spectra, or negative defects or scotomata [46]. Mood changes, lightheadedness, paresthesias, or a variety of other symptoms may be part of the aura. A large number of migraine subtypes and variants have been described. The recent international classification [43] has attempted to simplify the terminological confusion by dividing the many migraine subsyndromes into the two groups of migraine with and without aura. Criteria for the diagnosis of migraine without aura, formerly called "common migraine," are listed in Table 13-1. Migraine without aura is often bilateral, but the character of the pain usually remains throbbing, and the presence of nausea early in the attack helps to distinguish the syndrome from tension headache. Migraine with aura corresponds to the prior categories of "classic migraine." If the aura involves focal neurological symptoms, such as aphasia, confusion, weakness, or brainstem symptoms, then specific syndromes of "complicated migraine" are diagnosed. In general, the neurological symptoms occur during the aura and are followed by a throbbing, unilateral headache, though focal symptoms

Table 13-1. Criteria for diagnosis of migraine without aura (from the 1988 International Classification [43])

A. At least five attacks fulfilling B–D
B. Untreated headache duration 4–72 hours
C. At least two of the following characteristics:
   1. Unilateral location
   2. Pulsating quality
   3. Moderate to severe intensity
   4. Aggravation by physical activity
D. At least one of the following during headache:
   1. Nausea and/or vomiting
   2. Photophobia and phonophobia
E. Exclusion of other causes of headache by history, examination, laboratory tests, or lack of temporal relation to other cause of headache

may also occur during the headache phase. Criteria from the international classification for the diagnosis of migraine with aura are listed in Table 13-2.

The clinical phenomena of classic migraine are rich and fascinating. A number of specific types of migraine with aura have been described: hemiplegic migraine, ophthalmoplegic migraine, retinal migraine, basilar artery migraine, and confusional migraine. Hemiplegic migraine [47], usually a familial disorder, includes attacks of hemiparesis associated with headache, either as an aura or extending into the headache phase. The attacks can last for days and can occasionally produce a lasting deficit ("migrainous stroke"). Ophthalmoplegic migraine [48] is a similar syndrome in which a paresis of the third cranial nerve — occasionally accompanied by IV, VI, or other cranial nerve symptoms — is associated with the onset of the attack. In most cases, localized periorbital headache precedes the ptosis and diplopia, and the pupil is usually affected. Retinal migraine [49] refers to scintillations and other visual phenomena, occurring only in one eye, and usually followed by headache. Basilar migraine [50], described in 1961 by Bickerstaff, includes symptoms of vertigo, tinnitus, hearing loss, diplopia, binocular blurred vision or blindness, dysarthria, dysphagia, bilateral paresthesias or paresis, and decreased level of consciousness. Paroxysmal EEG discharges have been described during basilar migraine attacks, and anticonvulsants have sometimes proved effective in preventing attacks [51,52]. The relationship of basilar migraine to epilepsy, however, remains controversial, and some patients respond better to traditional antimigraine drugs than to anticonvulsants. Confusional migraine [53,54] is a syndrome seen mainly in children, in which a delirium or confusional state develops during the aura of a migraine attack. Bizarre perceptual distortions, referred to as the "Alice in Wonderland" syndrome, may occur during such attacks [55]. In adults, syndromes resembling transient global amnesia have been described with migraine attacks [56,57].

In addition to the varieties of classic migraine, several related migraine syndromes have been recognized. "Status migrainosus" [58] refers to prolonged states of headache, nausea, and vomiting lasting days or weeks. More commonly, an acute migraine is followed by a prolonged headache with features of tension or muscle contraction headache, often with associated

Table 13-2. Criteria for diagnosis of migraine with aura (from the 1988 International Classification [43])

A. At least two attacks fulfilling B
B. At least three of the following four characteristics:
  1. ≥1 reversible aura symptoms of focal cortical or brainstem dysfunction
  2. ≥1 aura symptom develops over >4 minutes or ≥2 symptoms occur in succession
  3. Aura does not exceed 60 minutes
  4. Headache follows aura within 60 minutes
C. Exclusion of other causes of headache by history, examination, laboratory tests, or lack of temporal relation to other cause of headache

tenderness of the scalp. "Migrainous stroke" refers to migraine syndromes followed by a permanent neurological deficit, and often changes of infarction on CT or MRI brain scans. Such stroke syndromes are rare in proportion to the frequent occurrence of migraines but are among the more common causes of stroke in young people [59,60]. A recent report included three patients in whom arteriography performed soon after the stroke demonstrated focal vasospasm [60]. The diagnosis of migrainous stroke, of course, requires exclusion of other causes of stroke, in addition to a history of classic migraine. A relationship between migrainous stroke and oral contraceptive use has been suspected [61]. Strokes related to venous sinus thrombosis also occur in women taking oral contraceptives. The new international classification [43] refers to status migrainosus and migrainous stroke as *complicated migraine,* a term used previously to mean any migraine syndrome accompanied by neurological symptoms other than visual.

Finally, a series of "migraine equivalents," or migraine syndromes without headache, have been described. These include benign positional vertigo, abdominal migraine, cyclical vomiting, and alternating hemiplegia of childhood [62]. All of these syndromes are more common in children than in adults, and the diagnosis is usually made with confidence only when a child with one of these syndromes then develops typical migraine headaches. A family history of migraine is also usually present. Fisher has also described migraine equivalents without headache, resembling transient ischemic attacks, in postmenopausal women [63].

In recent years, considerable knowledge has accumulated regarding the pathophysiology of migraine. The symptoms of throbbing pain and nausea have often been assumed to reflect dilatation of cerebral and meningeal vessels, while the aura was assumed to result from cerebral vasoconstriction. Among the sources of evidence for the vasoconstriction-vasodilatation theory were Wolff's studies of inhalation of amyl nitrate or carbon dioxide by migraineurs and observations of small vesssels in the bulbar conjunctiva during migraine attacks [3]. Early studies of cerebral blood flow by xenon inhalation techniques confirmed sequential reductions in flow during the aura, followed by increases in flow during the headache phase of classic migraine attacks [64]. Recent studies, however, have cast doubt on a simple vascular cause of the pain. Olesen, using intraarterial xenon infusions, has described a "spreading oligemia," or a wave of decreased blood flow, which often begins in the occipital lobes and then migrates forward at a rate of 2–3 mm/minute [65,66]. This rate of propagation corresponds well with maps of cortical discharge calculated from the "march" of visual auras in observant migraineurs, and it also corresponds with the rate of "spreading depression" produced by von Leao in experimental animals by electrical depolarization of the cerebral cortex [67]. Welch has reviewed evidence for spreading depression in migraine [68] and has recently detected changes in magnetic fields over the cerebral cortex in human migraineurs during attacks, confirming for the first time that spreading depression occurs in humans [69]. In Olesen's studies [65], the oligemia occurs not only during the aura but extends well into the headache phase, raising doubt that vasodilatation is the cause of headache pain.

Considerable evidence has pointed to abnormal neural activity in the brain as the root of the vascular changes. Monoaminergic pathways have been implicated, particularly the serotoninergic cells of the raphe nucleus of the brainstem, which project to the cerebral cortex, and the noradrenergic neurons of the locus ceruleus. Patients undergoing electrode placements in the periventricular grey matter of the midbrain for treatment of pain have described photophobia and throbbing head pain, reminiscent of migraine, suggesting that local neuronal firing can trigger migraine phenomena [70]. Firing of serotoninergic neurons in the raphe nucleus is regulated by local levels of serotonin. Reduced levels may precipitate firing and production of a migraine attack [71]. Moskowitz [72] has pointed to the role of the trigeminal nerve and its branches, which innervate cerebral vessels in the pia, and also the larger arteries of the circle of Willis. Stimulation of trigeminal fibers by the neuronal discharges of migraine may lead to release of substance P, dilatation of the affected vessels, and production of sterile inflammation in these vessels. Serotonin is found in trigeminal ganglia and may be involved in the vasodilatation, inflammation, and hyperesthesia produced locally. Serotonin may also be released as a result of platelet aggregation in migraine-afflicted vessels, though this source of serotonin is probably too small to account for the vascular changes. Stimulation of trigeminal fibers would be consistent with the unilateral distribution of migraine headaches, the presence of sterile inflammation around arteries following a migraine attack, and the combination of "posterior circulation" symptoms, such as scotomas and scintillations, with anterior head pain, since the ophthalmic division of the trigeminal nerve innervates the posterior cerebral and basilar arteries. The trigeminal/vascular mechanism links migraine to other causes of headache, such as meningitis, mass lesions with traction on the dura, and vasculitis, all of which involve stimulation of vascular trigeminal fibers and vasodilatation.

The treatment of migraine headache has three aspects: abortive, prophylactic, and nonpharmacological. Abortive treatments are designed to halt the progression of a migraine that has already begun, or to prevent the evolution of an aura into the headache phase. Ergot vasoconstrictors, such as ergotamine tartrate, administered as sublingual tablets, oral tablets (caffergot®), inhalers, or rectal suppositories, have a long tradition in migraine therapy. These drugs work both as vasoconstrictors and as serotonin blockers. Unfortunately, only a minority of migraine patients derive adequate relief from ergots alone. These drugs also cause acute vasoconstriction, leading in some patients to extremity cramps, nausea, and vomiting, and even anginal chest pain. Administration of these agents should be limited to three to four doses, equivalent to 2 mg of ergotamine tartrate per day, and 8–10 doses per week. A recent advance has been the use of dihydroergotamine, or DHE, given intravenously in a dose of

0.5–1.0 mg, often preceeded by 10 mg of metaclopramide (Reglan®), injected intravenously or intramuscularly to prevent nausea [73,74]. Intravenous DHE treatments are effective in over 50% of migraine attacks [74]. Recently, intravenous prochlorperazine (Compazine®) at a dose of 10 mg has also proved very effective in aborting migraine headaches [75]. Other alternatives in the abortive therapy of migraines include chlorpromazine or narcotic analgesics. DHE and prochlorperazine appear to be at least as effective as narcotics, without the potential for addiction, but intravenous medications require a visit to a doctor's office or emergency room.

Numerous drugs are employed in the prophylaxis of migraine headaches. Most were discovered fortuitously but fit in well with current theories of migraine pathogenesis. First, the drug methysergide, or Sansert®, has long been known to prevent migraines. Methysergide is now known to be a peripheral serotonin blocker but a central serotonin agonist. As a central agonist, it may decrease firing of the raphe cells and prevent migraine attacks. Methysergide is effective, but its use is limited by ergotlike side effects and by the long-term development of fibrous tissue hyperplasia, which can lead to renal failure. Doses are begun at 2 mg once or twice daily, and are increased to as much as four times daily. Even if the drug is effective, a drug-free period of at least 4 weeks should be planned every 6 months. A class of new drugs with serotonin blocking properties is undergoing clinical testing. The only other currently available serotonin blocker is cyproheptadine (Periactin®). This medication is sometimes effective in childhood migraine but is generally not useful in adults because of its sedative and appetite stimulant effects.

Propranolol (Inderal®) and other beta-blocking drugs are usually the first choice for migraine prophylaxis [76,77]. These drugs may block vascular beta-receptors, or they may have effects on the central noradrenergic pathway from the locus ceruleus. Propranolol is begun at 10–20 mg bid and advanced to as much as 160–320 mg daily, often in sustained-release preparations. Beta blockers may precipitate asthma and cause side effects of depression, lack of energy, bradycardia, and hypotension. Other beta blockers, such as timolol, nadolol, atenolol, and metoprolol, have been found to have comparable effectiveness as migraine prophylactic agents [78,79]. Clonidine (Catapres®), a centrally acting alpha-adrenergic agonist, has proved disappointing in migraine prevention.

Calcium-channel blockers are often used as second-line migraine prophylactic agents, after beta blockers. These drugs may also work either at vascular or neuronal sites; the exact mechanism is unknown. Verapamil (Isoptin®, Calan®) has been the most studied, in doses of 160–320 mg/day [80,81], but nifedipine, diltiazem, and most recently nimodipine [82] have been tried with varying success. These drugs all have a direct vasodilating effect, and they appear to trigger migraines in some patients.

The tricyclic antidepressants, especially amitriptyline, have considerable effectiveness in preventing migraine attacks. These drugs inhibit the reuptake of both norepinephrine and serotonin in nerve terminals. By increasing local levels of serotonin, they may reduce firing of the raphe neurons and decrease migraine attacks. One study showed no correlation between changes in depression scales and reduction in migraine frequency, suggesting that these drugs are not simply acting as antidepressants [83]. Monoamine oxidase inhibitors, such as tranylcypromine (Nardil®), also increase local levels of catecholamines. These drugs are also effective in preventing migraine, though they are less popular than tricyclics because of the need to maintain rigorous diets to prevent hypertension from tyramine-containing foods and beverages. One final psychotropic agent, lithium, may also have some effectiveness in migraine, though it is employed more in cluster headache.

In terms of practical migraine prophylaxis, drugs are used if the patient is experiencing more than one to two headaches per month of a disabling severity, and if simple measures such as stress reduction, biofeedback, and discontinuation of estrogen preparations have not helped. Propranolol or another beta blocker is usually the first choice, followed by verapamil or another calcium-channel blocker. Tricyclic antidepressants are usually tried third, with methysergide, MAO inhibitors, or lithium held in reserve for refractory cases. The great majority of migraine patients will respond to one or another of these agents.

Nonpharmacological migraine therapies include biofeedback and related relaxation techniques [84]. Other, experimental nonpharmacological techniques of migraine control, such as stellate ganglion blocks [85], epidural blood patches [86], and magnetic therapy, were discussed in Chapter 12.

CLUSTER HEADACHE

Though their clinical characteristics are quite distinct [87], cluster headaches, in older classifications, were considered variants of migraine. Older terms for this headache syndrome include histamine headaches, Horton's cephalgia, and Sluder's or sphenopalatine neuralgia. The term *cluster* refers to the tendency of these headaches to occur in flurries of episodes, each usually lasting a shorter duration than a migraine (usually 15–180 minutes), but recurring daily or multiple times per day for days or weeks, then disappearing as mysteriously as they came. Such clusters may occur every few months, or once every several years. The pain itself is sharp and severe, usually located around one eye, and associated with local autonomic signs, such as redness and tearing of the eye, ptosis, and nasal congestion. Patients often get up and pace during clusters, whereas migraine sufferers usually prefer to lie down in a quiet, dark place. The pain may be so severe as to drive patients to suicide. Cluster headaches frequently wake patients from sleep and may recur nocturnally for days on end. The patient population afflicted by cluster headaches also differs from that of migraine; clusters are more common in males than females, especially young and middle-aged males. *Chronic cluster headache* refers to sharp headache pains of similar location and associated autonomic signs, but occurring chronically over more than a year, with less than a 14-day remission [43].

Two localized headache syndromes resembling cluster headache have recently been distinguished. The first, chronic paroxysmal hemicrania, involves briefer and more frequent episodes of sharp unilateral or periorbital head pain, with associated autonomic signs similar to those of cluster headache [88]. These headaches, unlike cluster, are more common in women than men. The second, idiopathic stabbing or "ice pick" headache, involves stabbing pains, lasting less than a second, localized to the periorbital region, temple, or parietal scalp. These typically occur in migraine sufferers [89]. Both chronic paroxysmal hemicrania and idiopathic stabbing headaches respond well to indomethacin at a dose of 25 mg tid.

The treatment of cluster headache is often problematic. Abortive treatments include ergots or oxygen inhalation. Ergotamine taken at bedtime may prevent the nocturnal episodes. Prophylactic drugs with efficacy in cluster headache include methysergide, indomethacin, lithium, amitriptyline and related tricyclic drugs, and corticosteroids. Lithium is often especially effective in chronic cluster headaches [90]. Beta blockers and calcium-channel blockers are less effective than in migraine. Serial trials of these various drugs may be necessary.

CRANIAL NEURALGIAS

The final category of head pains, the cranial neuralgias and atypical facial pains, differ from the headache syndromes described in that they principally affect the facial structures rather than the head. Trigeminal neuralgia, or tic douleureux, refers to sharp, lancinating pains, lasting seconds at a time, localized within the distribution of one trigeminal nerve, and often triggered by touch on the face or temperature changes [91]. The syndrome is common in elderly persons. Diagnosis requires a normal examination, without evidence of abnormal trigeminal function other than pain, and without any other underlying neurological disorder. The cause of the pain is unknown, though pulsating arteries along the trigeminal nerve as it exits from the brainstem have been found by Janetta [92]. Medical treatment of tic douleureux involves carbamazepine (Tegretol®), which is usually quite effective. In refractory cases, tricyclic antidepressants, neuroleptics, and baclofen (Lioresal®) may reduce the pain somewhat. Surgical approaches include cutting the trigeminal ganglion, production of a radiofrequency lesion via a spinal needle in the trigeminal ganglion, or exploration of the trigeminal nerve in the posterior fossa with separation of the nerve from vascular structures. One variant of trigeminal neuralgia, Raeder's syndrome, involves the first division of the trigeminal nerve and thus produces pain in a similar distribution to cluster headache. Horner's syndrome is frequently associated. As in trigeminal neuralgia, carbamazepine appears to be especially effective [39]. As mentioned earlier, localized cranial neuralgias around the eye overlap with cluster headache.

CONCLUSIONS

Headache treatment is a challenging discipline for all physicians who want to help their patients. The empiric therapies of the past are being supplanted by specific drug treatments based on emerging information about the neurobiology of headache pain. New migraine prophylactic agents are being developed that promise to revolutionize this field. Nonpharmacological treatments are also expanding.

REFERENCES

1. Waters WE. 1975. Prevalence of migraine. J Neurol Neurosurg Psychiat 38:613–616.
2. Ziegler DK. 1985. Epidemiology of migraine. Headache 4:3–11.
3. Dalessio DJ. 1972. Wolff's Headache and Other Head Pain, 3rd ed. New York, Oxford University Press.
4. Lance JW. 1981. Headache. Ann Neurol 10:1–10.
5. Duffy GP. 1983. The "warning leak" in spontaneous subarachnoid hemorrhage. Med J Australia 1:514–516.
6. Leblanc R. 1987. The minor leak preceding subarachnoid hemorrhage. J Neurosurg 66:35–39.
7. Adams HP, Jergenson BD, Kassell NF, Sahs AH. 1980. Pitfalls in the recognition of subarachnoid hemorrhage. JAMA 244:794–796.
8. Allen GS, Ahn HS, Preziosi TJ, et al. 1983. Cerebral arterial spasm. A controlled trial of nimodipine in patients with subarachnoid hemorrhage. N Engl J Med 308:619–624.
9. Vermeulen M, Lindsey KW, Murray GD, et al. 1984. Antifibrinolytic treatment in subarachnoid hemorrhage. N Engl J Med 311:432–437.
10. Kassell NF, Torner JC. 1984. The international cooperative study on timing of aneurysm surgery — an update. Stroke 15:566–570.
11. Solomon RA, Fink ME. 1987. Current strategies for the management of aneurysmal subarachnoid hemorrhage. Arch Neurol 44:796–774.
12. Graff-Radford NR, Torner J, Adams HP, Kassell NF. 1989. Factors associated with hydrocephalus after subarachnoid hemorrhage. A report of the cooperative aneurysm study. Arch Neurol 46:744–752.
13. Aminoff MJ. 1987. Treatment of unruptured cerebral arterio-venous malformations. Neurology 37:815–819.
14. Brown RD, Wiebers DO, Forbes G et al. 1988. The natural history of unruptured intracranial arteriovenous malformations. J Neurosurg 68:352–357.
15. Ratzan KR. 1985. Viral meningitis. Med Clin NA 69:399–411.
16. Chun CH, Johnson JD, Hofstetter M, Raff MJ. 1986. Brain abscess. A study of 45 consecutive cases. Medicine 65:415–431.
17. Bredesen DE, Levy RM, Rosenblum ML. 1988. The neurology of human immunodeficiency virus infection. Q J Med 68:665–667.
18. Navia BA, Jordan BD, Price RW. 1986. The AIDS dementia complex. I. Clinical features. Ann Neurol 19:517–524.
19. Lew D, Southwick F, Montgomery MW, et al. 1983. Sphenoid sinusitis. A review of 30 cases. N Engl J Med 309:1149–1154.
20. Meyers BR. 1984. Bacterial sinusitis. J Family Practice 18:117–127.
21. Huston KA, Hunder GG. 1980. Giant cell (cranial) arteritis: A clinical review. Am Heart J 100:99–107.
22. Biller J, Asconape J, Weinblatt ME, Toole JF. 1982. Temporal arteritis associated with normal sedimentation rate. JAMA 247:486–487.
23. Moore PM, Cupps TR. 1983. Neurological complications of vasculitis. Ann Neurol 14:155–167.
24. Moore PM. 1989. Diagnosis and management of isolated angiitis of the central nervous system. Neurology 39:167–173.
25. Kaye BR, Fainstat M. 1987. Cerebral vasculitis associated with cocaine abuse. JAMA 258:2104–2106.
26. Mohr JP, Caplan LR, Melski JW, et al. 1987. The Harvard cooperative stroke registry: A prospective registry. Neurology 28:754–762.

27. Gorelick PB, Hier DB, Caplan L, Langenberg P. 1986. Headache in acute cerebrovascular disease. Neurology 36:1445–1450.
28. Ott KH, Kase CS, Mohr JP. 1974. Cerebellar hemorrhage: Diagnosis and treatment. A review of 56 cases. Arch Neurol 31:160–167.
29. Chester EM, Agamanolis DP, Banker BQ, Victor M. 1978. Hypertensive encephalopathy: A clinicopathologic study of 20 cases. Neurology 28:928–939.
30. Larson EB, Omenn GS, Lewis H. 1980. Diagnostic evaluation of headache. Impact of computerized tomography and cost-effectiveness. JAMA 243:359–362.
31. Ahlskog JE, O'Neill BP. 1982. Pseudotumor cerebri. Ann Int Med 97:249–256.
32. Corbett JJ, Thompson HS. 1989. The retional management of idiopathic intracranial hypertension. Arch Neurol 46:1049–1051.
33. Vicario S, Danzyl D, Thomas DM. 1982. Emergency presentation of subdural hematoma: A review of 85 cases diagnosed by computerized tomography. Ann Emerg Med 11:475–477.
34. Symonds C. 1962. Concussion and its sequelae. Lancet 1:1–5.
35. Levin HS, Mattis S, Ruff RM, et al. 1987. Neurobehavioral outcome following minor head injury: A three-center study. J Neurosurg 66:234–243.
36. Haas DC, Lourie H. 1988. Trauma-triggered migraine: An explanation for common neurological attacks after mild head injury. J Neurosurg 68:181–188.
37. Edmeads J. 1978. Headaches and head pains associated with diseases of the cervical spine. Med Clin North Ann 62:533–544.
38. Pfaffenrath V, Dandekar R, Pollmann W. 1987. Cervicogenic headache — The clinical picture, radiological findings and hypotheses on its pathophysiology. Headache 27:495–499.
39. Needham CW. 1978. Major cranial neuralgias and the surgical treatment of headache. Med Clin North Ann 62:545–557.
40. Reik L, Hale M. 1981. The temporomandibular joint pain-dysfunction syndrome: A frequent cause of headache. Headache 21:151–156.
41. Friedman AP. 1979. Characteristics of tension headache: A profile of 1,420 cases. Psychosomatics 20:451–461.
42. Saper JR. 1982. The mixed headache syndrome: A new perspective. Headache 22:284–286.
43. Olesen J. 1988. Classification and diagnostic criteria for headache disorders, cranial neuralgias and facial pain. Cephalalgia 8(Suppl 7):9–96.
44. Beaty ET, Haynes SN. 1979. Behavioral intervention with muscle-contraction headache: A review. Psychosom Med 41:165–180.
45. Olesen J. 1978. Some clinical features of the acute migraine attack. An analysis of 750 patients. Headache 18:268–271.
46. Hachinski VC, Porchawka J, Steele JC. 1973. Visual symptoms in the migraine syndrome. Neurology 23:570–579.
47. Glista GG, Mellinger JF, Rooke ED. 1975. Familial hemiplegic migraine. Mayo Clin Proc 50:307–311.
48. Friedman AP, Harter DH, Merritt HH. 1962. Ophthalmoplegic migraine. Arch Neurol 7:320–327.
49. Hedges TR. 1976. Isolated ophthalmic migraine in the differential diagnosis of cerebro-ocular ischemia. Stroke 7:379–381.
50. Bickerstaff ER. 1961. Basilar artery migraine. Lancet 1:1–15.
51. Camfield PR, Metrakos K, Andermann. 1978. Basilar migraine, seizures, and severe epileptiform EEG abnormalities. A relatively benign syndrome in adolescents. Neurology 28:584–588.
52. Swanson JW, Vick NA. 1978. Basilar artery migraine. 12 patients, with an attack recorded electroencephalographically. Neurology 28:782–786.
53. Gascon G, Barlow C. 1970. Juvenile migraine, presenting as an acute confusional state. Pediatrics 45:628–635.
54. Ehyai A, Fenichel GM. 1978. The natural history of acute confusional migraine. Arch Neurol 35:368–369.
55. Golden GS. 1979. The Alice in Wonderland syndrome in juvenile migraine. Pediatrics 63:517–519.
56. Olivarius B deF, Jensen TS. 1979. Transient global amnesia in migraine. Headache 19:335–338.
57. Caplan L, Chedru F, Lhermitte F, Mayman C. 1981. Transient global amnesia and migraine. Neurology 31:1167–1170.
58. Couch JR Jr., Diamond S. 1983. Status migrainosus: Causative and therapeutic aspects. Headache 23:94–101.

59. Spaccavento LJ, Solomon GD. 1984. Migraine as an etiology of stroke in young adults. Headache 24:19–22.
60. Rothrock JF, Walicke P, Swenson MR, et al. 1988. Migrainous stroke. Arch Neurol 45: 63–67.
61. Collaborative Group for the Study of Stroke in Young Women. 1975. Oral contraceptives and stroke in young women: Associated risk factors. JAMA 231:18–22.
62. Hockaday JM. 1988. Equivalents of migraine. In JM Hockaday (ed), Migraine in Childhood. London, Butterworths.
63. Fisher CM. 1980. Late-life migraine accompaniments as a cause of unexplained transient ischemic attacks. Can J Neurol Sci 7:9–17.
64. Sakai F, Meyer JS. 1978. Regional cerebral hemodynamics during migraine and cluster headaches measured by the ^{133}Xe inhalation method. Headache 18:122–132.
65. Olesen J, Larsen B, Lauritzen. 1981. Focal hyperemia followed by spreading oligemia and impaired activation of rCBF in classic migraine. Ann Neurol 9:344–352.
66. Olesen J. 1987. The ischemic hypotheses of migraine. Arch Neurol 44:321–322.
67. Leao AAP. 1944. Spreading depression of activity in cerebral cortex. J Neurophysiol 7:359–390.
68. Welch KMA. 1987. Migraine. A biobehavioral disorder. Arch Neurol 44:323–327.
69. Welch KMA. 1989. New frontiers in migraine pathogenesis. Paper presented at the symposium, Headache: Changing Perspectives and Controversies, Scottsdale, Arizona, January, 1989.
70. Raskin NH, Hosobuchi Y, Lamb S. 1987. Headache may arise from perturbation of brain. Headache 27:416–420.
71. Raskin NH. 1988. Headache, 2nd ed. New York, Churchill Livingstone.
72. Moskowitz MA. 1984. The neurobiology of vascular head pain. Ann Neurol 16:157–168.
73. Raskin NH. 1986. Repetitive intravenous dihydroergotamine as therapy for intractable migraine. Neurology 36:995–997.
74. Belgrade MJ, Ling LJ, Schleevogt MB, et al. 1989. Comparison of single-dose meperidine, butorphanol, and dihydroergotamine in the treatment of vascular headache. Neurology 39:590–592.
75. Jones J, Sklar D, Dougherty J, White W. 1989. Randomized double blind trial of intravenous prochlorperazine for the treatment of acute headache. JAMA 261:1174–1176.
76. Behan PO, Reid M. 1980. Propranolol in the treatment of migraine. The Practitioner 224:201–204.
77. Diamond S, Kudrow L, Stevens J, Shapiro DB. 1982. Long-term study of propranolol in the treatment of migraine. Headache 22:268–271.
78. Stellar S, Ahrens SP, Meibohm AR, Reines SA. 1984. Migraine prevention with timolol. A double-blind crossover study. JAMA 252:2576–2580.
79. Sudilovsky A, Elkind AH, Ryan RE, et al. 1987. Comparative efficacy of nadolol and propranolol in the management of migraine. Headache 27:421–426.
80. Solomon GD, Steel JG, Spaccavento LJ. 1983. Verapamil prophylaxis of migraine. A double-blind, placebo-controlled study. JAMA 250:2500–2502.
81. Markley HG, Cheronis JCD, Piepho RW. 1984. Verapamil in prophylactic therapy of migraine. Neurology 34:973–976.
82. Gelmers HJ. 1983. Nimodipine, a new calcium antagonist, in the prophylactic treatment of migraine. Headache 23:106–109.
83. Couch JR, Ziegler DK, Hassanein R. 1976. Amitriptyline in the prophylaxis of migraine. Neurology 26:121–127.
84. Fahrion SL. 1977. Autogenic biofeedback treatment for migraine. Mayo Clin Proc 52:776–784.
85. Parris WCV, Jamison RN, Lin SK, Kambam JR. Use of stellate ganglion blocks in treating unilateral migraine headaches. Presented to the American Society of Regional Anesthesia, San Francisco, CA, March 17–20, 1988.
86. Parris WCV. 1987. The use of epidural blood patch in treating chronic headache: Report of six cases. Can J Anaesth 34(4):403–406.
87. Duvoisin RC. 1972. The cluster headache. JAMA 222:1403–1404.
88. Sjaastad O, Dale I. 1976. A new (?) clinical headache entity: "Chronic paroxysmal hemicrania." Acta Neurol Scand 54:140–159.
89. Raskin NH, Schwartz RK. 1980. Icepick-like pain. Neurology 30:203–205.
90. Ekbom K. 1981. Lithium for cluster headache: Review of the literature and preliminary results of long-term treatment. Headache 21:132–139.

91. Fromm GH, Terrence CF, Maroon JC. 1984. Trigeminal neuralgia: Current concepts regarding etiology and pathogenesis. Arch Neurol 41:1204–1207.
92. Jannetta PJ. 1977. Observations on the etiology of trigeminal neuralgia, hemifacial spasm, acoustic nerve dysfunction and glossopharyngeal neuralgia. Definitive microsurgical treatment and results in 117 patients. Neurochirurgia 20:146–154.

14. THE ROLE OF SUBSTANCE P AND RELATED NEUROPEPTIDES IN CHRONIC PAIN MECHANISMS

WINSTON C.V. PARRIS

The management of chronic pain continues to be unsatisfactory and perplexing. The main reason for this inadequate state of affairs lies in the current poor comprehension of pain mechanisms. Several notable advances in understanding pain mechanisms have, however, been made recently. These advances lie in the area of the endogenous opioid system [1]; the role of stimulation in analgesia; and understanding of nociceptive modulating networks, including the periaqueductal gray area, the nucleus raphe-magnus, and the rostral ventral media medulla. Research in these areas, and also in the physiological properties of neurons in these nociceptive modulating nuclei, have provided a better understanding of pain mechanisms. When the possibility of bidirectional control of those neuropathways was considered rather than the traditional unidirectional control (which was purely inhibitory), it became clear that the roles of several neuropeptide systems were important. Many systems have been proposed as important in pain mechanisms. These include the serotoninergic system, the tachykinin system, the endorphin and enkephalin system, and the gamma-amino-butyric acid system, which all may play roles in the transmission and modulation of nociception. Peptidergic pathways constitute a large body of the central and peripheral nervous systems. These pathways may extend to regions modulating their primary effect at the spinal level or may extend to sensory pathways activated by nociceptive stimulation. The purpose of this chapter is to explore the role of substance P and related neuropeptides in the management of chronic pain.

Substance P belongs to a family of tachykinins [2] that have been isolated in the central and peripheral nervous systems of all vertebrate species and also in the epitheleal cells of the gastrointestinal tract. Substance P itself is an 11-amino acid neuropeptide that is found throughout the central and peripheral nervous system. The amino acid sequence of substance P and other members of the tachykinin peptide family are shown in Table 14-1. While the C-terminal fragment of the tachykinin molecule is very closely related to that of the other members of the tachykinin family, the N-terminal fragment of the individual molecule displays considerable variation in its amino acid composition. This variation of the amino acid composition of the N-terminal fragment accounts for the different functions of the individual members of the tachykinin family. Neuropeptides have specific functions that alter pathophysiological and even physiological responses in animals and may also serve as messenger molecules converting neurosignals into physiological responses. Their actions may be varied and complex. They may act either as neuromodulators or as neurotransmitters, and in the circulation they may have a "hormonal function."

History of substance P

Around 1930, a great deal of research involving biologically active, naturally occurring substances began to take place. One of the major reasons for this research activity was the development of useful pharmacological methods for analyzing biologically active extracts. These newly discovered techniques [3] produced many pharmacological discoveries, including the isolation of acetylcholine in the horse spleen. This finding provoked tremendous interest among contemporary pharmacologists who continued to attempt to validate several fundamental pharmacological hypotheses. Von Euler and Gaddum examined extracts of a variety of organs, including gut, brain, stomach, and lung tissue [4]. In 1934, they isolated an active substance in the form of a stable, dry powder known as preparation P. Subsequently, this active principle was called substance P, and it was first known for its effect on the rabbit jejunum.

Table 14-1. The tachykinin peptide family

Molluscan tachykinins	
Pyr-Pro-Ser-Lys-Asp-Ala-Phe-Ile-Gly-Leu-Met-NH$_2$	Eledoisin
Amphibian tachykinins	
Pyr-Ala-Asp-Pro-Asn-Lys-Phe-Tyr-Gly-Leu-Met-NH$_2$	Physalaemin
Pyr-Ala-Asp-Pro-Lys-Thr-Phe-Tyr-Gly-Leu-Met-NH$_2$	Lys^5,Thr^6-Physalaemin
Pyr-Pro-Asp-Pro-Asn-Ala-Phe-Tyr-Gly-Leu-Met-NH$_2$	Uperolein
Pyr----Asn-Pro-Asn-Arg-Phe-Ile-Gly-Leu-Met-NH$_2$	Phyllomedusin
Asp-Val-Pro-Lys-Ser-Asp-Gln-Phe-Val-Gly-Leu-Met-NH$_2$	Kassinin
Asp-Glu-Pro-Lys-Pro-Asp-Gln-Phe-Val-Gly-Leu-Met-NH$_2$	Glu^2,Pro^5-Kasinin
Asp-Pro-Pro-Asp-Pro-Asp-Arg-Phe-Tyr-Gly-Met-Met-NH$_2$	Hylambatin
Mammalian tachykinins	
Arg-Pro-Lys-Pro-Gln-Gln-Phe-Phe-Gly-Leu-Met-NH$_2$	Substance P

Subsequent research showed that substance P was present in a variety of other tissues, including the central nervous system. Pernow [5] showed in 1953 that the amount of substance P was greatly reduced in the aganglionic section of the intestine in Hirschsprung's disease. It has been established subsequently by Hokfelt that substance P normally occurs in high concentrations in Auerbach and Meissner plexuses. (It is these plexuses that are deficient in Hirschsprung's disease.)

In 1953, Fred Lembeck of the University of Graz, in Austria, demonstrated that the dorsal roots and vagus nerve were especially rich in substance P. This finding was later confirmed by Pernow in the same year. The difference in substance P content between the dorsal and the ventral roots became the basis for Lembeck's hypothesis [6] that substance P may be the neurotransmitter substance of the primary afferent (sensory) neuron. Later, it was shown that cutting the peripheral nerve altered the amount of substance P in the cut fragments, and that the amount of substance P was decreased in the peripheral portion of the cut nerve, while the central portion contained increased amounts of substance P [7]. Von Euler and Gaddum subsequently demonstrated that intraarterial injections of substance P produced various neurotropic effects in the brain of the cat and rabbit [4]. Further work on substance P led to the purification, isolation, and elucidation of its molecular structure by Chang and Leeman in 1970 [8]. Advances in the utilization of absorption chromatography using aluminum oxide facilitated this discovery, along with the associated advances made in radioimmunoassay techniques.

In an attempt to determine the relative activity of the different isolated extracts, these were originally assayed against a standard of isolated intestine. Their activity was also determined by their effect on rabbit blood pressure in the presence of atropine. These early experiments demonstrated that substance P lowered the blood pressure in laboratory animals and that this effect was due mainly to peripheral vasodilatation [9]. These studies confirmed the early findings of Fred Lembeck in 1953 when he made similar observations. Purified substance P extract produced significant vasodilatation when small amounts were injected intraarterially in human subjects. An extension of this work has led to the speculation that synthetic substance P antagonists may have a therapeutic role to play in chronic pain management and in the management of other pathophysiological states.

Substance P as a member of the tachykinin family

Peptidergic pathways constitute a large portion of the central and peripheral nervous system. These pathways include not only the sensory pathways involved in and activated by nociceptive stimulation, but also those pathways that modulate nociception at the spinal level. Peptidergic pathways are also involved in memory, learning, behavior, temperature, blood pressure regulation, and psychiatric disease. An analysis of the neuropeptides in the central nervous system shows that substance P, as a member of the tachykinin family of neuropeptides in its distribution, is ubiquitous in its location. It is present in most parts of the autonomic nervous system and in several areas within the central nervous system. Further, substance P is found in the enteric neuroplexus of the gastrointestinal tract and also in specific cells of the endocrine glands. In the gastrointestinal tract, substance P is known to influence the motility of the gastrointestinal system. The possible relationship between substance P and Hirschsprung's disease has already been mentioned [5].

It was believed initially that substance P was the only tachykinin in mammalian tissue. Although later, other tachykinins, including neurokinin A, neurokinin B, and neuropeptide K, were discovered. These findings will become very significant as analyses of substance P assume greater clinical significance. The presence of other neuropeptides with substance P-like immunoreactivity is important in laboratory methods involving substance P assays, especially if radioimmunoassay techniques or immunocytochemical techniques are utilized. All mammalian tachykinins share common C-terminal pentapeptide sequences and they all have a unique series of biological activities. Hokfelt has demonstrated the coexistence of substance P along with various neuropeptide neurotransmitters within the same neuron [10]: Cholecystokinin, a neuropeptide, has been shown to coexist with dopamine in mesencephalic cells; substance P and thyroid-stimulating hormone have been shown to coexist in the neurons of the medulla oblongata and vasoactive intestinal peptide; another neuropeptide had been shown to coexist with acetylcholine within autonomic ganglia. The physiological significance of the coexistence of these neuropeptides with the various neurotransmitters has not yet been elucidated. It seems clear that the co-occurence of these neuropeptides must have specific physiological and possibly pathophysiological implications.

While the mammalian substance P and other tachykinins may have relevance to pain management and other physiological functions, the use of the amphibian molluscan tachykinins as research tools should not be underestimated. Several members of the tachykinin family have been found in the octopod salivary glands and in the skin of amphibian organisms. Recent studies have also shown that substance P is present in coelenterates and (to make matters more confusing), it has also been demonstrated that the amphibian tachykinin, physalaemin, may be present in mammalian tissues [11]. As a consequence of these remarkable findings, it is clear that the various members of the tachykinin family may be found at both ends of the phylogenetic spectrum. There have been several explanations offered for these interesting findings. It is possible that the molecular structure of the peptide may have been changed during the evolutionary process and that certain portions of the molecular sequence may have been retained during the process of evolution. It is also possible that the tachykinins may have originated in unicellular organisms and that these neuropeptides have been maintained intact in higher organisms during the evolutionary process [12]. An alternative viewpoint is that the genes for these tachykinins developed in vertebrates and were introduced into unicellular organisms and multicellular invertebrates by plasmids. This theory cannot be validated until the appropriate genes have been demonstrated, isolated, and analyzed.

The amphibian tachykinins include physalaemin, kassinin, hylambatin, phyllomedusin, and others. The prototype of the molluscan tachykinin is eledoisin. The C-terminal fragment of all the tachykinin molecules is similar in all members of the family. While the N-terminal fragment displays considerable variation in its amino acid composition, it is this portion of the molecule that accounts for the differences in the biological activity of the individual tachykinins. The significance of eledoisin in the saliva glands of the mollusc, *Eledone moschata*, and also the significance of the neuropeptides in the skin of various amphibians is not clear [13]. Whereas these findings may be of no biological significance, they may, on the other hand, hold one of the great mysteries of biological function. As further methods of isolation, purification, and measurement of neuropeptides become available, it is very likely that these intricate mysteries may begin to unfold. Recent advances in radioimmunoassay techniques, and more specifically, recent advances in mass spectroscopy may possibly help to untangle some of these challenging problems and shed new light on the roles of neuropeptide tachykinins.

The potency of three typical tachykinins have been measured in various bioassay systems and compared to a standard of physalaemin. These bioassay systems included dog blood pressure, rabbit blood pressure, portal venous blood flow, hepatic artery blood flow, rabbit salivary secretion, guinea pig ileum, hamster urinary bladder, and rat colon, to name a few. The data obtained from these measurements suggest that there may be four different tachykinin subfamilies, each characterized by a set of distinct biological activities [14]. These activities include the following generalizations:

1. Substance P has the most pronounced action on blood pressure, vascular smooth muscle, and possibly on mammalian cerebral neurons.
2. Physalaemin and its group are the most potent stimulants of salivary, lacrimal, and pancreatic secretion, and have a powerful effect on amphibian and molluscan neurons.
3. Kassinin is characterized by poor action on blood pressure and salivary secretion, but has a potent effect on the smooth muscle of the gut and the urinary tract.
4. Eledoisin has a pronounced effect on stimulating smooth muscle of the gastrointestinal tract and of the urogenital system. It is also demonstrated to have a striking effect on central regulatory mechanisms of drinking behavior.

The above findings suggests that kassinin has the least stimulant effect on the various systems considered, but that its duration of action is more sustained than that of the other members of the tachykinin family.

It is very likely that the physiological and pathophysiological roles of substance P may have to be reexamined as more data on the other tachykinins and their relationship to substance P and to other neurotransmitters become available. Thus, it is prudent to analyze carefully the data obtained from the use of substance P as the sole representative of the tachykinin family, since these data may be meaningless, inasmuch as substance P may exist more naturally with the other tachykinins than in isolation. In that context, the data obtained from the nonmammalian tachykinins may in time provide very meaningful information on the role of substance P as a member of the tachykinin family.

Substance P as a possible neurotransmitter

There are several criteria that must be present in order to classify a compound as a neurotransmitter. These criteria include the presence of that compound in presynaptic neurons; the release of that compound in response to presynaptic stimulation; the presence of greater amounts of that compound in the dorsal root compared to the ventral root, and for that compound to exert an excitatory effect on spinal neurons. The role of substance P as a transmitter of primary afferent fibers has been already established. The precise mechanism of action of substance P as a neurotransmitter regarding its synthesis and its subsequent inactivation at the synaptic site has not yet been clearly elucidated. The ionic mechanisms involved and the electrical potentials associated with those mechanisms would also require further study. The work of Lembeck et al. has demonstrated that substance P appears to be an excitatory neurotransmitter of the spinal dorsal root fibers [15]. It is not clear whether substance P is a transmitter of some of the dorsal root fibers or of all the dorsal root fibers. It is also possible that there may be considerable species variability as far as that concept is concerned. As sophisticated immunohistochemical studies are developed, a clearer concept of substance P as a neurotransmitter should emerge. Hokfelt et al. have contributed much in that area and have demonstrated that only 10–20% of the neurons in rat spinal ganglia were substance P-positive [16]. Henry, using electrophoretically applied substance P, demonstrated excitation of the cat spinal neurons following activation induced by noxious stimuli applied to the skin [17]. The results of these studies demonstrated that substance P is related specifically to nociception. While one explores the possible sites of action of substance P as a neurotransmitter, it is also feasible that the dorsal root fibers may not be the site of action in some species, or certainly not the only site of action in other species. Otsuka has speculated that substance P may exert a direct depolarizing action at the spinal motor neuron level [18]. Siato has demonstrated that the antispasmodic agent, baclofen, (a known antagonist of the depolarizing action of substance P) blocked monosynaptic and polysynaptic reflexes, as well as the dorsal root potetial in the rat spinal cord, suggesting that substance P may play its neurotransmitter role as an excitatory transmitter at the spinal motorneuron level [19]. Further, Takahashi has demonstrated that the amount of substance P in the ventral horn is slightly reduced after section of the dorsal roots [20].

The excitatory role of substance P as a neurotransmitter has been compared extensively with the known excitatory neurotransmitter, L-glutamate. Konishi reported that the time course of depolarization of motor neurons was slightly slower when substance P was applied to the isolated rat spinal cord than when L-glutamate was added to the same region [21]. The reason for this delay may have been due to diffusion of substance P through the spinal cord tissue. Henry showed that substance P had a synergistic effect on the excitatory properties of L-glutamate when added to the cat spinal neurons [22]. Further work by Konishi showed that this synergism was not initially present, but rather when substance P and L-glutamate were applied together to the motor neuron in the isolated rat or frog spinal cord, a simple additive effect was produced [23]. Much more work needs to be done in order to evaluate the precise role of substance P as a neurotransmitter and even to compare its mechanism to some selective cholinergic mechanisms.

The effect of capsaicin on substance P
Capsaicin is an extract of red pepper and is chemically trans-8-methyl-N-vanillyl-6-nonenamide. This extract forms the pungent and blistering factor in the red pepper. Joo, Szolcsanyi, and Jansco [24], have exploited the unique pharmacological properties of this compound and used it as a research tool to explore the role of substance P as a neurotransmitter in nociceptive stimuli. In so doing, they showed that capsaicin, when administered chronically to adult rats, may cause selective damage to unmyelinated afferent fibers and may subsequently produce a long-lasting analgesic response to chemical irritants. Jessell concluded that this response was due to the depletion of substance P from the dorsal horn by capsaicin [25]. Further Jansco, Szolcsanyi, et al. demonstrated that a single treatment of capsaicin to newborn rats produced permanent damage to the smaller-caliber sensory fibers producing permanent analgesia to heat and chemically induced pain in these animals [26]. These observations of Jansco were subsequently duplicated by Holzer [27] and Nagy [28]. The mechanism by which capsaicin produces analgesia and associated depletion of substance P in primary afferent nerves has led several researchers to conclude that substance P is a neurotransmitter of nociception. Unfortunately, this explanation is not completely correct, since it has been demonstrated by other workers that capsaicin affects not only the unmyelinated fibers in peripheral nerves, but also unmyelinated autonomic fibers, the small-cell population of the dorsal root ganglia, and small-diameter myelinated fibers (A-delta) [29]. It is possible that all those fibers may be involved in pain transmission and modulation. In a detailed study, Helke et al. [57] demonstrated that capsaicin (50 mg/kg) administered subcutaneously to neonatal rats produced a marked decrease in substance P levels in the dorsal roots, and to a lesser extent in the dorsal horn, but that the levels in the ventral horn were

unaffected. The same studies also showed that somatostatin (another neuro-peptide found in the central nervous system) is significantly decreased in the dorsal root following treatment with capsaicin. These studies demonstrate that the original premise that capsaicin might represent a specific antagonist to substance P-containing afferent fibers, is no longer accurate. The current thought is that capsaicin antagonizes not only substance P but other neuropep-tides, including, somatostatin. Thus, these apparent properties of capsaicin have been utilized not only as a research tool in exploring pain mechanisms in sensory nerves, but also as a drug (zostrix and axain ointment) for treating intractable pain in patients with postherpetic neuralgia and reflex sympathetic dystrophy. Its clinical efficacy in these conditions is still under review.

Release and inactivation of substance P

In 1956, Angelucci demonstrated that there was significant substance P-like activity in the perfusate of the frog spinal cord [30]. Otsuka showed subse-quently that repetitive stimulation of the dorsal roots of the perfused isolated spinal cord of the newborn rat produced a marked increase in substance P-like immunoreactivity in the perfusate of that preparation [31]. These workers further showed, by contrast, that when a similar preparation was perfused with a low-calcium, high-magnesium solution (producing complete block of synaptic transmission), the same repetitive stimulation of the dorsal root no longer produced a significant change in substance P immunoreactivity. This situation was completely reversed when the spinal cord preparation was perfused with a solution containing a high-potassium concentration, produc-ing a large increase in the release of substance P-like immunoreactivity. These studies by Otsuka were subsequently duplicated by Iversen [32] and demon-strated that substance P is released predominantly from the dorsal roots of the spinal cord.

Neurotransmitter substances are usually inactivated by two mechanisms: a reuptake phenomenon similar to the inactivation of norepinephrine and an enzymatic biodegradation similar to acetylcholine. Understanding of the effect of substance P on its receptors in the central nervous system, and of its inactivation and biodegradation, has been hampered by unsatisfactory labora-tory methods to track these processes. Hanley et al. described techniques based on a neurophysiological approach to study the action of substance P on central nervous system receptors [33]. Further work on the development of a radioli-gand receptor binding assay using H^3-labeled substance P has facilitated modest gains in that process. When slices of rat spinal cord substantia nigra and hypothalamus were incubated with I^{125}-labeled substance P, no accumu-lation of the substance P in these tissues was detected. Segawa et al. have demonstrated the presence of substance P-inactivating enzymes systems in various regions of the spinal cord [34]. These regions include the basal ganglia and the hypothalamus. The inactivating substance P enzyme has been extracted,

Table 14-2. Distribution of immunoreactive peptide
transmitter and hormonal substances in mammalian tissues

Substance	Locations
Enkephalins (derivatives of proenkephalin)	Substantia gelatinosa, many parts of CNS, GI tract, CSF, blood
Endorphins (derivatives of pro-opiomelanocortin)	Hypothalamus, thalamus, brain stem, adrenal medulla lungs, placenta, GI tract, CSF, blood
Dynorphin (derivatives of prodynorphin)	Posterior pituitary, duodenum
Tachykinins (derivatives of preprotachykinin)	Primary afferents, many parts of CNS, GI tract, CSF, blood, saliva, pericardial fluid
Vasoactive intestinal peptide (VIP)	Postganglionic cholinergic neurons, some sensory neurons, hypothalamus, cerebral cortex, GI tract, periaqueductal grey matter.
Calcitonin gene-related protein (CGRP)	Endings of primary afferent neurons, sensory nerves
Somatostatin (SRIF)	Hypothalamus, many components of the CNS, GI tract, blood

purified, and found to be a neutral metalloenzyme. This metalloenzyme has been found in the membranes of the brain and has been demonstrated to cleave and inactivate substance P by possibly utilizing an endopeptidase action. This enzyme appears to be specific for substance P and may play a major role in its metabolic degradation. As more work to find specific inhibitors of substance P is done, agents that are antagonists to substance P-inactivating enzymes may be discovered. The therapeutic implications of these possible findings are very exciting and may lead to better understanding of pain mechanisms; they may also provide pharmacological tools to treat various pain syndromes.

Other neuropeptides in the central nervous system

In addition to the traditional neurotransmitters (acetylcholine, amino acids, monoamine) present in the brain, there are several neuropeptides [2] that are present in smaller amounts than amines. These include enkephalins, endorphins, dynorphins, tachykinin, vasoactive intestinal peptide (VIP), calcitonin gene-related peptide (CGRP), cholecystokinin, and somatostatin (Table 14-2). These neuropeptides may be classified according to their anatomical, functional, or structural characteristics. For example, the hypothalamic-releasing hormones include thyrotropin-releasing hormones and the corticotropin-releasing hormones, while the pituitary peptides include endorphin and adrenocorticotropic hormone. The gastrointestinal peptides include cholecystokinin, substance P, and somatostatin, while a miscellaneous group includes bradykinin, carnosine, calcitonin gene-related peptide, and sleep peptides. Some of the neuropeptides show similarities in their amino acid sequences with their precursor propeptides. It is likely that most of the neuropeptides may be derived from a precursor proopiomelanocortin (POMC), while some members of the endophin family of neuropeptides derive from other precursors, including proenkephalin and prodynorphin. This ancestral relationship may thus form a basis for classification. Some neuropeptides have been classified according to their bioassay techniques, and their names still reflect physiological functions or the specific sites of their physiological action. These neuropeptides include vasoactive intestinal peptide and cholecystokinin. It is clear that these diverse systems of classification may be very confusing and misleading. The large number of neuropeptides that have been discovered, and those yet to be discovered, suggests that a more efficient and practical mechanism of classification should be sought.

Somatostatin is a neuropeptide that is found in the central nervous system and appears to have some opioid activity. It is a 14–amino acid compound, which may have an agonist-antagonist effect at the opioid receptor level. Chrubasik et al. have demonstrated that somatostatin, when injected into the epidural space, may be used to manage postoperative pain [35]. These same workers have also demonstrated that somatostatin may have a place in the management of pain in patients with terminal cancer [36]. Parris et al. have shown in a small study that intravenously administered somatostatin appears to decrease substance P activity in human subjects [37]. There is considerable controversy regarding the inhibitory and excitatory effects of somatostatin on neurons. Parris et al. have also demonstrated that somatostatin may be utilized to treat carcinoid syndrome in the perioperative period [38]. This activity, in addition to the other gastrointestinal and endocrine functions of somatostatin, makes it difficult to pinpoint a specific neurogenic action in the presence of all those other functions of somatostatin.

Vasoactive intestinal peptide is widely distributed in the nervous system. It is extremely abundant in the sensory fibers and the autonomic fibers of human skin. This neuropeptide is a 28–amino acid compound that was originally isolated from the gastrointestinal tract. Vasoactive intestinal peptide has been demonstrated to be a potent vasodilator, like substance P. It is concentrated in large quantities in the sacral segments of the spinal cord, and it has been postulated to play a significant role in the neurotransmission involving visceral afferents [39]. Consequently, it may play a role in peristalsis, digestion, and the absorptive functions of the gastrointestinal tract. Yaksh et al. have demonstrated that stimulation of the sciatic nerve with intensities adequate to activate the nonmyelinated afferent fibers, and possibly the small–diameter myelinated fibers, produces a release of vasoactive intestinal peptide [40].

Calcitonin gene–related peptide (CGRP), like substance P and vasoactive intestinal peptide, is a potent vasodilator. Calcitonin gene–related peptide increases substance P release in vitro and has been demonstrated by Le Greves [41] to be a potent inhibitor of substance P degradation. Moskowitz has shown that in patients with migraine headaches there is an increase in calcitonin gene–related peptide in the cerebral vessels [42]. It has also been demonstrated that intrathecally administered calcitonin gene–related peptide lowers the nociceptive threshold for mechanical stimulation and also increases the excitability of the nociceptive reflex in cats. These and other studies appear to support the hypothesis that calcitonin gene-related peptide facilitates nociceptive transmission from peripheral pain receptors to the spinal cord.

It appears that all the above-mentioned neuropeptides may play a role in pain perception, pain modulation, and pain regulation. The mechanisms by which they accomplish these different functions are varied and possibly interrelated. The levels at which these various actions are accomplished may also vary, and in some cases the location may be the same. As newer techniques for isolating and measuring these compounds are discovered, greater understanding of the role of neuropeptides in general, and substance P in particular, may be made.

Clinical implications of substance P in pain management

The evidence that substance P is a neurotransmitter released from the peripheral branches of primary afferent nerves is very good, even if not totally conclusive. There is very little doubt that substance P is released from the central terminals of primary afferent neurons, producing an excitatory effect on the spinal dorsal horn neurons. Significant advances in understanding the functions of substance P have been made by using substance P antagonists. As more of these antagonists are developed and utilized, greater information on the precise role of substance P-mediated potentials in the spinal cord and other regions of the central nervous system may be elucidated. It is very likely that substance P might be co-released from selective primary afferent nerve terminals in the dorsal horn together with some unidentified fast-acting neurotransmitter. Many speculations on this and other possibilities involving the actions of substance P, either alone or in relationship with other neurotransmitters, make the future very exciting for research in this area. The fact that the highest concentration of substance P is found in the substantia nigra is clearly significant. In this region of the midbrain, the major output includes dopaminergic neurons. The major inhibitory inputs are gamma-amino butyric acid fibers, while the major excitatory inputs are substance P fibers. In view of the possible relationship and effects of the dopamine system of the substantia nigra in certain neurological disease processes, there is room for pharmacological manipulation of the function of that region of the brain by substance P-related "agonist and antagonist" using drugs and appropriate therapeutic modalities.

The intense interest in pain has been highlighted by the developing importance of neuromodulators and neurotransmitters. The role of nociceptive stimulation involving peptidergic pathways and their modulating effect at the spinal level provides a sound basis for the clinical significance of the neuropeptides. The continued discovery of opioid neuropeptides, including the endorphins, dynorphins, leucine-enkephalin, methionine-enkephalin, and their various precursor compounds, has contributed meaningfully to the advances in pain research. The locations of these opioid neuropeptides in the various regions of the brain suggest that these compounds are very important in the modulation of nociception. The works of Yaksh et al. [43] have demonstrated that enkephalin when injected using micropipettes into the periaqueductal graey area, have profound analgesic activity. Further, Iversen has demonstrated that enkephalin and other opioid receptors are to be found in the interneurons of the dorsal horn of the spinal cord [44].

More evidence for the analgesic role of the opioid neuropeptides was demonstrated by Han and Xie, who showed that dynorphin and other opioid neuropeptides were important mediators for electroaccupuncture analgesia in the rabbit spinal cord [45]. These and other studies on the spinal localization of the opioid neuropeptides and their analgesic effect may play an important role in modulating pain transmission in the substantia gelatinosa. Although the specific mechanisms of these hypotheses remain unclear, it is very likely that the basic hypothesis is sound. Research tools in helping to advance these hypotheses, and in some cases to explain them, have been implemented by capsaicin (the substance that depletes substance P in peripheral nerves) and by substance P antagonists, together with in-vitro studies and perfusate preparations.

As more knowledge and data on the involvement of the neuropeptides in pain mechanisms, pain transmission, and pain modulation become available, and as the techniques involving these studies become more specific, some of the complex mysteries of chronic pain may become better understood. Significant difficulties still remain in the solution of these problems. These difficulties remain because pain in the human subject is so complex and is influenced by several subjective and objective factors, including the behavioral, environmental, cultural, emotional, disease states, genetic factors, and unfortunately, secondary gain. Data from the animal model, and their correlation to the human model, needs to be interpreted very carefully. Deductions and conclusions ought to be considered appropriately, and several factors have to be taken into account before these conclusions can be made. Several problems inherent to the neuropeptides compound the difficulties of that major task. These problems include the multifunctional role of the neuropeptides, including the gastro-intestinal, circulatory, and endocrine effects that may make correlation between the levels of the neuropeptides and any specific neural activity very difficult to interpret. Another major problem of the neuropeptides is the lack of precise information regarding their origin in the cerebrospinal fluid or in the plasma. This lack of information makes it difficult to correlate any change in neuropeptide concentration to a given pain stimulus or to a given specific neurophysiological event. Notwithstanding, it is appropriate to speculate that the levels of the neuropeptides in the various body fluids (cerebrospinal fluid, saliva, and plasma) may be a correlate, or even a biological marker, of pain. If this assumption is tenable, then the same premise may allow the assessment of a particular therapeutic modality to be followed by evaluation of the levels of neuropeptides in individual body fluids.

Most neuropeptides that have been found in the central nervous system have also been isolated in these cerebrospinal fluids [46]. The cerebrospinal fluid serves as a medium where substances are released from the central neurons and where substances not metabolized in the cerebrospinal fluid may accumulate. The level of any substance, including the neuropeptides, in the cerebrospinal fluid would depend on the rate of its biosynthesis and also on the rate of release, dilution, its inactivation, and subsequent biodegradation in the cerebrospinal fluid compartment. The precise mechanism would vary according to the individual neuropeptide. There are some neuropeptides that may be passively secreted into the cerebrospinal fluid, while others may be actively produced in that region. In spite of the unclear relationship between the neuropeptides and the cerebrospinal fluid, there is still a compelling inclination to make a correlation between cerebrospinal fluid neuropeptide concentrations and certain acute and/or chronic pain syndromes. Akil et al. have helped demonstrate that there are significant increases in beta-endorphin-like immunoreactivity in the human ventricular spinal fluid following analgesic electrical stimulation [47]. Almay et al. showed that the cerebrospinal fluid substance P levels of chronic low back pain patients are significantly lower than the cerebrospinal fluid substance P levels of healthy human volunteers [48]. Within that group of patients, they showed that substance P levels were significantly lower in patients with neurogenic back pain than in patients with idiopathic back pain. However, both groups of patients, that is, neurogenic and idiopathic back pain patients, had lower cerebrospinal fluid substance P levels than healthy human volunteers. Vaeroy et al. showed that patients with fibromyalgia had elevated cerebrospinal fluid substance P levels and that these patients also had a high incidence of Raynaud's phenomenon [49]. Correspondingly, low levels of beta-endorphins in cerebrospinal fluid have been found in patients with chronic nonspecific headache when these patients were compared with normal patients. Further documentation of the relationship between the neuropeptides and disease states was provided by Tamsen et al., who showed that the postoperative demand for analgesics after major surgery correlates directly with preoperative levels of cerebrospinal fluid endorphins [50]. Thus, the relationship between neuropeptides, notably the opioid neuropeptides, and substance P levels in the cerebrospinal fluid appears to correlate with chronic pain, although the precise pathophysiological significance of this observation remains to be elucidated.

In reviewing the work of Almay et al. showing the relationship between cerebrospinal fluid substance P levels and chronic back pain, Parris et al. [51] sought to avoid using such an invasive approach (lumbar puncture) to determine neuropeptide levels. Instead, they used saliva as the body fluid in which to measure substance P. Since the presence of substance P in saliva had never been documented, the first task was to demonstrate the presence of substance P in saliva. In this regard, a number of healthy volunteers donated saliva and blood for substance P analysis. The saliva was immediately frozen and stored at −70°C until extraction. The blood was centrifuged immediately so as to minimize hydrolysis by endopeptidase. This centrifugation process took place in a refrigerated centrifuge and was followed by immediate freezing and storage at −70°C until extraction. The technique for extraction, purification, and radioimmunoassay of substance P was that described by Yanaihara et al. [52,53].

The results of these preliminary studies showed that the dilution curve for the saliva extract was indistinguishable from the substance P standard curve. The implication of this finding is that the saliva extract contains a substance P-like compound that is immunologically identical to substance P (Figure 14-1). The results also showed that the saliva and plasma substance P levels in the chronic back pain patients were both lower than the corresponding levels of substance P in healthy human volunteers (Figure 14-2). Further, the results showed that the saliva substance P levels, expressed on the basis of ng/mg of protein, were appropriately 100 times higher than corresponding levels in plasma in both patient groups (healthy human volunteers and chronic back pain patients) [51].

One may speculate as to the significance of these findings. It is tempting to suggest that substance P might be a correlate, or possibly a biological marker, of chronic back pain. However, the origins and functions of neuropeptides in plasma are, at best, unclear. The biogenesis, release, dilution, and subsequent biodegradation of substance P in the plasma has not yet been elucidated completely. It is also known that circulating neuropeptides are not able to

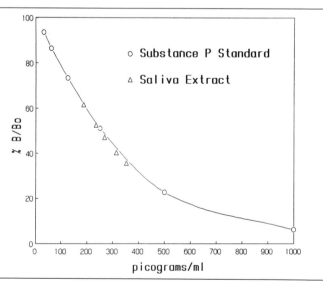

Figure 14-1. Correlation between saliva extract and substance P dilution curves. (Reprinted with permission).

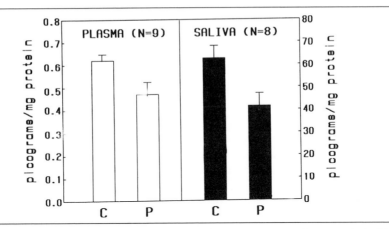

Figure 14-2. Comparison of mean (±SEM) levels of immunoreactive substance P in healthy volunteers (C) and chronic pain patients (P). (Reprinted with permission).

cross the blood-brain barrier in any significant quantities, and it is further believed that low concentrations of neuropeptides that cross the blood-brain barrier may do so as a function of the lipophilicity of specific neuropeptides. The origin of the high concentration of substance P in saliva is not known at this time. The half-life of neuropeptides in plasma is very short, and the levels in relation to these short half-lives make meaningful interpretation difficult.

There are several substances that are known to antagonize the action of substance P. Although these substances have not yet been utilized clinically, they have been known to be effective in laboratory preparations. Examples of these substances that are substance P antagonists [54] include adenosine monophosphate and trimethaphan camphorsulfonate (Arfonad®). Their effect has been shown on the guinea-pig ilium. The antispasmodic compound, baclofen (Lioresal®) has been demonstrated to antagonize the depolarizing action of substance P on rat spinal motor neurons. Baclofen also reduces the depolarizing action of L-glutamate, which is known to be an excitatory transmitter [55]. This intriguing characteristic of baclofen has been exploited and utilized epidurally in clinical trials to treat pain in human subjects. Clearly, as more work on the substance P antagonists [56] is done and more advances are made, the clinical utilization of these discoveries would be be very effective in chronic pain management.

In conclusion, it is clear that the neuropeptide era promises to be an exciting and productive one that should have a profound effect on our understanding of neurochemical transmission. The consequences of research in this area are likely to have a radical impact on pain management and to play a big role in unlocking some of the mysteries of chronic pain. As more current data are accumulated linking the interrelationships between substance P (and the other neuropeptides) and the endogenous opioid compounds, parallel clinical strategies should develop in helping to solving many problems associated with the treatment of pain syndromes.

ACKNOWLEDGMENTS

The author would like to thank Drs. Brian Sweetman and David McGrath for their editorial assitance.

REFERENCES

1. Krieger DT. 1983. Brain peptides: What, where and why? Science 222:975–985.
2. Barker JL. 1976. Peptides: Roles in neuronal excitability. Physiol Rev 56:435–452.
3. Basbaum AI, Fields HL. 1984. Endogenous pain control systems: Brainstem spinal pathways and endorphin circuitry. Annu Rev Neurosci 7:309–338.
4. von Euler US, Gaddum JH. 1931. An unidentified depressor substance in certain tissue extracts. J Physiol (London) 72:74–87.
5. Pernow B. 1953. Studies on substance P — purification, occurrence, and biological actions. Acta Physiol Scand 29(Suppl. 105):1–90.
6. Lembeck F. 1953. Zur Frage der zentralen übertragung afferenter impulse. III. Mitteilung. Das vorkommen und die bedeutung der substanz P in den dorsalen wurzeln des ruckenmarks. Naunyn-Schmiedebergs Arch Exp Pathol Pharmakol 219:197–213.
7. Erspamer V. 1981. The tachykinin peptide family. Trends Neurosci 4:267–269.
8. Chang MM, Leeman SE, Niall HD. 1971. Amino-acid sequence of substance P. Nature New Biol 232:86–87.
9. Gaddum JH, Schild H. 1934. Depressor substances in extracts of intestine. J Physiol (London) 83:1–14.
10. Hökfelt T, Kellerth JO, Nilsson G, Pernow B. 1975. Substance P: Localization in the central nervous system and in some primary sensory neurons. Science 190:889–890.
11. Deininger PL, Daniels GR. 1986. The recent evolution of mammalian repetitive DNA elements. Trends Genet 2:76–80.
12. Tatemoto K, Lundberg JM, Jornvall H, Mutt V. 1985. Neuropeptide K: Isolation, structure and biological activities of a novel brain tachykinin. Biochem Biophys Res Commun 128:947–953.
13. Konishi S, Otsuka M. 1971. Actions of certain polypeptides on frog spinal neurons. Jpn J Pharmacol 21:685–687.
14. Said SI, Mutt V. 1970. Polypeptide with broad biological activity: Isolation from small intestine. Science 169:1217–1218.
15. Lembeck F, Zetler G. 1971. Substance P. In JM Walker (ed), International Encyclopedia of Pharmacology and Therapeutics, Vol. 1. Oxford, Pergamon, pp. 29–71.
16. Hökfelt T, Kellerth JO, Nilsson G, Pernow B. 1975. Experimental immunohistochemical studies on the localization and distribution of substance P in cat primary sensory neurons. Brain Res 100:235–252.
17. Henry JL, Krnjevic K, Morris ME, 1975. Substance P and spinal neurones. Can J Physiol Pharmacol 53:423–432,
18. Otsuka M, Konishi S. 1974. Electrophysiology of mammalian spinal cord in vitro. Nature 252:733–734.
19. Saito K, Konishi S, Otsuka M. 1975. Antagonism between Lioresal and substance P in rat spinal cord. Brain Res 97:177–180.
20. Takahashi T, Otsuka M. 1975. Regional distribution of substance P in the spinal cord and nerve roots of the cat and the effect of dorsal root section. Brain Res 87:1–11.
21. Konishi S, Otsuka M. 1974. The effects of substance P and other peptides on spinal neurons of the frog. Brain Res 65:397–410.
22. Henry JL. 1976. Excitation of spinal nociceptive neurons by substance P (abstr.). Nobel Symp. 37, Substance P, Stockholm, pp. 29–31.
23. Konishi S, Otsuka M. 1974. Excitatory action of hypothalamic substance P on spinal motoneurones of newborn rats. Nature 252:734–735.

24. Joo F, Szolcsanyi J, Jansco-Gabor A. 1969. Mitochondrial alterations in the spinal ganglion cells of the rat accompanying the long-lasting sensory disturbance induced by capsaicin. Life Sci 8:621–626.

25. Jessell TM, Iversen LL, Cuello AC. 1978. Capsaicin-induced depletion of substance P from sensory neurones. Brain Res 152:183–188.

26. Szolcsanyi J. 1977. A pharmacological approach to elucidation of the role of different nerve fibers and receptor endings in mediation of pain. J Physiol (Paris) 73:251–262.

27. Holzer P, Jurna I, Gamse R, Lembeck F. 1979. Nociceptive threshold after neonatal capsaicin treatment. Eur J Pharmacol 58:511–514.

28. Nagy J, Hunt SP, Emson PC, Iversen LL. 1982. Fluroide-resistant acid phosphatase containing neurones in dorsal root ganglia are separate from those containing substance P or somatostatin. Neuroscience 7:89–97.

29. Holzer P. 1988. The sensory-efferent function of capsaicin-sensitive sensory nerve endings: Involvement of tachykinins, and other neuropeptides. Neuroscience 24:739–768.

30. Angelucci L. 1956. Experiments with perfused frog's spinal cord. Br J Pharmacol 11:161–170.

31. Otsuka M, Konishi S. 1976. Release of substance P-like immunoreactivity from isolated spinal cord of newborn rat. Nature 264:83–84.

32. Iversen LL, Jessell T, Kanazawa I. 1976. Release and metabolism of substance P in rat hypothalamus. Nature 264:81–83.

33. Hanley MR, Iversen LL. 1980. In SJ Enna, HI Yamamura (eds), Neurotransmitter receptors Part I. Amino Acids, Peptides, and Benzodiazepines. London, Chapman and Hall, pp. 71–103.

34. Segawa T, Nakata Y. 1976. Substance P in rabbit brain and spinal cord: Regional and subcellular distribution and evidence for lack of high-affinity uptake system. Jpn J Pharmacol 26(Suppl.):100p.

35. Chrubasik J, Meynadier J, Scherpereel P, Wunsch E. 1985. The effect of epidural somatostatin of postoperative pain. Anesth Analg 64:1085–1088.

36. Chrubasik J, Meynadier J, Blond S, Scherpereel P, Ackerman E, Weinstock M, Bonath K, Cramer H, Wunsch E. 1984. Somatostatin, a potent analgesic. Lancet 2:1208–1209.

37. Parris WCV, Kambam JR, Naukam RJ et al. 1988. The effect of somatostatin on plasma substance (SP) in carcinoid syndrome. Regul Pept 22:142.

38. Parris WCV, Oates J, Kambam J et al. 1988. Pre-treatment with somatostatin in the anesthetic management of a patient with carcinoid syndrome. Can J Anaesth 35(4):413–416.

39. Basbaum AI, Glazer EJ. 1983. Immunoreactive intestinal polypeptide is concentrated in the sacral spinal cord: A possible marker for pelvic visceral afferent fibers. Somatosens Res 1:69–82.

40. Yaksh TL, Abay EO II, Go VLW. 1982. Studies on the location and release of cholecystokinin and vasoactive intestinal peptide in rat and cat spinal cord. Brain Res 242:279–290.

41. Le Greves P, Nyberg F, Terenius L, Hokfelt T. 1985. Calcitonin gene-related peptide is a potent inhibitor of substance P degradation. Eur J Pharmacol 115:309–311.

42. Moskowitz MA. 1984. The neurobiology of vascular head pain. Ann Neurol 16:157–168.

43. Yaksh TL, Tyce GM. 1979. Microinjection of morphine into the periaqueductal gray evokes the release of serotonin from spinal cord. Brain Res 171:176–181.

44. Iversen LL, Nagy J, Emson PC, Lee CM, Hanley M, Sandberg B, Ninkovic M, Hunt S. 1981. Substance P, enkephalins and the problems of pain. In L Stjarne, P Hedqvist, H Lagarcrantz, A Wenmalm (eds), Chemical Transmission 75 Years. New York, Academic Press, pp. 501–512.

45. Han J-S, Xie G-X. 1984. Dynorphin: Important mediator for electroaccupuncture analgesia in the spinal cord of the rabbit. Pain 18:367–376.

46. Jessel TM. 1982. Substance P in nociceptive sensory neurons. In Substance P in the Nervous System. Ciba Foundation Symposium, No. 91, London, Pitman, pp. 255–258.

47. Akil H, Richardson DE, Barchas JD, Li CH. 1978. Appearance of beta-endorphin-like immunoreactivity in human ventricular cerebrospinal fluid upon analgesic electrical stimulation. Proc Natl Acad Sci USA 75:5170–5172.

48. Almay BGL, Johansson F, Von Knorring L, Le Greves P, Terenius L. 1988. Substance P in CSF of patients with chronic pain syndromes. Pain 33:3–9.

49. Vaeroy J, Helle R, Forre O, Kass E, Terenius L. 1988. Elevated CSF levels of substance P and high incidence of Raynaud's phenomenon in patients with fibromyalgia: New features for

diagnosis. Pain 32:21–26.
50. Tamsen A, Sakurada T, Wahlstrom A, Terenius L, Hartvig P. 1982. Postoperative demand for analgesics in relation to individual levels of endorphins and substance P in cerebrospinal fluid. Pain 13:171–183.
51. Parris WCV, Kambam JR, Naukam RJ, Sastry BVR. 1990. Immunoreactive-substance P is decreased in saliva of patients with chronic back syndromes. Anesth Analg 70:63–67.
52. Yanaihara C, Sato H, Hirohashi M, et al. 1976. Substance P radioimmunoassay using N-tyrosyl-substance P and demonstration of the presence of substance P-like immunoreactivities in human blood and porcine tissue extracts. Endocrinol Jpn 23:457–463.
53. Incstar, Corp. Substance P by radioimmunoassay. Revised 10/86, Part #10393. Stillwater, MN, Incstar, Corp.
54. Stern P, Huković S. 1961. Specific antagonists of substance P. In P Stern (ed), Symposium on Substance P, 83–88. Sarajevo, Sci. Soc. Bosnia Herzegovina, 143 pp.
55. Davidoff RA, Sears ES. 1974. The effects of Lioresal on synaptic activity in the isolated spinal cord. Neurology 24:957–963.
56. Phillis JW. 1976. Is -(4-chlorophenyl)-GABA a specific antagonist of substance P on cerebral cortical neurons? Experientia 32:593–594.
57. Helke CH, Dimicco JA, Jacobowitz DM, Kopin IJ. 1981. Effects of capsaicin administration to neonatal rats on substance P content of discrete CNS regions. Brain Res 222:428–431.

15. CURRENT THERAPY OF REFLEX SYMPATHETIC DYSTROPHY

NEAL M. GOLDBERGER AND WINSTON C.V. PARRIS

The first description of severe, sustained pain and concomitant limb atrophy following peripheral nerve injury was by Denmark [1] in 1813. More complete documentation was provided by Mitchell [2] in 1864 when he treated traumatic limb injuries that occurred during the Civil War. The term *causalgia* came into use in the late 1860s, and was derived from the Greek words *kausos* and *algos*, meaning "heat" and "pain," respectively [3]. Mitchell was able to document clearly the clinical presentation of causalgia but was not able to find an effective treatment. Much later in the 20th century, the role of the sympathetic nervous system was elucidated, and evidence of the therapeutic efficacy of surgical sympathectomy in treating causalgia was demonstrated in the 1930s. What has followed since that time has been the development of a multitude of theories and as many treatments, all attempting to explain the complex pathophysiology of the sympathetic nervous system and pharmacologic mechanisms to control its function. Some of these mechanisms and therapies will be discussed later in this chapter.

It is important to define terminology as it applies to the spectrum of sympathetic disease. The terms *causalgia* and *reflex sympathetic dystrophy* are often incorrectly assumed to be interchangeable. Causalgia refers to the clinical syndrome that develops after the direct injury of a nerve. What usually follows is dysfunction of the sympathetic nervous system resulting in dystrophic and neuropathic changes in the affected region (usually an extremity). In reflex sympathetic dystrophy, the clinical syndrome is similar, but there is no known direct nerve injury. Roberts [4] suggests that the clinical similarity between reflex sympathetic dystrophy and causalgia is such that the term *sympathetically mediated pain* may be a general description of a sympathetic nervous system disease process that includes causalgia and reflex sympathetic dystrophy as components. There are many other pain syndromes that would fall under this categorization of sympathetically mediated pain. These include posttraumatic pain syndrome, mimo causalgia, minor causalgia, minor traumatic dystrophy, shoulder hand syndrome, shoulder atrophy, and posttraumatic edema. For the purpose of this chapter, the term *reflex sympathetic dystrophy* will be used to describe these syndromes. However, the term *sympathetically mediated pain* may best describe the role that the sympathetic nervous system plays in the development of pain, autonomic dysfunction, and the dystrophic changes that subsequently occur.

CLINICAL FEATURES

Patients with sympathetically mediated pain may present after a major or minor traumatic injury. However, there are patients who have the classical features of reflex sympathetic dystrophy without any history of trauma. Only a small percentage of all injuries will result in the development of reflex sympathetic dystrophy syndrome, and the predisposing factors are not particularly well understood. These factors may include 1) the presence of a painful injury, 2) susceptibility of the sympathetic nervous system, which includes hereditary factors and personality traits, and 3) an abnormal sympathetic reflex, which may include inappropriate stages of healing [5,6].

Patients often report the onset of pain soon after injury. This pain continues until it reaches an extreme intensity within days to weeks, and may be described by the patient as a constant burning sensation in the region of injury. This is often accompanied by a deep throbbing or crushing sensation. The intensity of pain may seem to be out of proportion to the severity of injury. The pain is often noted by the patient to be continuous, with extreme aggravation of the symptoms caused by motion, touching, or emotional excitement. Kleinert et al. has described the progression of reflex sympathetic dystrophy through three stages [7]:

1. *Vasodilation.* This includes increased blood flow to the region, with burning pain and dysesthesia. Skin temperature is elevated and accelerated nail and hair growth are present with localized edema, dry scaly skin, and decreased movement [8].
2. *Vasoconstriction.* This phase is characterized by increased hypersensitivity and burning pain, lowered skin temperature, decreased hair and nail growth, hyperhydrosis, and cyanotic skin coloration. Emotional changes may occur with seclusion and marked protection of the extremity [9].
3. *Atrophic phase.* Decreased hypersensitivity, normalization of blood flow and temperature, smooth, glossy skin, abnormal sweating, and osteoporosis [10].

The distribution of pain in reflex sympathetic dystrophy does not follow a dermatomal pattern. In true causalgia, pain may follow the distribution of a single peripheral nerve. In reflex sympathetic dystrophy, pain will follow an arterial (or vascular) distribution that does not correlate with dermatomal or peripheral nerve anatomy. The absence of radicular symptoms associated with hyperpathic pain may suggest the possibility of a reflex sympathetic dystrophy diagnosis.

Patients may present for treatment in any of the three previously described phases. Clinical experience suggests that early intervention in the clinical course provides for better therapeutic and functional results [11]. The chances of satisfactory patient recovery after the onset of reflex sympathetic dystrophy diminish markedly after a 6-month period. It must be noted, however, that patients with reflex sympathetic dystrophy may have spontaneous resolution of their pain syndromes, and some authors speculate this may occur in 50% of patients [12,13]. Thus, it is expedient to promote early diagnosis and treatment of the syndrome because one cannot predict the patients who will not have spontaneous remission [14].

PATHOGENESIS

Many theories have evolved to describe the mechanism of reflex sympathetic dystrophy development and the protracted severe pain syndrome that follows. There is much ongoing discussion about particular mechanisms and physiological models, but none really offers a completely satisfactory explanation. There is also a great deal of research activity surrounding the rationale of the different pain mechanisms postulated and therapeutic strategies used in the management of reflex sympathetic dystrophy.

The possible role of the sympathetic nervous system in disease was first described in the 17th century by Willis [15]. In the 1700s, Winslow [16] used the term *sympathetic* to indicate the nervous structure involved in maintaining "sympathy" or "harmony." Thus, the integrated function of the sympathetic nervous system in homeostasis was conceptualized. It was also noted that the sympathetic nervous system was involved in sensation. This was further elucidated by Claude Bernard [17] in the 1800s.

Despite knowledge of the sympathetic nervous system for over 150 years, progress in understanding its role in the development of pain syndromes has been slow. In fact, it is unclear at present whether sympathetic blockade by local anesthetics affects sympathetic afferent or efferent nerve fibers. It has been suggested that sympathetic afferents may modulate nociceptive stimuli prior to entering the dorsal horn of the spinal cord. Sympathetic efferents provide evidence for the "vicious" cycle of response to painful stimuli [18]. Painful stimuli cause increased activation of the sympathetic efferents, which produces further vasoconstriction, ischemia, and some of the chronic dysfunctional and structural changes associated with reflex sympathetic dystrophy [19]. Some investigators have hypothesized concepts such as post-traumatic peripheral tissue abnormalities or sensitization of central nociceptive neurons in the etiology of reflex sympathetic dystrophy. The role of wide dynamic range neurons and the effect of sympathetic efferents was hypothesized by Roberts [4] as a possible mechanism of action.

Doupe et al. [20] have suggested the possibility of an artificial synapse occurring between the sympathetic and somatic sensory nerves after nerve injury. This theory does not explain the fact that while pain begins almost immediately after an injury in reflex sympathetic dystrophy, the known histological nerve changes associated with nerve injury require a substantially longer period of time to evolve. This is substantiated by the fact that it takes myelin several days before histological manifestation of degeneration becomes evident. In addition to the many hypotheses that include changes associated with the peripheral nervous system, there are theories that involve the central nervous system as well. Melzack and Wall proposed a gate control pain mechanism, which suggests that pain impulses reaching the brain must surpass a critical level [21]. It has also been shown that loss of afferent stimulation from peripheral nerves can cause spontaneous firing of neural impulses from the dorsal horn of the spinal cord: This results in nociception. Thus, nociception may in fact originate in the dorsal horn and possibly elsewhere along the neuraxis. Higher structures may therefore affect dorsal horn firing by sending information down descending pathways. The higher centers have their own input from peripheral afferents and therefore may be affected by peripheral stimulation. This is one possible explanation for the effectiveness of transcutaneous electrical nerve stimulation (TENS) in the management of reflex sympathetic dystrophy. Thus, the pathogenesis of reflex sympathetic dystrophy is at present unclear, although there are many theoretical hypotheses that may explain certain facets of this syndrome.

DIFFERENTIAL DIAGNOSIS

Thorough history taking and meticulous physical examination are important ingredients in the evaluation and diagnosis of the reflex sympathetic dystrophy patient. There are several disorders that may mimic reflex sympathetic dystrophy and the differential diagnosis is complex. Ofter, there is a "grey" area and it is difficult to rule out completely a sympathetically mediated process. Primary injury may be present with a superimposed reflex sympathetic dystrophy. Many painful entities have several pathways of neurological involvement [22]. Thus, an assessment of the role that the sympathetic nervous system plays must be elucidated.

Some patients with persistent pain after an injury or surgery may be referred to a pain control center or pain clinic for evaluation and treatment. The customary postsurgical pain after an operative procedure, e.g., hernia, may last as long as 6 weeks, so a precise determination of time after injury is an important historical point. There may be a surgical or posttraumatic somatic nerve injury that is primarily responsible for the complaint of pain. Patients who present with joint pain should be investigated for inflammatory processes.

Extreme tenderness over extremities should be investigated for the possibility of local myofascial pain with its associated trigger points. The skeletal system should be examined physically and radiologically so as to avoid misdiagnosing fractures and other structural abnormalities.

Raynaud's disease or phenomenon may cause vascular constriction of one or of all distal extremities. This disease (just as reflex sympathetic dystrophy) does respond positively to sympathetic blockade and calcium-channel blockers, but the response to treatment is variable and unpredictable. It is, however, possible to have both Raynaud's and a secondary reflex sympathetic dystrophy simultaneously in the same patient.

In an attempt to assess the role of the sympathetic nervous system in a particular pain process, the following steps may be taken:

1. Patient evaluation to rule out the possibility of other significant pathology causing pain. For example, if a patient presents with unilateral back pain, one must rule out myofascial pain, a herniated disc, or such less common diagnostic entities as metastatic carcinoma (e.g., prostate, ovary). Initial comprehensive evaluation of the chronic pain patient with appropriate ancillary investigations should facilitate the diagnostic process.
2. Attempt to define the mechanism of the underlying pain syndrome.
3. Use of differential spinal or diagnostic blocks.
4. Trial of sympathetic blocks may be performed (i.e., stellate ganglion or lumbar sympathetic blocks).

The assessment of the sympathetic nervous system by differential block may be accomplished as follows. For the patient who has lower extremity pain, it may be possible to differentiate sympathetic, somatic, or a central etiology for pain by performing a differential spinal block with preservative-free normal saline and varying concentrations of procaine [23]. There is, however, some controversy concerning the effectiveness of interpreting the results of a differential spinal block, since subjective evaluation is required. There are several practical drawbacks to using the differential spinal block. The procedure is time consuming, it is unwieldy to implement, and it may provide unreliable information that could be misleading. Another technique may be used to differentiate sensory, motor, and sympathetically mediated pain. This is a differential epidural block and is utilized by observing the onset of pain during "block regression." This block is performed by placing a catheter in the epidural space and dosing with 3% 2-chloro-procaine (Nesacaine®). Block regression is noted by observing the onset of pain complaints and by correlating the presence of motor, sensory, or sympathetic block. Another option for assessing sympathetic function is by performing an appropriate sympathetic block and noting the degree of relief that the patient experiences. This technique, however, does not rule out a placebo response.

DIAGNOSTIC TESTING

As mentioned earlier, it is appropriate to obtain studies that will allow one to rule out other causes of pain. Radiographic studies demonstrate acute injury, swelling, osteoporotic change, or fracture. Computerized tomography scans may further define anatomical abnormalities resulting from vascular effects induced by the reflex sympathetic dystrophy. Three-phase bone scanning may also be used to assist in the diagnosis of reflex sympathetic dystrophy [24]. The early-phase ^{99}Tc diphosphate bone scan may demonstrate increased blood flow in particular areas, while the late phase scan highlights increased isotope concentrations around the joints of the affected limb [25]. These scans have a variable sensitivity (approximately 60–90%) but a high specificity (92–98%). Another diagnostic test for reflex sympathetic dystrophy is the skin electro-potential response using a modified electrocardiograph. This experimental device is able to document differences in both the magnitude and duration of skin electrical potentials [26]. The investigators state that this test is very specific for reflex sympathetic dystrophy, but it has not achieved widespread use.

Thermography may be regarded as a specific and accurate indirect correlate of sympathetic function [27]. Thermography involves the ability to obtain a display of skin surface temperature. This is recorded in a color scheme fashion such that a particular temperature is matched to a particular color. Thus an outline of the extremity or the region examined is obtained that contains color gradients along a color continuum. It is therefore possible to compare symmetric portions of the body in an effort to find hypothermic or hyperthermia areas. Skin temperature asymmetry may be ascribed directly or indirectly to differences in regional skin perfusion. This may reflect changes in sympathetic nervous activity. For example, if a patient presents with a complaint of unilateral lower limb pain, and thermography demonstrates relative hypothermia of that extremity as compared to the opposite extremity, then the diagnosis of reflex sympathetic dystrophy becomes very likely. Thermography may be performed after sympathetic blockade and may demonstrate hyperthermia of the blocked extremity and thus correlate with successful sympathetic block. Some controversy exists regarding the reliability and diagnotic reproducibility of thermography. This is mainly due to variations in the equilibration process (which is very vital to ensure accuracy and standardization) of thermography.

TREATMENT OF REFLEX SYMPATHETIC DYSTROPHY

There continues to be much controversy over the treatment of reflex sympathetic dystrophy. Much of this controversy stems from empiric results in selected patients. There are few prospective well-designed, controlled studies of reflex sympathetic dystrophy therapy. The wide variety of treatments available, coupled with the diversity of the backgrounds of the treating physicians (family practitioners, orthopedists, neurologists, neurosurgeons, anesthesiologists, and psychiatrists), do not allow for easy evaluation of the efficacy of individual treatment modalities.

In this section, the management approach taken at the Vanderbilt University Pain Center will be reviewed. At this center, a multidisciplinary approach is undertaken with the anesthesiologist functioning as the primary physician directing the medical evaluation. The patient is also interviewed and evaluated by a clinical psychologist, physical therapist, and a nurse algologist. Initially, the patient is evaluated by the anesthesiologist, who obtains a thorough history and performs a physical examination. At this time, a patient–physician interaction is cultivated and subsequently nurtured. The patient is scheduled for appropriate thermography, interacts with the nurse algologist, and views a pain video for informational and educational purposes. After discussions by members of the pain team, the medical director/anesthesiologist meets with the patient and his or her family to discuss the diagnosis and its implications, therapeutic options, and a strategy of management. At this meeting, informed consent is obtained for the designated treatment. The customary therapeutic options for the average patient include sympathetic blocks, adjuvant medications, psychological interactions, biofeedback, and intensive physical therapy. The patient may be started on a treatment course that allows emotional issues to be addressed and aggressive physical therapy started at a relatively early point in time. Improving the range of motion of the affected limb or region is an important aspect of care that is emphasized very early in the treatment course [28].

The importance of initiating sympathetic blockade early in the management of these patients must not be underestimated. Interruption of the sympathetic reflex via ganglionic or intravenous block procedures are both diagnostic and therapeutic. Performed early after injury, sympathetic blockade was reported to be extremely beneficial [29]. The pain cycle may be interrupted by local anesthetic-induced block of the sympathetic ganglia. Although this is usually temporary (i.e., local anesthetics have a defined duration of action), there may be changes in the intensity of neural activity that occur long after cessation of local anesthetic action [30]. This may explain the rationale for patients who obtain long-lasting or permanent pain relief following a series of sympathetic blocks long after the local anesthetic action has ceased.

Sympathetic blockade may be induced by the placement of local anesthetic agents in the proximity of the sympathetic ganglia. The stellate ganglion is used for sympathetic blockade of the head, neck, upper extremity, and upper chest, while the lumbar sympathetic ganglia are used for lower extremity sympathetic blockade. In addition, the celiac plexus may be used in patients with sympathetically mediated pain between the fourth and tenth thoracic dermatomes, which correlates with visceral pain problems. These blocks can be effectively administered by an anesthesiologist trained in pain management. A thorough understanding of principles of cardiopulmonary resuscitation and knowledge of resuscitation equipment is essential and medicolegally prudent prior to the administration of nerve blocks. Use of 0.25% bupivacaine in volumes of 10 ml for the stellate ganglion, 20 ml for the lumbar sympathetic ganglia, and 30 ml for the celiac plexus has provided excellent sympathetic blockade without undesirable concurrent motor weakness. This is ideal for outpatient use.

It is also possible to block afferent and efferent sympathetics of the upper extremity by brachial plexus and intravenous regional (Bier) sympathetic blocks and corresponding lower extremity sympathetics by epidural, subarachnoid, and intravenous regional (Bier) sympathetic blocks. These approaches allow easier and safer use of continuous local anesthetic infusions for patients who require intense inpatient therapy coupled with continuous sympathetic block. Combining continuous infusions with active physical therapy may resolve a reflex sympathetic dystrophy that has been refractory to outpatient management [31].

Other therapies for reflex sympathetic dystrophy have been investigated as well. For the patient who does not respond to a sympathetic block series, there are alternative therapies. In 1974, Hannington-Kiff [32] introduced the technique of intravenous regional sympathetic blockade using guanethidine. Guanethidine displaces noradrenaline from storage sites in sympathetic nerve endings and further inhibits its reuptake. This causes a depletion of noradrenaline at the postganglion sympathetic nerve endings. Several prospective studies [33] were undertaken and this therapy was recommended for patients presenting with Stage II or Stage III reflex sympathetic dystrophy. Parenteral guanethidine is not currently available for commercial use in the United States (preliminary investigative reports suggest that it should be available shortly), but it is widely used in Europe and Canada.

The use of intravenous reserpine by Bier block in reflex sympathetic dystrophy has also been investigated [34]. Chinuard et al. [35] reported that the use of 1 mg of reserpine in 50 ml of saline for upper extremity blocks and 2 mg of reserpine in 100 ml of saline for lower extremity blocks relieved symptoms in 20 of 25 patients after a Bier procedure with a tourniquet time of 15 minutes. No side effects of the medication were noted in that study. Unfortunately, because reserpine is not widely used as an antihypertensive agent anymore, the drug is no longer manufactured in the United States and is therefore not available for routine use in reflex sympathetic dystrophy.

Investigators have used such drugs as pure beta-blockers [36], labetolol [37] (combined beta- and alpha-adrenergic antagonist), calcium-channel blockers [38], bretylium [39], and clonidine [40]. These techniques have theoretical pharmacological mechanisms that would allow for diminished activity of the sympathetic nervous system in the region of block. However, the efficacy of these therapies in prospective studies is yet to be determined. These techniques may offer some advantage for the patient who has not responded to an initial sympathetic block series. Oral nifedipine 10 mg four times daily has been used and may hold promise for patients who have not responded to conventional therapy [38].

The use of oral cortiocosteroids in Stage I reflex sympathetic dystrophy has been a common therapy for many years [41]. With more detailed understanding of the anatomy and physiology of newer spinal cord receptors (particularly corticosterone and glucocorticoid receptors), there may be greater validity to this therapy. Dirksen et al. [42] described his modification, i.e., epidural steroid injection, in the clinical improvement of a patient who previously was treated with direct sympathetic blockade and intravenous guanethidine without effect. The systemic effects of high-dose steroids include many undesirable side effects, but this is not seen with epidural steroid (methyl-prednisolone) injection. The efficacy of this therapy needs to be evaluated further.

The use of surgical sympathectomy in the treatment of reflex sympathetic dystrophy used to be more commonly utilized than at the present time. Abram [43] suggests that in order to benefit from this therapy patients should meet the following criteria:

1. The patient should receive pain relief from previous sympathetic blocks.
2. Pain relief should last as long as the vascular effects of the blocks.
3. Placebo should provide no pain relief.
4. Severe behavioral dysfunction and secondary gain should be excluded prior to treatment.

Neurolytic sympathetic blocks may be occasionally considered for patients with intractable pain due to reflex sympathetic dystrophy [44] and who have met the above-mentioned criteria. This technique is, however, associated with many unacceptable complications and is almost obsolete. Neurolysis of the stellate ganglia cannot be performed because of the anatomical proximity of the brachial plexus, spinal cord, and vascular structures (including vertebral and carotid arteries).

A cornerstone of pharmacological therapy has been the use of tricyclic antidepressant drugs [45]. These may be used singly or with nonsteroidal antiinflammatory agents [46]. This combination of therapy has been found by several investigators to produce pain relief and improvement in sleep patterns. There are many reports of low-dose tricyclic antidepressants producing effective pain control. The tricyclic antidepressant drugs may cause sedation and such anticholinergic side effects as dry mouth, weight gain, palpitations, and arrhythmias. Their mechanism of action may be by blocking the reuptake of noradrenalin and serotonin. It is known that pain modulation involves the action of several vasoactive substances, including noradrenalin and serotonin. The complex pharmacology of both the tricyclic antidepressant drugs and their neuronal activity is being actively investigated. Suffice it to say that tricyclic antidepressants coupled with nonsteroidal antiinflammatory drugs provide pharmacological changes that may augment the response of a patient to sympathetic blockade and physical therapy.

Transcutaneous electrical nerve stimulation (TENS) has been suggested to be helpful in the management of reflex sympathetic dystrophy [47]. Many investigators have found that use of TENS may provide short-term analgesia, which allows for concomitant aggressive physical therapy. In some other clinical situations, TENS may aggravate the patient's pain and therefore has limited application.

There are many potential therapies for treatment of reflex sympathetic dystrophy. The consensus for rational therapy among most algologists today is to use a multidisciplinary approach to pain management, with comprehensive evaluation, psychological assessment, thermographic evaluation, appropriate nerve block therapy, group therapy, patient education, aggressive physical therapy, and vocational therapy when applicable. Patients may be started on a regimen of tricyclic antidepressant drugs (with or without sedative effects depending upon their individual sleep pattern) as well as concomitant supplementation with nonsteroidal antiinflammatory medication. Response to nerve blocks is recorded and a progressive plan is implemented based upon response. While most patients improve with this therapy, the ones who fail may be candidates for intravenous regional Bier blocks, with or without an appropriate adrenergic blocking agent, steroids, and lidocaine. Oral nifedifine or phenoxybenzamine [48] may be used in resistant cases.

New therapies are constantly being investigated. Recent pathophysiological data [49] from the central pain signaling hyperexcitability of various neurones of the spinal cord suggest that preoperative nerve blocks and nerve blocks immediately postinjury may diminish or prevent the development of neuropathic or sympathetically mediated pain. The placement of dorsal column stimulators has been found to be helpful in some patients with refractory pain secondary to reflex sympathetic dystrophy. A modality that is increasingly used in Europe and may hold promise is magnetic field therapy, which is currently under investigation in the United States. A variety of pharmacological agents, including new narcotic analgesics, nonsteroidal antiinflammatory drugs, serotonin antagonists, alpha-adrenergic antagonists, substance-P antagonists, and centrally acting drugs, are constantly being investigated for their efficacy in treating reflex sympathetic dystrophy. An equally large number of modalities, including nerve blocks, surgical procedures, and hyperstimulation techniques (TENS, acupuncture, low-power laser modulation, magnetic therapy, etc.), are also utilized (clinically and experimentally) to treat reflex sympathetic dystrophy. The importance of continued investigation of these various treatment modalities cannot be overestimated.

CONCLUSIONS

Much has been learned about the pathophysiology of reflex sympathetic dystrophy in the past several years. The causes of reflex sympathetic dystrophy are yet unclear, although basic science research is starting to unravel the mysteries of sympathetic neurotransmission and the neuropharmacological interactions present in dysfunctional sympathetic nerves. Many beneficial changes have occurred in the clinical management of patients with reflex sympathetic dystrophy. The advent of multidisciplinary pain clinics has allowed for the integration of information and treatment modalities. The diagnosis of this syndrome is now facilitated by the use of such modalities as thermography, electrogalvanic skin response, and radionucleide bone scans. New pharmacological therapies, such as beta-blocking drugs, calcium-channel blocking agents, and bretylium tosylate, are being investigated. Other non-pharmacological approaches, such as physical therapy, biofeedback, and magnetic field therapy, are currently being evaluated. The clinical approach to diagnosing and managing reflex sympathetic dystrophy will change in the future as more relevant information becomes available.

REFERENCES

1. DeSaussure RL. 1978. Causalgia. Clin Neurosurg 27:626–636.
2. Thompson JE. 1979. The diagnosis and management of post-traumatic pain syndromes (causalgia). Aust NZ J Surg 49:299–304.
3. Headley B. 1987. Historical perspective of causalgia, management of sympathetically maintained pain. Phys Ther 67(9):1370–1374.
4. Roberts WJ. 1986. A hypothesis on the physiological basis for causalgia and related pains, Pain 24:297–311.
5. De Takats G. 1937. Reflex dystrophy of the extremities. Arch Surg 34:939.
6. Fontaine R, Herrmann L. 1933. Posttraumatic osteoporosis. Ann Surg 17:26.
7. Kleinert HE, Norberg H, McDonough JJ. 1980. Surgical sympathetomy: Upper and lower extremity. In GE Omer et al. (eds). Management of Peripheral Nerve Problems. Philadelphia, W.B. Saunders, pp. 285–302.
8. Jaeger B, Singer E, Kroening R. 1986. Reflex sympathetic dystrophy of the face. Report of two cases and a review of the literature. Arch Neurol 43(7):693–695.
9. Mitchell SW, et al. 1864. Gunshot wounds and other injuries of nerves. Philadelphia. J.B. Lippincott.
10. Sudeck P. 1900. Ueber die acute enzundliche knochenatropie. Arch Klin Chir 62:147.
11. Bonica JJ. 1979. Causalgia and other reflex sympathetic dystrophies. In JJ Bonica, JC Lebeshand, P Albefessard (eds), Advances in Pain Research and Therapy, Vol. 3. New York, Raven Press.
12. Sunderland S. 1976. Pain mechanisms in causalgia. J Neurol Neurosurg Psychiatry 39:471–480.
13. Abram SE, Anderson RA, Muitra-D'Cruze AM. 1981. Factors predictory short-term outcome of nerve blocks in the management of chronic pain. Pain 10:323–330.
14. Stanton-Hicks, Janig, Boas. 1989. Reflex Sympathetic Dystrophy. Boston, Kluwer Academic Publishers, pp. 165–172.
15. Willis T. 1672. De Anima Brutorum (De Scientia Seu Cognitone Britorum). London. Davis.
16. Winslow JB. 1732. Exportim Anatomique de la Structure du Corps Humain. Paris. Duprey et Desessartz.
17. Bernard C. 1858. Leçons sur la Physiologies et la Pathologie, du Système Nerveux. Paris. Bailliere.
18. Bonica JJ. 1953. The Management of Pain. Philadelplhia, Lea & Febiger.
19. Schwartzman RJ, McLellan TL. 1987. Reflex sympathetic dystrophy, a review. Arch Neurol 44:555–561.
20. Doupe J, Cullen CR, Chance GQ. 1944. Post traumatic pain and causalgia syndromes. J Neurol Neurosurg Psych 7:3348.
21. Melzack R, Wall PD. 1965. Pain mechanisms: A new theory. Science 150:971–979.
22. Raja SN, Meyer RA, Campbell JN. 1988. Peripheral mechanisms of somatic pain. Anesthesiology 68:571–590.
23. Winnie AP, Collins JJ. 1968. The pain clinic: I, Differential neural blockade in pain syndromes of questionable etiology, Med Clin North Am 52:123–124.
24. Demangeat JL, Constatinesco A, Brunot B, Foucher G, Farcot JM. 1988. Three-phase bone scanning in reflex sympathetic dystrophy of the hand. J Nucl Med. 29(1):26–32.

25. Holder LE, Machennes KE. 1984. Reflex sympathetic dystrophy in the hand: Clinical and scintographic criteria. Radiology 152:517–522.
26. Cronin KD, Kirsner RL, Fitzroyy VP. 1982. Diagnosis of reflex sympathetic dysfunction, use of the skin potential response. Anesthesia 37(8):848–852.
27. Lightman HI, Pochaczevsky R, Aprin H, Ilowite NT. 1987. Thermography in childhood reflex sympathetic dystrophy. J Pediatr 111(4):551–555.
28. Rowlingston JC. 1983. The sympathetic dystrophies. Int Anesthesiol Clinic 21:117–129.
29. Boas RA, Hatangdi VS, Richards EG. 1976. Lumbar sympathectomy, a percutaneous chemical technique. In JJ Bonica D Albe-Fessard (eds), Advances in Pain Research and Therapy, Vol. 1. New York, Raven Press, pp. 685–689.
30. Lankford LL. 1983. In CM Evants (ed), Reflex Sympathetic Dystrophy in Surgery of the Musculo Skeletal System. Edinburgh, Churchill Livingstone.
31. Raj PP. Personal communication.
32. Hannington-Kiff JB. 1974. Intravenous regional sympathetic block with guanethidine. Lancet 1:1019–1020.
33. Driessen JJ, et al. 1983. Clinical effects of regional intravenous guanethidine (Ismelin) in reflex sympathetic dystrophy. Acta Anesthesiol Scan 27:505–509.
34. Glynn CJ, Basedow RW, Walsh JA. 1981. Pain relief following postganglionic sympathetic blockade with intravenous guanethidine. Br J Anaesthesia 53:1297–1302.
35. Churnard, et al. 1981. Intravenous reserpine for treatment of reflex sympathetic dystrophy. South Med J 74(12):1481–1484.
36. Sensen G. 1974. Propranolol for causalgia and Sudeck's atrophy. JAMA:227–327.
37. Parris WCV, Harris R, Lindsey K. 1987. Use of intravenous labetolol in treating resistant reflex sympathetic dystrophy. Pain 4:S206.
38. Prough DS, McLeskey CH, Poehling GG, Koman LA, Weeks DB, Whitworth T, Semble EL. 1985. Efficacy of oral nifedipine in the treatment of reflex sympathetic dystrophy. Anesthesiology 62(2):796–799.
39. Ford SR, Forrest WH Jr., Eltherington L. 1988. Treatment of reflex sympathetic dystrophy with intravenous regional bretylium. Anesthesiology, 68(1):137–140.
40. Glynn CJ, Jones PC. 1990. An investigation of the role of clonidine in the treatment of reflex sympathetic dystrophy. In Stanton-Hicks, Jänig, Boas (eds), Reflex Sympathetic Dystrophy. Boston, Kluwer Academic, pp. 187–196.
41. Chreslensen K, Jensen EM, Naer I. 1982. The reflex dystrophy syndrome response to treatment with systemic corticosteriods. Acta Chir Scan 148:653–655.
42. Dirksen R, Rutgers MJ, Collen JM. 1987. Cervical epidural steroids in reflex sympathetic dystrophy. Anesthesiology 66(1):71–73.
43. Abram SE. 1986. Pain of sympathetic origin. In P Raj (ed), Practical Management of Pain, 451–463, Chicago, Yearbook Medical Publishers.
44. Loh L, Nathan, PW. 1978. Painful peripheral states and sympathetic blocks. J Neurol Neurosurg Psychiat 41:661–671.
45. Schwartzman RJ, McLellan TL. 1987. Reflex sympathetic dystrophy, a review. Arch Neurol 44:555–561.
46. Casey KL. 1986. Toward a rationale for the treatment of painful neuropathies. In R Dubner, GF Gebhart, MR Bond (eds), Proceedings of the Vth World Congress on Pain. Amsterdam, Elsevier, pp. 165–174.
47. Meyer GA, Fields HL. 1972. Causalgia treated by selective large fibre stimulation of peripheral nerve. Brain 95:163–166.
48. Ghostine SY, et al. 1984. Phenoxybenzamine in the treatment of causalgia. J Neurosurg 60:1263–1268.
49. Cook AJ, Woolf CJ, Wall PD, et al. 1987. Dynamic receptive field plasticity in rat spinal cord dorsal horn following C-primary afferent input. Nature 325:151–153.

16. DIFFERENTIAL DIAGNOSIS OF PAINFUL CONDITIONS AND THERMOGRAPHY

WILLIAM B. HOBBINS

Thermography is used for qualifying and quantifying thermal changes in the skin. All the basic thermal observations of the skin that have been made by isolated thermometer or thermal sensors are applicable.

The present measurement methods allow for simultaneous regional measurement. Thus, autonomic vasomotor function of the three cutaneous nerves of the hand can be measured precisely and territorial boundaries of each nerve delineated "objectively" rather than subjectively.

Autonomic efferent sympathetic function is recorded by thermography. Afferent C-fiber nociceptive spinal recruitment of efferent function can also be demonstrated. Cutaneous projected referred pains can be recorded as vasomotor responses.

This chapter on thermography will cover the following areas: history, equipment, protocols, thermal pain differentials, autonomic function tests, and advantages of thermography in anesthetic management of pain with regional blocks.

HISTORY

Since the time of Egyptian papyrus recordings, humankind has associated illness and injury with temperature changes. It has been reported that early Egyptians distinguished between general fever and inflammation by using different words for systemic hyperthermia and local heat associated with inflammation. Although the finger was used as a sensor in Egyptian time, the

Greeks were credited with using wet mud applied to a "suffering surface" to determine temperature variation. The first area to dry was designated the warmest. Around 400 BC, Hippocrates wrote, "In whatever part of the body excess of heat or cold is felt, the diagnosis is there to be discovered."

At the end of the 1500s, Galileo reintroduced the thermoscope, which had been developed in the second century AD by Heron in Alexander. In the 17th and 18th centuries, respectively, the German physicist Fahrenheit and the Swedish astronomer Celsius calibrated the instruments used today to measure the heat of our body and the environment. In 1860, a German named Wunderlick recorded human temperature in both health and disease states. By flattening the end of the "thermoscope," he tried to measure human skin temperature and made observations that are still correlative today. The measurements were not thought significant, however, due to factors of environment and surface control problems causing flaws in accuracy [1].

The conceptual evolution of fire as one of the four basic elements (with air, water, and earth being the others) to our present understanding of fire as heat transfer occurred in the 18th and 19th centuries in Bath, England.

In a series of experiments, William Herschel and his son, John, observed and recorded infrared waves — the heat transfer wavelength of the electromagnetic spectrum. This finding was made during William Herschel's work with prisms and thermometry to determine which color was the warmest. During this experiment, a thermometer recorded the higher temperature and was red in color when randomly placed. Thus, the term *infrared* was coined and is now known as a wavelength between 0.7 and 1000 microns of the electromagnetic spectrum. The younger Herschel made the first "thermogram" by placing black soot of a lamp on photographic film to which alcohol was applied while infrawavelengths were passing through it. The alcohol removed the black soot by a process of evaporation, showing the white areas to be the hottest [2].

With the invention of an electronic sensor of infrared electromagnetic waves and the production of the first telethermographic machine by Barnes, the development of thermography was revolutionized. During the Second World War, an elaboration of this technology was utilized to view troop operations and the location of artillery at night. Thermography was also used extensively in the Second World War and the Korean War. On this continent, the first medical application of thermography is attributed to Dr. Ray Lawson of McGill University in Montreal. He did extensive primary work measuring the surface temperature of the skin against the temperature of the arteries and veins in patients with breast cancer. Dr. Lawson came to the conclusion that there was a direct correlation between skin temperature and vascular temperature [3].

EQUIPMENT

At the present time, there are many manufacturers of electronic thermographic equipment. The oldest in continuous service is AGEMA, a Swedish corpora-

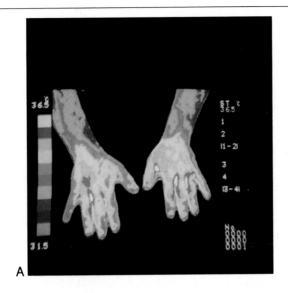

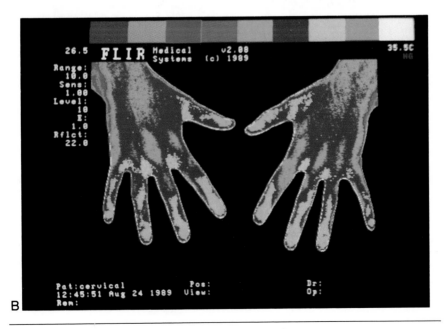

Figure 16-1. Electronic thermograms. A: Slow scan; B: real time.

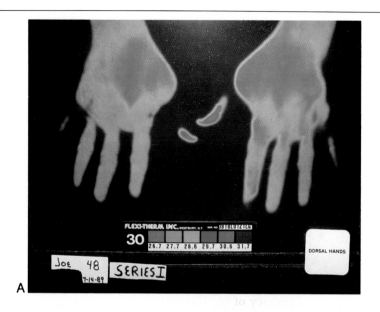

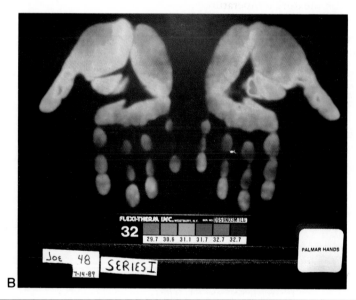

Figure 16–2. Liquid crystal thermograms. Scale of color in Celsius.

tion. Inframetrics, Hughes Aircraft, Flir Aircraft, Dorex, Clearwater Computers, and Bales are the major providers of such equipment operating in the United States today.

There are two major methodologies of electronic scanning (Figure 16-1). One uses multiple scans per second, which are computerized into an image and often recorded on videotapes. The second methodology involves a slow scan using 3–4 seconds to scan an area to get an actual recovery of the infrared data that is recorded as hard data. The basic differences in the performance of the two has to do with the fact that, in the real time or fast scan, one can watch an object, such as an athlete, in motion. In the present displays, however, a certain amount of noise is present in the resultant picture. The slow scan allows one to observe a given object in a steady state and its transformation as long as the subject has no motion. This is much more responsive to imaging and the finer anatomy, such as the face and hands. With the discovery of cholesterol crystals, an additional method of regional temperature measurement has been established. These crystals have physical characteristics that can be used to measure temperature. The basic crystals used are cholestrol esters and were originally derived from the fat of Australian sheep. There are over 300 of these crystals. Each crystal is identified by the temperature at which a reflective light shows a color change from red to blue when heated. This transformation results from a twisting and contraction of the crystal when exposed to heat. The accuracy of these crystals is a constant physical characteristic and can measure temperature to 0.10°C. When used initially in medical thermography, these crystals were applied directly to the skin, overlaid upon skin that had been painted black. The resulting pattern would then provide a "heat map" picture. However, with further research, the crystals were applied to elasticized black mylar sheets attached to a box frame. Dr. Phillip Meyers, a radiologist in New Orleans, Louisiana, patented a device that has made it possible for these liquid crystals to be used against curved surfaces by stretching them across such a box. With a fixed hard mylar surface on the viewing side, he was able to inflate these boxes and have the expanded latex crystal sheets conform to the curvatures of most areas of the body [4] Figure 16-2.

In 1976, with the enactment of medical device laws, the FDA grandfathered electronic thermography as a medical device for temperature measurement. Liquid crystals, however, prior to 1978, were used exclusively in Europe, and not approved for medical temperature measurement in the United States. In 1978, after extensive hearings and investigation, the FDA finally approved liquid crystal technology as an accurate measure of regional skin temperature in human medicine [5].

Isolated skin temperature measurement bulb thermometers and electronic sensors continue to be used. Liquid crystal thermography is limited by size of contact area and the size of the detector. Electronic thermography images the surface of the body related to distance and focal length and width of the lens. A hand-held infrared bulometer manufactured by Linear Laboratories is accurate to 0.10°C with an observed area of 1 cm. This can measure localized areas without contact. For point skin temperature measurements, the infrared bulometer has excellent accuracy.

PROTOCOLS FOR SCREENING AND STUDY

There are two types of methods of skin temperature measurement. Liquid crystal thermography is well adapted to screening. This strategy can be used in the examining room or operating room to measure regional temperature as a part of a neurological workup. No preparation is needed, except to apply the device to the area of complaint. Liquid crystal thermography can also the used in vascular and plastic surgery, suspected venous thrombosis, and dermatological conditions. Dramatic asymmetries suggest a need for complete thermography study. It has been shown that the human surface temperature is normally symmetrical. Table 16-1 is a consolidation of the data of Uematsu [6]. Any temperature asymmetry of greater than 0.6°C is considered significant and needs correlation clinically [7]. Established protocols for thermographic studies have been established by the American Academy of Thermology [8]. Other thermographic societies have addressed these matters as well. Two major areas other than proper equipment have been addressed in the protocols. Room preparation and patient instructions are most important and are summarized. The room should be made windowless and illuminated by fluorescent lights. The temperature should be maintained at 20°C and air flow should be without drafts. The patient should have clean skin, with no creams or powders. Exposure to ultraviolet infrared, diathermy, and TENS therapy should be avoided. Vasomotor drugs — nicotine, phenothiazines, calcium blockers, and alcohol — should be restricted. Patients should be disrobed in a consistent fashion.

The examination is performed on a segmental basis: cervical, thoracic, or lumbar. Additional protocols for cranial/facial studies, peripheral neuropathies, and vascular studies have been described.

A cervical exam includes regional temperature measurement of the posterior neck and superior shoulders; lateral oblique shoulders; right and left lateral upper arms; posterior, lateral, anterior, and medial forearms; and dorsal and ventral aspects of the hands.

A thoracic exam includes posterior views from C8 to T8 (upper posterior view) and T8 to L2 (lower posterior view), upper and lower lateral flanks, as well as anterior views of the upper chest, and the upper and lower abdomen.

A lumbar exam includes posterior lumbar views from L1 to the inferior gluteal area. Thermal focus exams are made by increasing the refinement of the warmest emission. The remainder of the exam involves the right and left oblique buttocks, lateral thighs, anterior and posterior thighs, lateral, anterior, and posterior lower legs, and the dorsal and plantar (ventral) feet views.

Cranial facial exams include frontal, oblique, and lateral facial views. Frequently with liquid crystal, the frontal and mental areas must be examined separately. With electronic equipment, the views must be taken perpendicular to the major surface.

The above-described studies are taken after equilibration, i.e., 10–15 minutes of the patients being exposed, while completely undressed, to the 20°C temperature for surface cooling.

Table 16-1. Normal thermographic measurements: Thermal symmetry of the skin

Confidence factor: Body segment	50% x^a	 sd^a	84% +1sd	98% +2sd	98% +2sd	98% +2sd[b]
Forehead	0.12	0.093	0.22	0.30	0.3	0.5
Cheek	0.18	0.186	0.37	0.56	0.6	0.7
Chest	0.14	0.151	0.19	0.34	0.4	0.9
Abdomen	0.18	0.131	0.31	0.44	0.5	0.3
Cervical spine	0.15	0.091	0.24	0.33	0.4	0.6
Thoracic spine	0.15	0.092	0.24	0.33	0.4	0.3
Lumbar spine	0.25	0.201	0.45	0.65	0.7	0.7
Scapula	0.13	0.108	0.24	0.35	0.4	0.5
Arm — biceps	0.13	0.119	0.25	0.37	0.4	0.3
Arm — triceps	0.22	0.155	0.38	0.54	0.6	0.6
Forearm — lateral	0.23	0.198	0.43	0.63	0.7	0.8
Forearm — medial	0.32	0.158	0.48	0.64	0.7	1.0
Palm — lateral	0.25	0.166	0.42	0.59	0.6	0.6
Palm — medial	0.23	0.197	0.43	0.63	0.7	0.6
Fingers — average	0.38	0.064	0.44	0.50	0.5	1.0
Thigh — anterior	0.11	0.085	0.20	0.29	0.3	0.7
Thigh — posterior	0.15	0.116	0.27	0.39	0.4	0.4
Knee — anterior	0.23	0.174	0.40	0.57	0.6	0.6
Knee — posterior	0.12	0.101	0.22	0.32	0.4	0.4
Leg — anterior	0.31	0.277	0.59	0.87	0.9	0.9
Leg — posterior	0.13	0.108	0.24	0.35	0.4	0.4
Foot — dorsum	0.30	0.201	0.50	0.70	0.7	0.6
Foot — heel	0.20	0.220	0.42	0.64	0.7	0.7
Toes — average	0.50	0.143	0.64	0.78	0.8	1.4
Trunk — average	0.17	0.042	0.21	0.25	0.3	
Extremities — average	0.20	0.073	0.27	0.34	0.4	

[a] Uematsu. 1985. Symmetry of skin temperature comparing one side of the body to the other. Thermology 1:4–7.

[b] Uematsu et al. 1986. Reproducibility of skin temperature symmetry during a one year period. In Abernathy and Uematsu (eds), Medical Thermology.

UPPER EXTREMITY			TRUNK				LOW EXTREMITY			
$\overline{X}$	+1s	+2s		$\overline{X}$	+1s	+2s		$\overline{X}$	+1s	+2s
50%	84%	98%	Cumulative	50%	84%	98%	Cumulative %	50%	84%	98%
Scapula		0.5°C	Forehead			0.7°C	Thigh			0.7°C
Triceps		.6	Cheek			.7	Knee			.6
Biceps		.3	Chest			.9	ant. Leg			.9
Forearm outer		.8	Abdomen			.3	dors. Foot			.6
	inner	1.0	Cervical			.6	Post. Thigh			.4
Palm	median	.6	Thoracic post.			.3	Popliteal			.4
	ulnar	.6	Lumbar			.7	Calf			.4
Fingers		1.0					Heel			.7
							Toes			1.4

From Abernathy, Uematsu 1986. Medical Thermology pp. 111–112, with permission.

Present observations suggest that the immediate pictures, followed by the "equilibrated" series at 15 minutes, may have the greatest significance, thus demonstrating the cooling down rates and territorial changes. As this is a functional measurement, more than one observation should be taken to confirm asymmetric findings. Some investigators perform these additional studies on subsequent dates but any exam must be confirmed. Autonomic challenge may be required in many observations and will be discussed at length later in this chapter.

BASIC NEUROPHYSIOLOGY OF SKIN THERMAL REGULATION

By weight, the skin is one of the largest organs of the body and its major function is thermal regulation of the body. This function is centrally controlled by the spinal cord from T2 to L2. In this area of the cord are contained the preganglionic cell bodies. The regulation of these cell bodies stems from central descending control and other neurochemical influences. Spinalized humans use the latter mechanism for fever production or oblation. Fever is produced by vasoconstriction of the blood flow in the papillary dermis [9].

The dermis is an excellent substance for heat transfer. It has an emissivity of 0.98, thus approaching a perfect black body (a theoretically perfect absorber of all incident radiation).

The skin is therefore an efficient "space suit" and prevents loss of heat from the body when its vascular compartment is empty. It has been shown that heat from sources deeper than the dermis, or 0.6 cm, will not be apparent on the surface [10]. Dermal circulation is controlled by shunts in the transverse subdermal vascular anatomy. The presence or absence of dermal papillary circulation allows heat from the core to be convected to the exterior or conserved for the core. This is the main control of central core temperature.

This mechanism is entirely controlled by the postganglionic cell body and its axon in each cutaneous distribution of the peripheral nerve. This axon influences the alpha receptors in the smooth muscle shunts. The postganglionic cell is normally controlled by the preganglionic cell and axon. The

Table 16-2. Basic physiology of cutaneous thermal asymmetries

Hyperthermia	Hypothermia
1. Loss of sympathetic fiber (postganglionic) function	1. Increased sympathetic fiber (postganglionic) function
2. Blockade of alpha receptor in dermal vessel[a]	2. Hypersensitization of alpha receptor in dermal vessel[b]

[a] Common substances that block the alpha receptors are substance P, as occurs in antidromal sensory fiber stimulation; histamines; prostaglandins; and nearly all substances from mast cells and bradykinins involved in tissue injury.
[b] Hypersensitization occurs in denervation. Denervation is thought to allow the receptor to be more sensitive to circulating noradrenalin in the denervated area. (This explains the thermal equilibration that occurs with time in denervation.) Thus, continued thermal loss from the core in the affected cutaneous area is prevented.

neurochemical reaction at this level is acetylcholine and nicotinic substances [11]. Recent evidence suggests that postganglionic cell receptors are also sensitive to opioids. These opioids appear not to affect vasomotor function but the associated pain syndrome [12].

Thus it has been confirmed (Ochoa) that there are two major causes of skin hyperthermia and two major causes of hypothermia (Table 16-2) [13]. In a clinical situation, the skin temperature symmetry or asymmetry depends on the postganglionic function and the involved alpha receptor. With this basic concept, thermal changes can be used in the differential diagnosis of many diseases and injuries. Thermography completes the neurological examination of peripheral nerve function.

DIFFERENTIAL DIAGNOSIS OF PAINFUL CONDITIONS
Two major classes of thermographic responses can be made by mechanisms that cause either hyperthermia, isothermia, or hypothermia: 1) recruitment of the efferent sympathetic system; 2) direct sympathetic fiber neuropathy in the spinal nerves. These divisions are purely arbitrary in that recruitment occurs in peripheral neuropathy, as well as root and pathologies. Differential diagnosis of pain syndromes [14] thus can be further defined as

1. Referred pains — somatovisceral cutaneous responses (Head, recruitment)
2. Autonomic defense pain (recruitment)
3. Peripheral neuropathic pain; nerve root and peripheral nerves (both recruitment and neuropathy of the sympathetic nervous system)

REFERRED PAIN
Referred pain is defined in this context as the recruited efferent sympathetic response, secondary to a nociceptive C-fiber or afferent sympathetic signal. The unmyelinated C-fiber travels into the paravertebral sympathetic nerves and enters the spinal cord through the dorsal ganglion, where the cell body is located. This cell connects with a polymodal cell in the lateral spinal area. At some spinal level, this polymodal neuron connects to a preganglionic sympathetic cell. The recruited preganglionic sympathetic fiber then signals a specific postganglionic system to create a cutaneous vasomotor response. This response is usually hyperthermia in referred pain. These cutaneous areas are specific [15,16] and are referred to as Head zones (Table 16-3). Referred "visceral" pain has a localized hyperthermia in the paresthesia area of cutaneous projection.

This same recruited sympathetic referral is in place for "somatic" nociception of the muscles, ligaments, joints, bones, and all somatic organs [17,18]. Each organ refers its pain to a cutaneous area; the referral "territories" of perceived pain and the cutaneous changes are that of hyperthermia and electrical resistance changes [19,20]. Kellegren recorded "cutaneous" maps of segmental interspinous ligaments referral zones after stimulating nociceptions

Table 16-3. Cutaneous referral area: Area of perceived pain with associated cutaneous paresthesia that can be manifested objectively

Organ of origin	Sympathetic pathway	Sympathetic ganglion	Area of thermal response
Heart	Cardiac	Th1–Th5	Thorax and inner upper arm
Asc. aortic arch (aneurysm)	Cardiac	Th1, Th2	Right shoulder and neck
Gallbladder	Right splanchnic	Th7–Th9	Above umbilicus on right side
Pancreas	Splanchnic	Th7–Th9	Anterior upper abdomen, occasionally through to back
Lower esophagus, gastric cardia, duodenal cap	Splanchnic	Th7	Region of xiphoid
Duodenum	Splanchnic	Th7–Th10	Midline and deep, from xiphoid to umbilicus
Jejunum, ileum	Splanchnic	Th10	Region of umbilicus
Appendix	Splanchnic	Th11, Th12	Right lower quadrant of abdomen (2nd stage pain)
Upper colon	Splanchnic	Th11–L1	Side of abdomen below umbilicus
Kidney pelvis	Lower splanchnic	Th10–L1	Region of costovertebral angle, occasionally to glans penis
Ureter	Renal, spermatic, and hypogastric plexus	Th11–L1	Lateral border of rectus muscle, suprapubic region up to umbilicus, groin, down the leg, occasionally to glans penis
Bladder fundus	Hypogastric	Th11–L1	Suprapubic region
Testis	Spermatic plexus	Th10	Groin
Uterine fundus	Superior hypogastric plexus	Th11–L1	Lower lateral quadrants of abdomen
Ovary, fallopian tube	Along ovarian arteries	Th10	Small of back, also lateral to and below umbilicus

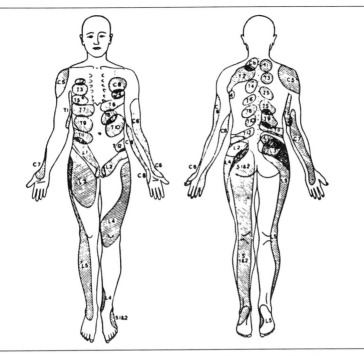

Figure 16-3. Maps showing the segmental reference of deep pain resulting from stimulation of interspinous ligaments. The numbers identify the region to which pain was referred from injecting hypertonic saline into the cervical (C), thoracic (T), lumbar (L), and sacral (S) ligaments. The segmental zones resemble but are not identical to the dermatomes (Kellgren).

by injecting 6% saline into spinal vertebral lamina (Figure 16-3). He established the same zones for many of the major muscles [21]. The somatic referral areas are also thermographically hyperthermic. These hyperthermic areas are unresponsive to sympathetic stimulation [22]. This provides further evidence for preganglionic recruitment. Travell and Simmons [23] also showed this recruited referral area. Trigger points are tender but are not thermographically involved unless the "referred" pain territory includes the irritable focus anatomically.

Recent studies with magnetic resonance imaging (MRI) [24] of lumbar back-pain patients have shown Kellgren pain referrals for anterior ligaments, and lateral and central disk. These are the same areas of referral as for posterior radiculopathy. Radiculopathies present as cold areas, whereas thermography in these somatic referrals should theoretically be "hot." Such thermographic correlations have yet to be made. Thus thermography with "referred" visceral-somatic pain will demonstrate a specific cutaneous reference zone. These areas will be hot and unresponsive to sympathetic stimulation testing [25,26].

AUTONOMIC DEFENSE PAIN

The second major correlative thermographic differential diagnosis is that of sympathetic maintained pain (SMP) responses. These are initially normal core protective responses, but with persistence of this normal reflex they become the basis of this syndrome [27,28].

In response to any injury or disease, the sympathetics take a reflexive position of vasoconstriction in the majority of individuals. Thus, a large territorial recruitment of cutaneous sympathetic response occurs and is usually hypothermic. We find that insignificant or significant injuries may immediately result immediately in level 1 or 2 reflex sympathetic dystrophy syndrome (RSDS) [29]. These responses are normal but may persist after their proper response time. Roberts has shown that such reflexes can and do sensitize other receptive anatomy peripherally. This sequence then continues until the cycle is interrupted [30]. Thermography will classify the vasomotor response of RSDS [31]. Most of the responses are "cold" and are indicative of increasing vasoconstriction. A small percentage are hot or vasodilated [32]. Some anesthesiologists use this differential as an indication for entirely different therapies [33].

Each individual's response to a thermal challenge is unique. In a study of breast skin temperature of women with hands placed in ice water, the individual responses were varied. Both hands were placed in floating ice water for 45 seconds, and breast thermograms were taken before and after the cold challenge. The majority of the women (64%) had a decrease of 1°C of the breast territory immediately, and 8% had a paradoxical of increase in recorded temperature. The remainder showed no change [34].

This phenomenon occurs in SMP syndromes and in other nociceptive phenomena. This may explain why some patients respond to various therapies while others do not. Because thermography can, for example, evaluate a vasoconstrictive area's response to stellate ganglion blocks, it can be used to adapt treatment to an individual's particular pattern of response. Thermography records regional and neural unresponsive areas precisely, and these often correspond to the pain perceptive area. For example, in response to a sympathetic nerve block, a whole hand may vasodilate, except for the entire ulnar cutaneous distribution. This is noteworthy and provides valuable information on sympathetic function of the ulnar nerve. Thermography records accurately the effect of therapy on the vasomotor response of RSDS as complete or incomplete, and helps to explain objectively individual benefits or lack of benefits from a specific therapy. It also will help influence supplemental therapy.

PERIPHERAL NEUROPATHIC PAIN

Peripheral nerves may be classed as "organs" and show similar "organ"-type referral pains as any other "organs." Thermography has been shown to have an unique correlative finding in radiculopathy, defining radiculopathy as root pathology. These findings are different from peripheral neuropathy and cannot be interpolated.

ROOT ENTRAPMENT

Pochaczevsky, Meyers, and Wexler initially observed a phenomenon that has been verified as present 80–90% of the time in radiculopathy [35]. This phenomenon has two parts: One is a dorsal skin temperature change of hyperthermia at the appropriate spinal segmental level. It has been shown that the hyperthermic strip on the dorsal skin has no cutaneous autonomic function [22]. This is an "organ-like" referral from the root. The other is a hypothermic pattern in the "projected pain" area in the extremities (thermatomes [36]). The specific cutaneous nerve distribution is usually included in this hypothermic observation. This is an extremely helpful physiological finding in confirming root pathology. These data are similar to the histamine skin test for root "avulsion" compared to peripheral nerve injury.

Peripheral nerve findings (distal from the dorsal ganglion) are extremely important, and various thermographic phenomena have been demonstrated. The most specific is denervation hyperthermia. This has been recorded with specific nerve blocks, transection, and neurectomies [37–39]. In addition, metabolic neuropathies — such as diabetic, alcoholic, or leprotic etiologies — have been recorded. These show hyperthermic areas in patchy areas before confluence. Brand also observed that hyperthermia preceded insensate status in leprosy by 6 months [40], and studies of diabetic preinsensate and insensate feet have also confirmed these associations [41].

Peripheral neural entrapments have various stages of thermographic findings and other observed changes until complete denervation. For example, the median nerve may show SMP with total hand vasoconstriction. In some cases the vasoconstriction may be limited to median nerve distribution. Median nerve cutaneous distribution becomes "hot," when there is progression to denervation. The entire hand and forearm can become "hot," but this is considered an atypical SMP response of recruitment and may be a level 1 or 2 RSDS.

In carpal tunnel syndromes, disturbed autonomic response to temperature challenge or other autonomic challenges occurs. It has been shown that immersion of the hands in 4°F water for 20 minutes will show the autonomic dysfunction during the recovery period. Thermograms are taken until the pre-immersion thermal image occurs in the contralateral hand [42].

Thus autonomic function of peripheral nerves can be recorded with thermography. Ochoa has also observed antidromic sensory nerve phenomena and recently described the ABC syndrome (angry backfiring C-nociceptive nerve fiber syndrome) [43]. He continues to study peripheral nerve function with thermography, thus further classifying the neuropathies and neuropathic pain [44].

SPINAL CORD

Spinal cord injury with quadriplegia shows vasoconstriction below the sensate area. It has been reported that equilibration occurs after 7 days. Recovery prior to 7 days indicates a better prognosis for sensory and motor recovery [45–47]. Additional findings have been shown with syringomyelia and the distinct shape of a syrinx [48]

Differential diagnoses can be stereotyped as follows: 1) localized thermographic hyperthermia is correlated with somato-visceral cutaneous referral. 2) Regional or territorial asymmetries are associated with SMP syndromes, often preceding RSDS. 3) Specific cutaneous nerve distribution thermographic changes are associated with various neuropathies. These can be hot or cold, or isothermic under standard thermographic conditions.

A study of 600 consecutive subacute or chronic pain syndromes showed 45% referral syndrome, 33% sympathetic recruitment, and 30% neuropathic. The total percentage is more than 100% because of combinations of the associated pain syndrome [49].

AUTONOMIC FUNCTION TESTS

Thermography measuring autonomic vasomotor response is not a static or fixed exam, but a dynamic one. In a standard exam, an area of asymmetry of decreased or increased heat on the body surface is primarily related to the sympathetic function. Because of this control, when an area of asymmetry is found, an autonomic challenge test is indicated. In certain cases, when the standard exam findings are symmetrical, a possible abnormal sympathetic response will only be ruled out with autonomic function testing. This is performed by stimulating the autonomic system. The following outline presents various types of thermographic autonomic challenge tests [50,51]:

1. Warm bath — indirect
2. Ice water immersion — indirect
3. Cold bath — direct
4. Ischemic challenge
5. Sympathetic ganglion block
6. Epidural block
7. Hyperoxia
8. Hypercarbia

On the day of such challenge exams, a standard control exam of the area of interest should be performed. Proper patient preparation with general precautions should be taken. The oral temperature should be recorded at the beginning and the end of the procedure. This helps to determine the patient's subsequent response to the challenge. The thermographic room temperature is controlled between 20 and 22°C, and all air draughts are eliminated. The

Table 16-4. Autonomic challenge tests

	Warm Bath	Ice immersion	Cold bath	Ischemic test	Ganglion block	Epidural block
Area as interest shows vasoconstriction	X			X	X	X
Area as interest shows vasodilatation		X	X		X	X
	A	B	C	D	E	F

Selecting the right challenge is important. The significance of each response must be correlated to the clinical picture.

patient should be adequately undressed. The proper selection of autonomic challenge test should then be made (Table 16-4).

Each of these exams should be correlated with the patient's change in symptoms, if any. Specific protocols for each challenge test can be found in Table 16-5 [50].

THERMOGRAPHIC ADVANTAGES FOR THE ANESTHESIOLOGIST

Anesthesiologists are important team players in pain management, and in many areas of the country are leading the way in caring for chronic pain patients. They will need thermography. There are practically no reliable objective measures of chronic pain, but thermography provides some objective recording for comparison. Thermography can contribute to two areas in patient care: 1) Diagnosis can be subclassified. 2) Management and results can be documented. Table 16-6 provides an outline of the advantages of thermography for regional anesthesiologists [52].

CAUSE OF THERMOGRAPHIC ASYMMETRIES OTHER THAN PRIMARY AUTONOMIC FUNCTION

Arterial vascular occlusion, venous thrombosis, lymph edema, and various dermatological conditions may alter dermal temperature and interfere with neurogenic thermographic correlation. With arterial disease, lack of dermal perfusion is seen initially and collateral circulation in the skin is seen later [53–55]. Venous obstruction causes a distal hyperthermia in anatomical correlation with venous drainage [56,57]. Varicose veins that are closer than 0.6 cm to the skin surface may be clearly visualized. Edema in the skin prevents full dermal papillary vascular blood flow and is seen as cold territorial areas.

Any lesion of the skin that is vascular, neoplastic, or metabolic may create positive thermographic findings [58–60]. Any condition or factor that changes

Table 16-5. Autonomic challenge test protocol

WARM BATH

1. A container large enough for immersion of each hand or foot or both hands or feet should be filled with 40°C water.
2. If the area of interest is in the upper half of the body, use the feet; if the area of interest is in the lower half of the body, use the hands.
3. A vasodilatation should be noted starting at 10 seconds in the area of interest. Immersion can continue until there is no further change in the uninvolved side.

ICE IMMERSION

1. The containers are filled with water and floated with ice.
2. The hands or feet are placed in the ice water for 45 seconds. This time span causes pain in most subjects. Some may insist on removing the extremit(ies) before 45 seconds because of pain. If there is no response in 45 seconds, continue immersion for a full 2 minutes.
3. Immediate vasoconstriction should occur in the extremity of interest or in the trunk surfaces. (No facial change should occur, thus the forehead is a good reference.)
4. Caution should be taken if there is a history of hypertension.

COLD BATH

1. A container large enough for immersion of each hand or foot or both hands or feet should be filled with 10°C water.
2. The extremities of interest, hands or feet, (such as in carpal tunnel diagnosis) should be placed in this bath for 20 minutes. (This is done after the baseline exam.)
3. Upon removal of the hands or feet from the bath, thermograms are taken at 5-minute intervals until they return to the baseline examination. If, after 30 minutes, this return to prechallenge has not occurred, it is recorded and the examination is stopped. This must be done bilaterally and simultaneously.

ISCHEMIC TEST

1. Baseline thermographic examinations of the extremities are taken.
2. The extremity of interest has a tourniquet (blood pressure cuff) applied and raised to above systolic pressure. It is allowed to remain on for 15 minutes.

ISCHEMIC TEST (CONTINUED)

3. During this ischemic period, the thermograms are taken at 5-minute intervals bilateraly.
4. Thermograms are taken at once and at 1-minute intervals after release of the tourniquet. This is continued until the baseline returns or until the maximum vasodilatation is noted. (The patient may not vasoconstrict for some time. Follow-up is optional.)

SYMPATHETIC GANGLION BLOCK

1. Baseline examination should be taken before block. (If the block will be done at another location, this baseline should be done within 24 hours.)
2. Following the stellate or paravertebral ganglion block, thermograms should be performed unchallenged within 6 hours.
3. Follow-up examinations for persistence of the changes can be performed as clinically indicated. (This will often predict the necessity of further blocks before clinical condition.)

EPIDURAL BLOCK

These can be performed and may change the thermographic findings by blockade of the dorsal root afferents. However, these are difficult to correlate to autonomic function. When used therapeutically for relief of pain, thermographic monitoring is indicated. Areas of sympathetic vasoconstriction will become isothermic but not hyperthermic, as with a ganglion block.

HYPEROXIA

The patient is given 100% oxygin for 5 minutes. Thermograms are taken at 3-minute intervals until return to prehyperoxia level. Expected response should be vasoconstriction, best recorded in the frontal area.

HYPERCARBIA

The patient is given 5% carbon dioxide for 3 minutes. Thermograms are taken at 3-minute intervals until return to prehypercarbia levels. Expected response should be vasodilatation.

Paradoxical reactions have been recorded in narcolepsy, cluster headache, vascular headache, and drug responses, thus further classiffying headaches.

Table 16-6. Thermography for regional anesthesiologists

Thermography — Diagnosis and correlation	Thermography — Management

1. Records the sympathetic response to nociception of:
  a) Nerve pathology
  b) Somatic nociception
    1) Muscle, ligament, joint, and bone injury
    2) Monoplegia, paraplegia, quadriplegia
    3) Old locomotor problems (polio, arthrosis)
    4) Facilitation
  c) Idiopathic responses to
    1) Injury
    2) Immobilization
    3) Disease
2. Classifies type of sympathetic response
  a) Location
    1) Ipsilateral
    2) Contralateral
    3) Bilateral
  b) Extent
    1) Localized
    2) Regional
      i) Peripheral
      ii) Central
  c) Temperature
    1) Hypothermia
    2) Hyperthermia
  d) Function
    1) Presence of sympathetic function
    2) Absence of sympathetic function
	1. Record clinical course
	  a) Progression of thermographic signal
	  b) Regression of thermographic signal
	  c) Recurrence of thermographic signal
	2. Monitoring diagnostic and therapeutic blocks
	  a) Show completeness — success or failure
	  b) Differentiate response
	    1) Postganglionic fiber
	    2) Receptor sensitivity
	  c) Compare epidural and postganglionic responses
	  d) Record direct nerve blocks
	3. Record medication effects
	  a) Complete response
	  b) Incomplete response
	  c) Functional response
	4. Monitor clinical course after block
	  a) Isothermic stability
	  b) Functional changes

the emissivity or conductive quality of the dermis will also affect the thermogram. These factors include creams, ointments, and powders.

CONCLUSIONS

Thermography is an objective measurement of skin temperature on a territorial basis. The skin temperature is directly and exclusively a measure of blood flow in the dermis. This circulation brought to the surface from the core will be recorded as temperature and can approach core temperature. The sympathetic efferents and the dermal alpha receptors are responsible for the dermal blood flow and thus the observed temperature.

Major "recruitments" of the sympathetics occur in referred pain and in SMP and RSDS. The "somato-visceral" cutaneous pain referrals produce local hyperthermia. In SMP syndromes, territories are spinally recruited, resulting in vasodilation or vasoconstriction as a basic defense mechanism.

Other than these "recruitments," the major thermographic findings are of various neuropathies. Thus, the postganglionic axon portion of the peripheral nerves will show different thermal responses to various injuries and diseases of the nerves. These will be recorded in the cutaneous territories of each nerve.

Thermography is a simple, convenient method of documenting skin blood flow. The recording is necessary for a complete neurological exam showing autonomic function. It is also an objective monitor for any manipulation of the nervous system for the control and relief of pain that results in autonomic challenge.

REFERENCES

1. Bar-Sela A. 1986. The history of temperature recording from antiquity to the present. In Medical Thermology. Washington D.C. American Academy of Thermology, pp. 1–6.
2. Putley EH. 1982. History of infrared detection — Part I. Infrared Physics vol. 22:125–131.
3. Lawson RN. 1956. Implications of surface temperatures in the diagnosis of breast cancer. Cana Med Assoc J 75:309.
4. Goodley PH. 1983. Thermography. JAMA 249:1003–1004.
5. Yin L. 1984. FDA's role in medical thermography. In Thermal Assessment of Breast Health. London, MTP Press, pp. 18–25.
6. Uematsu S, Braden E, Brelsford K, Russett M, Trattner M, Wolfe F, Wursta J 1986. Reproducibility of skin temperature symmetry during a one year period. Medical Thermology. Washington, D.C., American Academy of Thermology, pp. 99–114.
7. Feldman F, Nickoloff EL. 1984. Normal thermographic standards for the cervical spine and upper extremities. Skeletal Radiol 12:235–249.
8. Pochazevsky R, Abernathy M, Borten M, Fischer AA, Goodman PH, Haberman J, Uematsu S. 1986. Technical guidelines for thermography. Edision 2 Thermography 2(2):108–112.
9. Appenzeller O. 1986. Clinical Autonomic Failure. Amsterdam, Elsevier Science Publishers.
10. Nilsson SK. 1974. Surface temperature over an artificial source. Phys Med Biol 19(5):677–691.
11. Schmidt R, Schmidt G, Thews G. Springer-Verlag, 1983. Human Physiology. New York, p. 115.
12. Arias L, Schwartzman R, Bartkowski R, Tom C, Grossman K. 1989. Sufentanil stellate ganglion injection in the treatment of refactory Rfl sympathetic dystrophy. Regional Anesthesia 14(2):90.
13. Hobbins WB. 1986. Basic concepts of thermology and its application in the study of the sympathetic nervous system. Presented at The Second Albert Memorial Symposium in Washington, D.C., September 17, 1986, in press.
14. Hobbins WB. 1982. Thermography and Pain. In Biomedical Thermology. New York. Alan R. Liss, pp. 361–375.
15. Head H. 1983. On disturbances of sensation with especial reference to the pain of visceral disease. Brain 16:1–133.
16. Ghyton AC. 1981. Somatic sensations. Basic Human Neuro-physiology. Philadelphia, W.B. Saunders, pp. 125–129.
17. Schmidt RF, Thews G. 1983. Somatovisceral sensibility, cutaneous senses, proprioception, pain. Human Physiology, Berlin, Springer-Verlag, pp. 211–233.
18. Willis WD. 1985. Nociceptors. The Pain System. Basel, S. Karger, pp. 60–61.
19. Richter, CP. 1929. Nervous control of electrical resistence of the skin. Bull John Hopking Hosp 45:56–74.
20. Riley LH Jr., Richter CP. 1975. Uses of the electrical skin resistance method in the study of patients with neck and upper extremity pain. John Hopking Med J 137:67–74.
21. Kellgren JH. 1937–1938. Observations on referred pain arising from muscle. Clin Sci 3:176.
22. Green J, Becker C, Green S, Hazelwood C. 1986. Sympathetic skin responses correlated with abnormal infrared thermogram in patients with low back pain and radiculopathy. Academy of Neuro-Muscular Thermography.
23. Travell J, Simons D. 1983. Background and principles. In Myofascial Pain and Dysfunction: The Trigger Point Manual. Baltimore, Williams & Wilkens, 2:5–44.

24. Jinkins JR, Whittemore AR, Bradley WG. 1989. The anatomic basis of vertebrogenic pain and the autonomic syndrome associated with lumbar disk extrusion. Am J Radiol 152:1277–1289.

25. Hobbins WB. 1973. Thermography in general surgical practice. In Proceedings of the American Thermography Soc, AGA, pp. 67–92.

26. Hobbins WB. 1982. Thermography and pain. Biomedical Thermology. New York, Alan R. Liss, pp. 361–375.

27. Uematsu S. 1984. Telethermography in the diagnosis of the reflex sympathetic dystrophy. In Recent Advances in Medical Thermology. New York, Plenum Press, pp. 379–395.

28. Uematsu S, Hendler N, Hungerford Long DM, Ono N. 1981. Thermography and electromyography in the differential diagnosis of chronic pain syndromes and reflex sympathetic dystrophy. Electromyog Clin Neurophysiol 21:165–182.

29. Racz G, Lewis R Jr., Fabian G. 1986. Therapeutic approaches to reflex sympathetic dystrophy of the upper extremity. Clin Iss Region Anesth 1(2).

30. Roberts WJ, Fogleson ME. 1986. A neuronal basis for sympathetic maintained pain. Thermology 2(1):2–6.

31. Hobbins WB. 1988. RSDS and thermography. Reflex Sympathetic Dystrophy Syndrome Association Digest 1.

32. Hobbins WB. 1984. Thermography of the breast — a skin organ. In Thermal Assessment of Breast Health. Lancaster, England, MTP Press, pp. 37–48.

33. Filner B. 1989. Role of myofascial syndrome treatment in the management of reflex sympathetic dystrophy syndrome. First International Symposium of Fibromyalgia, Minneapolis, MN.

34. Hobbins WB. Thermographic autonomic challenge. Unpublished data.

35. Pochazevsky R, Wexler CE, Meyers PH, Epstein JA, Marc JA. 1982. Liquid crystal thermography of the spine and extremities — its value in the diagnosis of spinal root syndrome. J Neurosurg 56:386–395.

36. LeRoy P. 1988. Thermatomes. INITIAL, Thermal Image Analysis, Inc., Madison, Wisconsin 9(3):2.

37. Ochoa JL, Torebjork E, Marchettini P, Sivak M. 1985. Mechanisms of neuropathic pain: Cumulative observations, new experiments, and further speculation; In Advances in Pain Research and Therapy, Vol. 9. New York, Raven Press, pp. 431–450.

38. Comstock W, Ochoa J, Marchettini P. 1986. Neurogenic warming of human hand provinces by activation of the unmylinated population of single skin nerve fascicles. Society for Neuroscience 1986 abstract form.

39. Uematsu S. 1985. Thermographic imaging of cutaneous sensory segment in patients with peripheral nerve injury. J Neurosurg 62:716–720.

40. Ebner JD, Brand P. 1973. Thermography — an index to tissue repair in splinting the insensitive hand: Preliminary case review. Proceedings Annual Meeting of the American Thermographic Society, June 23–24, 1973, Gloucester, MA.

41. Stess RM, Sisney PC, Moss KM, Graf PM, Louie KS, Gooding GAW, Grunfeld C. 1986. Use of liquid crystal thermography in the evaluation of the diabetic foot. Diabetes Care 9(3):267–272.

42. Lerman, VJ. 1985. Cold test with serial thermography (CTST) in the evaluation of the peripheral nerve lesion. Presented at XIIIth World Congress of Neurology, Hamburg, September 1–6, 1985.

43. Ochoa J. 1984. The newly recognized painful ABC syndrome: Thermographic aspects. Thermology, vol. 2. pp. 65–107.

44. Ochoa J. 1986. Personal correspondence to Council of Scientific Affairs of the AMA.

45. Normell LA. 1974. The cutaneous thermoregulatory vasomotor response in health subjects and paraplegic men. Scand J Clin Lab Invest Suppl33:1–41.

46. Sherman RA, Ernst JL, Markowski J. 1986. Relationships between near surface blood flow and altered sensations among spinal cord injured veterans. Am J Phy Med 65(6):281–297.

47. Ishigaki T, Kobayashi H, Asai H, Sakuma S, Sakai M. 1986. Thermography of spinal cord lesions. In Biomedical Thermology. New York, Alan R. Liss, 6(1):95–96.

48. Ishigaki T, Sakuma S, Okae S, Asai H, Shinamoto K. 1986. Infrared imaging in syringeomyelia: Correlation with the laterality of the syrinx. Thermology 1(3):135–141.

49. Hobbins WB. 1987. Differential diagnosis of somatic pain by thermography. Presentation at the Fifth World Congress on Pain (International Association for the Study of Pain), Hamburg,

Germany, August 22–27, 1987.
50. Hobbins WB. 1986. Protocol for autonomic challenge test. INITIAL, Thermal Image Analysis, Inc., Madison, WI; Special Issue. pp. 4–6.
51. Govindan S. 1989. Facial protocol for differential correlation of various headache response. INITIAL, Thermal Image Analysis, Inc, Madison, Wisconsin 10(2):4.
52. Hobbins WB. 1989. Thermography for regional anesthesiologists. INITIAL; 10(2):5.
53. Abernathy M, O'Doherty D. 1978. The diagnosis of carotid artery insufficiency by infrared thermography. Circulation 28:31.
54. Karpman HL, Sheppard JJ, Clayton JC, Kalb IM. 1976. The use of thermography in a health care system for stroke. In S Uematsu (eds), Medical Thermography, Theory and Clinical Applications. Los Angeles, CA, Brentwood Publishing pp. 85–98.
55. Winsor T. 1971. Vascular aspects of thermography. J Cardiovasc Surg (no) 12:379–388.
56. Pochaczevsky R, Pillari G, Feldman F. 1981. Liquid crystal contact thermography of deep venous thrombosis. Am J Radiol 138:717–723.
57. Lindhagen A, Bergqvist D, Hallbook T, Lindroth B. 1982. After-exercise thermography and prediction of deep vein thrombosis. Br Med J (Clin Res) 284:1825–1826.
58. Stuttgen G. 1984. Temperature changes in skin disease. In EFJ Ring, B Phillips (eds), Recent Advances in Medical Thermology. New York. Plenum Press, pp. 121–129.
59. Miki Y, Matsuda K, Matsui K. 1982. Infra-red thermography in dermatology. Acta Thermographica 7(2):45–50.
60. Gautherie M, Grosshans E, Fattal M. 1985. Thermal assessment of malignant melanomas and other skin tumors based on the use of flexible liquid crystal films and a standardized protocol of interpretation. Thermology 1(1):20–25.

17. PSYCHOLOGICAL ASSESSMENT AND TREATMENT OF CANCER PAIN

MARTHA W. DAVIS, LEANNE WILSON AND THOMAS G. BURISH

The fear of cancer is largely the fear of pain. The reason is clear: Most cancer patients will experience pain either as a result of the disease process itself or as a result of the diagnostic and treatment procedures to which they are subjected. Given that approximately 30% of Americans will develop cancer [1], it is therefore not surprising that cancer pain has been described as one of the most pressing problems facing society today [2].

Most pain associated with cancer is the result of one or more of three processes. First, pain may develop from the disease process itself, as in tumor infiltration of the skeletal system, compression of nerves, or inflammation due to tumor growth. Second, pain may result from diagnostic procedures, such as bone marrow aspirations, or from treatment procedures, such as surgery, radiation, or chemotherapy. Finally, pain is affected by one's psychological state: Anxiety, depression, and other negative effects frequently accompany cancer and are known to be associated with an increased perception of pain [3–5].

Cancer pain is treated in a variety of ways, ranging from narcotic medications to special surgical procedures. Because these procedures often do not totally control pain and may have unpleasant side effects [6], psychological approaches to cancer pain management have been explored. The purpose of this chapter is to describe briefly several types of psychological interventions that are used to treat cancer pain. Because of space limitations, we have not attempted to provide either an exhaustive review of the clinical literature or a methodologically critical analysis of the research literature. Rather, the chapter provides a general summary of the most commonly used psychological interventions for both children and adults, the common mechanisms that may account for their effectiveness, and recommendations for their clinical implementation.

Two points should be emphasized about using psychological approaches to treat cancer pain. First, all cancer patients should receive educational and supportive interventions as a part of their pain treatment. In a general sense, these interventions might be subsumed under "psychological" techniques; however, they are not reviewed in this chapter. Second, effective cancer pain management is best achieved through a multidisciplinary approach that incorporates several different types of treatment approaches. From a clinical perspective, it is the combined impact across modalities, not the main effect of any one modality, that is of greatest importance. Thus, although this chapter focuses solely on psychological procedures, ultimately it is their adjunctive use with other pain control techniques, not their isolated impact, that is most important.

PSYCHOLOGICAL INTERVENTIONS FOR PEDIATRIC CANCER PATIENTS

Acute procedural pain

Psychological interventions for pediatric cancer pain have focused primarily on invasive treatment procedures, particularly bone marrow aspirations, venipunctures, and lumbar punctures. Because of the invasive and repeated nature of these procedures, and because many pediatric patients have a limited understanding of the nature or rationale for the treatment, pediatric patients often consider the treatment more painful than the disease [7–9]. Psychological approaches to reducing procedural pain include hypnosis, relaxation and imagery, cognitive techniques, and techniques that combine cognitive and behavioral strategies.

Hypnosis and relaxation/imagery techniques

A number of clinicians and researchers have explored the use of hypnotic and relaxation/imagery procedures for the reduction of procedural pain and distress in pediatric cancer patients. Children have been considered good candidates for hypnotic procedures because of their natural interest in and facility for fantasy and imaginative activities [10,11]. The use of progressive muscle relaxation training or other "nonhypnotic" relaxation procedures are less common in pediatric populations, especially at younger ages, though components of relaxation are often included in hypnotic procedures. Specifically, hypnosis for older children and adolescents usually includes inducing a physically relaxed state with suggestions for calm breathing, relaxation of muscle groups, the imagining of a peaceful and relaxing scene, and suggestions for comfort and pain reduction. However, younger children, usually below age ten, are commonly given a different type of hypnotic induction for dealing with painful medical procedures in which the therapist actively participates in creating, describing, and elaborating on an active story or fantasy (e.g., developing a fantasy of a superhero conquering pain), often weaving into the story information about the procedure taking place and giving indirect suggestions to promote comfort and active coping. A focus on passive or active muscular relaxation, closed eyes, and imagining relaxing scenes are used little or not at all.

Much of the research on hypnosis with pediatric cancer patients is anecdotal or uncontrolled, but generally positive in outcome [11,12]. In a quasi-experimental study with two treatment groups, Zelter and LeBaron [13] gave pediatric patients undergoing bone marrow aspirations and lumbar punctures either hypnosis or simple distraction with deep breathing. Results indicated that hypnosis significantly reduced self-reported pain, as compared to preintervention levels, for both medical procedures, while distraction and deep breathing significantly reduced pain only during the bone marrow aspirations.

In a more recent and rigorously designed study, Kuttner, Bowman, and Teasdale [14] assigned patients aged 3–10 years undergoing bone marrow aspirations to one of three conditions: 1) hypnosis; 2) deep breathing and distraction with toys, books, questions, or physical activities such as blowing bubbles; or 3) no psychological intervention. Their inclusion of young children is noteworthy in light of research suggesting that children under age seven exhibit and report a higher level of distress during invasive medical procedures than do older children [15,16]. Results indicated that for children under age seven, hypnosis was significantly more effective in reducing pain than the other two conditions. For children age seven and older, both intervention conditions were equally effective and superior to the control condition in reducing pain.

In summary, both clinical reports and some research data suggest that hypnotic and relaxation/imagery procedures can be effective in reducing procedural pain in pediatric cancer populations.

Cognitive coping strategies

Children who have difficulty with the imaginative aspect of hypnosis may still derive pain-reducing benefits from other types of cognitive activities. Generally these activities are aimed at either diverting attention away from the painful procedure through distraction or providing a way for the child to alter his or her appraisal of the situation through self-instructional strategies.

Distraction can be highly effective in reducing pain [17], especially when the child finds the task engrossing and sufficiently challenging or difficult that attentional effort is required. Children can often be helped to focus their attention away from a painful procedure by focusing on external objects, such as exciting toys, or by concentrating on internal tasks, such as mental arithmetic. Ross and Ross [18] reported on a 9-year-old who spontaneously used such a strategy:

I counted everything in the [examination] room if it was shiny or not shiny and I made it like a game, like the shinies team against the not shinies team and the shinies won. You have to count real fast so you can't think about what they [emergency room personnel] are doing.

The little research that has been done with nonhypnotic distraction for treating procedural pain in pediatric cancer patients [13,14] supports these general assertions.

In addition to distraction, self-instructional strategies that involve having a child rehearse and apply a set of statements aimed at both reducing anticipatory anxiety and coping with the painful procedures have been used to reduce pain. In general, self-instructional strategies involve helping a child to develop a set of positive and reassuring statements. The child is helped to memorize the statements and rehearse them subvocally or aloud any time he or she *thinks* about the impending procedure. During the actual procedure, the child is coached to continue with internal self-instruction and is given ample encouragement and help in doing so.

Although controlled research on the effectiveness of these procedures in reducing pain due to invasive procedures in pediatric cancer patients has not been reported, their use in other contexts and their ready application to the cancer setting suggests that they may be highly effective with procedures such as bone marrow aspirations, especially as part of a multicomponent treatment package.

Cognitive-behavioral strategies

Perhaps the most carefully conceptualized and empirically supported approach for procedural pain in pediatric cancer patients is an intervention package developed by Jay and her colleagues [18,19]. The package includes five primary components: 1) filmed modeling of an age-appropriate model undergoing the invasive procedure (e.g., bone marrow aspiration); 2) simple breathing exercises during which the children are instructed to take deep breaths and then exhale slowly (as if they were a big tire); 3) emotive imagery/distraction, which varies depending on the child's interests (for example, for young children an absorbing story incorporating themes of mastery and adventure may be developed and told to the child during the procedure); 4) reinforcement for doing what is asked (for example, often children are shown a small trophy and told that they can earn it by lying still during the procedure and doing their breathing exercises); and 5) behavioral rehearsal during which the therapist gives the child a doll and instructs him or her to "play doctor" by carrying out each step of the procedure on the doll, including practicing the coping strategies. Although the general components are the same for each child, the procedure is always tailored to meet the developmental level, abilities, and needs of the particular patient.

In a well-controlled clinical study of this procedure, Jay and her colleagues

[19] compared their cognitive-behavioral intervention package to a pharmacological intervention (oral Valium) and an attention control condition (watching
cartoons) on 56 leukemia patients who ranged in age from 3 to 13. The three
interventions were delivered in a randomized sequence within a repeated-
measures, counterbalanced design. Results indicated that children exhibited
significantly lower behavioral distress, pain ratings, and pulse rates when they
were in the cognitive-behavioral condition than when they were in the attention control condition. When they were in the Valium condition, the children
exhibited no significant differences from when they were in the cognitive-
behavioral condition, except that they had lower diastolic blood pressures.
These data suggest that the psychological intervention was generally as effective as the pharmacological treatment in reducing procedural distress. However, the effects of the cognitive-behavioral intervention did not carry over to
subsequent bone marrow aspirations, suggesting that the structure and guidance provided by the therapist before and during the procedure were essential
for its success.

Chronic pain
In addition to pain caused by invasive procedures, pediatric cancer patients
sometimes experience constant or chronic pain that is related directly to their
disease. Fortunately, it is currently believed that such pain is not common in
pediatric cancer patients. Children tend to have less cancer-caused pain than
adults, because they tend to have leukemias rather than solid tumor carcino-
mas of organ systems (e.g., stomach, lung, breast, ovary), as are found in
older populations. Acute leukemia is sometimes accompanied by moderate
pain during periods of relapse, but rarely produces severe, long-lasting pain. In
a survey of the prevalence and nature of pain among 139 pediatric and
adolescent cancer patients, Miser and his colleagues [20] reported that the
preponderance of pain was treatment related and acute. Only seven patients
were identified as having chronic pain.

On the other hand, it is well known that medical staff have often believed
incorrectly that children do not experience pain to the same degree as adults
and that they recover from painful experiences more quickly [21]. Moreover,
research suggests that when physicians do prescribe analgesics for the relief of
pain, they often underestimate the dosage that is needed [6], perhaps because
they fear long-term neurological damage from such medication use [7].

Although no rigorously controlled research has been reported on the use of
behavioral procedures for reducing chronic pain in pediatric cancer patients,
research on such approaches in other settings offers several suggestions. Clearly,
in such contexts psychological approaches should be viewed as adjunctive to
pharmacological treatment. The psychological procedures should address
both pain-perception regulation and pain behavior regulation [22]. Pain-perception regulation involves the teaching of skills to reduce perceived pain and
distress. For example, case study reports [10] with cancer children suggest that

hypnosis and relaxation/imagery can help to reduce chronic pain. Because of the constant nature of the pain, children benefit most if they are able to learn and use self-hypnosis or self-administered approaches, and if they are given regular reinforcement for the use of such coping strategies [10,23].

In addition to reducing the perception of pain, it is often important to reduce pain-related behaviors, such as withdrawal from activities, excessive crying, or acting out. Such behaviors are all too readily reinforced, often inadvertently, by the child's parents and family members who are sympathetic to the pain and are trying to do all they can to make the child more comfortable. When such pain behaviors develop, an operant approach to behavior change might have the most impact.

An operant approach to pain behavior management often includes reinforcement for substitute behaviors that are more appropriate and healthy. For example, one might set up a schedule whereby the child receives positive reinforcement for exercise or time spent out of bed. The reinforcement, which might vary from child to child and should be chosen in consultation with the parents, needs to be clearly specified. The goals should be modest enough initially that the child can readily earn rewards. Parents might increase their attentiveness and verbal reinforcement when the child is engaging in nonpain behaviors and reduce them for pain behaviors. Punishment also can be effective, if correctly used, for reducing pain behaviors, especially when used in conjunction with positive reinforcement for appropriate nonpain behaviors. However, punishment is a more controversial procedure, often disliked by parents, that is best not used initially in most cases. Clearly, any operant plan needs to be carefully designed in conjunction with, and explained carefully to, the child's parents and family members. Unless they support and cooperate with the plan, it is unlikely to succeed and may actually exacerbate pain behavior.

Summary

A number of different approaches have been found to modulate pain and distress for pediatric cancer patients. The particular method of pain control chosen should be based on a number of factors, including relevant developmental considerations, the child's physical and emotional status, whether the child has developed his or her own pain management approach, and if so, what it is and how effective it is. The willingness of the child's parents to learn and support the use of a psychological intervention is of particular importance.

The literature suggests that with the high-intensity pain and anxiety associated with painful medical procedures such as bone marrow aspirations, the therapist, or perhaps a medical professional or trained parent, needs to take an active role in structuring the intervention and coaching the child through the procedure, rather than teaching the child an exclusively self-help technique. This is especially true for children less than 7 years of age who are generally dependent on adults for direction and emotional support and who are more anxious and frightened by the procedures than older children. Preadolescents and adolescents are developmentally capable of and often interested in mastering techniques such as self-hypnosis or cognitive approaches exemplified by self-instruction. They also are better able to understand the medical necessity of the procedures. However, even older children are likely to require considerable help and support when dealing with either high-intensity acute or chronic pain.

PSYCHOLOGICAL INTERVENTIONS FOR ADULT CANCER PATIENTS

In contrast to the pediatric cancer pain literature, psychological interventions with adult cancer patients have focused primarily on chronic pain resulting from disease progression or medical treatment, rather than on acute procedural pain. Side effects associated with cancer treatment procedures, such as nausea and vomiting, fatigue, and weight loss, have been given considerable research and clinical attention but are not the focus of this chapter. However, the psychological interventions used for adult cancer pain are fundamentally similar to those used for these side effects with pediatric patients and include hypnosis, relaxation training, cognitive-behavioral strategies, and operant conditioning.

Hypnosis

Hypnosis was one of the first psychological treatments used for cancer pain in adults and remains one of the primary intervention strategies. When used with adults, hypnosis does not refer to a specific psychological procedure, but rather is used to describe a number of interventions that redirect the attentional focus of the patient. Hypnotic techniques generally include procedures aimed at producing deep physiological relaxation, heightened suggestibility, and enhanced imagery [24]. Suggestions of comfort, well-being, control, and attentional redirection or reinterpretation are given to decrease the perception of pain. In an attempt to avoid the negative views that some individuals have toward the word *hypnosis*, some researchers have used these hypnotic procedures with patients but have renamed them *passive relaxation training* [25].

A review of the literature suggests that the majority of published reports using hypnosis to alleviate chronic cancer pain have been either editorial or anecdotal in nature or have used uncontrolled designs [26–32]. Overall, these reports have suggested that hypnosis can be effective in reducing cancer pain. In a more convincing controlled study, Spiegel and Bloom [33] randomly assigned 44 women experiencing pain from metastatic breast cancer to one of three conditions: 1) a support group that met weekly for 90 minutes, 2) a similar support group that also received a 10-minute self-hypnosis exercise, and 3) a no psychological intervention control condition. Results indicated that patients who received the psychological interventions reported experiencing significantly less pain than patients in the control condition; the support group that received hypnosis reported less pain than the support group without hypnosis, but the difference was not significant.

Overall, clinical reports, case histories, and scant controlled research suggest that hypnosis can be an effective procedure for reducing cancer-related pain in adult patients.

Biofeedback

Biofeedback is the process of using special instrumentation to teach a person to control a biological response that is usually not under voluntary control or for which voluntary control has been lost. The goal is often to allow a person to change the response in such a fashion as to reduce a medical condition or symptom, including pain. Although biofeedback has frequently been studied in normal and select pain populations [34], there is little published data on its efficacy in reducing cancer pain.

In one of the few studies that has been reported, Fotopolos and her colleagues [35] administered EMG and skin temperature biofeedback to 12 cancer patients who had been in pain for an average of 12.1 months and were using both narcotic and non-narcotic analgesics without adequate pain relief. Unfortunately, only five patients completed the biofeedback training. Of these, two had significant pain relief in the laboratory setting and were able to generalize this relief to their home environments and to decrease their analgesic use. Of the remaining three subjects, two reported no change in pain and one reported an increase in pain and analgesic use.

In our view, based on pain research in other medical areas and on the little research that is available in the cancer area, it is likely that biofeedback can help in some cases to reduce cancer-related pain in adults. However, biofeedback is a comparatively expensive behavioral intervention that can be impractical to administer within a cancer treatment setting. Moreover, there is little evidence that biofeedback is significantly more effective than more readily available and easily administered behavioral techniques. Overall, therefore, we are not enthusiastic about its use in the cancer setting.

Relaxation training

Progressive muscle relaxation training was first developed by Jacobson [36] and later modified by a number of researchers and clinicians [37]. It involves having patients sequentially tense and relax various muscle groups throughout the body and concentrate on the contrast between feelings of tension and relaxation. In addition, patients are often instructed in deep breathing and are given guided relaxation imagery in order to focus their attention on pleasant and relaxing scenes. Interestingly, although relaxation training is often included as a component in multimodal pain-reduction treatment packages, there is little research on its use alone as a pain-reduction technique for adult cancer patients. Most of the published reports that do exist, although positive in their recommendations, are editorial-type articles without controlled research [38–

40]. In a quasi-experimental design, Graffam and Johnson [41] reported having 30 cancer patients listen to two tapes using a counterbalanced design. The first tape was a recording of music with guided relaxation imagery; the second was a recording of music with progressive muscle relaxation training. Results indicated that after listening to either tape, patients reported feeling significantly less pain and distress. Interestingly, however, the large majority of patients (77%) preferred the relaxation training tape.

Overall, there are insufficient data to confirm that relaxation training by itself is or is not an effective adjunctive procedure for reducing cancer pain. However, given the ample literature that supports its use in other aversive contexts, and its frequent inclusion in multimodal treatment packages, it is likely that relaxation training can, in fact, be a useful pain-relieving strategy. However, we suspect that the literature reflects long-standing clinical wisdom: Relaxation training is best used as an adjunctive procedure in combination with other psychological and pharmacological strategies, rather than as a solitary technique, for the reduction of cancer-related pain in adults.

Cognitive-behavioral strategies

Cognitive-behavioral strategies have proven effective in reducing procedural pain for pediatric cancer patients and in a variety of medical settings involving adult patients including surgery, endoscopic diagnosis, and non-cancer-related chronic pain [42,43]. It is therefore not surprising that cognitive-behavioral interventions have been suggested for treating adult cancer pain. In fact, Payne and Foley [40] have suggested that cognitive-behavioral interventions are one of the most important advances in the treatment of cancer pain. In spite of these collateral data and encouraging admonitions, there is relatively little controlled research on the use of cognitive-behavioral strategies for the reduction of pain in adult cancer patients, and what research has been conducted usually lacks rigorous methodological controls [44].

When cognitive-behavioral techniques have been recommended [43,45,46], they have typically included a variety of different components, including 1) constructing and repeating positive self-statements, as well as eliminating maladaptively distorted thoughts that can lead to negative emotions; 2) gaining relevant procedural and sensation information; 3) learning distraction techniques to redirect attention on more pleasant and relaxing situations; 4) learning specific coping strategies, such as progressive muscle relaxation training, self-hypnosis, or biofeedback-assisted relaxation; 5) receiving increased social support, often from family or former cancer patients; 6) rehearsing the coping strategies and other stress-reducing procedures; and 7) setting realistic goals for improvement.

Perhaps the most rigorous test of cognitive-behavioral interventions to reduce cancer pain is being undertaken by Syrjala and her colleagues [personal communication, October 1989]. Syrjala's cognitive-behavioral procedure involves four components: 1) constructing positive self-statements, and identifying and avoiding negative ones; 2) daily goal setting; 3) distraction; and 4) relaxation plus imagery. Thus far, the investigators have randomly assigned over 50 bone marrow transplant patients to 1 of 4 conditions: the combined cognitive-behavioral intervention, relaxation plus imagery, supportive contact, and treatment-as-usual control. Preliminary results suggest that patients in all three treatment groups are experiencing less pain than patients in the treatment-as-usual control group. Of the treatment groups, patients in the cognitive-behavioral group appear to be receiving the most benefit. Although encouraging, it must be emphasized that these results are preliminary and involve less than half of the intended patient sample.

Overall, researchers and clinicians are in strong agreement that cognitive-behavioral strategies can be highly effective adjunctive procedures for the control of cancer-related pain in adults. However, controlled research to support this assertion is lacking, though important work is now underway and appears to be providing positive results.

Operant strategies

The operant model of behavior proposes that pain is a set of observable responses (e.g., crying, limping, requesting medication) that may in part be a consequence of reinforcement or secondary gain (increased attention, special favors) [47]. As described earlier for pediatric patients, operant techniques are often used when specific pain behaviors are developed that have negative or unwanted consequences. For example, a mastectomy patient may complain of excessive pain to avoid physical therapy or resuming old responsibilities. In some cases, for example those of patients near death, one might often conclude that there is little value in trying to reduce or change pain behaviors through operant techniques, preferring rather to treat the behaviors in other ways or simply to tolerate or overlook them. In other cases, as described below, however, it is neither in the patient's nor others' best interests to do so.

When incorporating operant procedures into the pain modification process, three steps should be followed [43]. First, the behavior to be increased, decreased, maintained, or eliminated should be clearly identified and defined. Second, the therapist should identify reinforcers that are appropriate for the individual and for altering the target behavior. Finally, the therapist should have sufficient control over the setting to be able to regulate the reinforcements according to the preset plan. Usually this last requirement involves gaining cooperation from both the medical staff and the patient's family.

Most operant research is done as a case study or with small groups of patients, although often with adequate experimental controls. An example of a well-controlled single-subject study was reported by Redd [48] on a 64-year-old male with metastatic cancer. Within 3 weeks of hospitalization, the patient complained of intense pain and spent 60% of his waking time crying, moaning, and yelling. Narcotics appeared to have little impact. Eventually, the patient's behavior became disruptive to the other patients on the floor and to the medical staff. In addition, the patient also reported increased general distress and contemplated suicide. Even though the patient was judged to be terminal, an operant procedure was designed. It included a differential reinforcement procedure by which social stimulation was withdrawn from the patient whenever he began to cry in the absence of any discernible problem. When the patient ceased crying, he was given generous social attention. By the tenth day of the intervention, the patient had virtually discontinued crying and had increased his conversation time with others significantly. He thus was not only much less disruptive to others but was enjoying his family and friends much more than previously. These results were maintained over a 6-week follow-up period.

In summary, the considerable amount of operant research outside the cancer area, and that which has been reported within the cancer area, suggest that operant strategies can be highly effective in altering pain-related behaviors.

Summary

Psychological interventions for adult cancer pain have focused primarily on chronic pain due to the disease or its treatment, and secondarily on acute pain resulting from aversive procedures. In general, reports on the use of these interventions have been anecdotal and highly subjective, and have not included well-controlled empirical data. However, the results have not changed when well-controlled experimental designs have been used: Overall, the data are positive and suggest that procedures such as hypnosis, relaxation training, biofeedback, cognitive-behavioral strategies, and operant conditioning can be effective adjunctive techniques for reducing cancer-related pain in adults.

MECHANISMS OF ACTION

Most of the pychological interventions discussed in this chapter share common characteristics that might ultimately be largely responsible for their effectiveness. Although adequate research has not been conducted on these potential "mechanisms of action" to prove that they produce the treatment effect, their commonality across interventions, combined with suggestive research that has been conducted [49], does support their likely role in affecting treatment outcome. The three major shared characteristics are cognitive distraction, relaxation, and mastery/self-efficacy.

Hypnosis, relaxation training, biofeedback, cognitive strategies, and cognitive-behavioral approaches all include an element of cognitive distraction. During these procedures patients redirect or divert their attention from the painful situation to something more pleasant, such as relaxation instructions, pleasant imagery, positive self-statements, or a feedback signal. It is assumed that this attentional redeployment captures a significant portion of one's attentional capacity, thereby reducing the amount that can be used to attend to and process painful or anxiety-producing stimuli [50,51]. There is ample research to suggest that simple cognitive distraction can be effective in reducing pain [17].

A second element common to many psychological procedures is increased relaxation. Either directly through instructions or indirectly by attentional diversion, most of the psychological procedures described in this chapter decrease autonomic arousal, muscle tension, anxiety, and other negative affects, and increase feelings of relaxation and well-being. Each of these factors is believed to reduce perceptions of pain [52,53]. It is also possible that either because of the improved state of the patient or because they participate in the intervention, family members' levels of anxiety and other negative emotions also may decrease as a result of the psychological interventions, and that this, in turn, might further reduce the patient's distress and pain. For example, there are ample data to suggest that the anxiety levels of the parents of pediatric cancer patients undergoing aversive medical procedures are highly related to the anxiety levels and pain behaviors of their children [16,54]. This notion is sometimes referred to as the contagion hypothesis and has received empirical support [55], although there are also contradictory research findings [15]. Overall, however, it is well established that many psychological interventions produce increased relaxation in the patient and sometimes in family members, and that increased relaxation is associated with reductions in perceived pain.

A third common element of many of the psychological interventions is the promotion of a sense of self-efficacy, mastery, and control. In the face of an uncertain prognosis, repeated noxious medical treatments, and a general lack of an ability to help oneself, psychological interventions may give patients an opportunity to exercise some control over the situation. Achieving a sense of self-control can be an important factor in reducing pain in cancer patients [56,57]. Self-control allows a patient to develop a sense of mastery or efficacy, and feel better able to cope with unexpected difficulties or adverse situations. By learning self-relaxation, positive self-statements, techniques for controlling and redirecting one's attention, and altering one's physiological responses, cancer patients can come to believe that they have control over some aspects of the treatment and their internal responses to that treatment. In the end, these increased positive beliefs and outlooks might account for some of the treatment effect.

DISCUSSION

Most cancer patients will experience pain either as a result of their disease or its treatment. In a majority of cases, this pain will be accompanied by, and may be exacerbated by, a significant amount of psychological distress. Given this ubiquitous and multifaceted problem, it is not surprising that most cancer patients will benefit from a multimodal intervention approach aimed at reducing their pain and improving their psychological state. Within this setting, psychological treatments, used primarily as adjunctive procedures along with analgesic medications and other medical interventions, can play an important role.

Although there is ample theoretical and clinical support for the use of psychological interventions to reduce cancer pain, there is unfortunately little controlled research to support and define their treatment effect. However, what research or commentary does exist is overwhelmingly positive, and these reports are supported empirically by collateral research in other areas which suggests that psychological interventions can be highly effective in reducing both the perception of pain and the negative behaviors that often accompany it.

Although in general we are supportive of the use of psychological interventions in the cancer setting, it is important to emphasize that their application often requires considerable ingenuity and flexibility, and that in some situations they should not be used at all. For example, although biofeedback may be effective in reducing pain and increasing relaxation, its use in a hospital setting with an ill patient who is on narcotic analgesia may be impractical or inefficient. Reliance on other psychological procedures may be preferable. A child with an intense anticipatory fear of bone marrow aspirations may profit from a cognitive-behavioral approach, but the therapist may not have ample time to administer this involved intervention at each clinic visit. It may be necessary to train parents or nurses to administer some or all of the intervention if it is to be effective. In some cases, the administration of psychological interventions for pain management should be combined with more general psychological support and counseling to deal with other, more pressing psychological problems that may exist and be contributing to the pain. There are also patients who are not motivated or capable of using psychological interventions. Such patients may have limited ability to concentrate or visualize, have religious objections to various approaches, or be severely incapacitated by their disease. In such cases it would not be helpful to introduce psychological interventions, and it may be harmful to use them if their application delays the use of other more potent interventions.

When psychological interventions are used, it is important that they not be introduced to a patient in a way that reduces their potential impact. For example, sometimes psychological interventions are not tried until standard medical pain treatments have failed to produce adequate results. This late introduction of psychological procedures may suggest to the patient that these are the "last resort" approach, or that the medical staff have determined that the pain must at least in part be "psychological" or simply "in their head." In other cases, psychological interventions may not be requested until the patient has already been put on high levels of narcotic medications or is in intense pain. Such circumstances do not facilitate the learning or the administration of psychological procedures, especially those that involve learning some skill through regular practice (such as relaxation training) or that require considerable concentration or other types of cognitive involvement. In such cases, it is helpful if the patient is able to learn the intervention or practice the approach before he or she is suffering from intense pain or under heavy medication. Each of these examples suggests that it is best to include the psychologist as part of the treatment team so that the psychological interventions can be appropriately integrated into the overall pain management program.

ACKNOWLEDGMENTS
The authors thank Karen Syrjala and Robert Jamison for their helpful comments on an earlier draft of the manuscript. The writing of this manuscript was supported in part from grant PBR-29 from the American Cancer Society.

REFERENCES

1. American Cancer Society. 1989. Cancer Facts and Figures: 1989. New York, American Cancer Society.
2. Bonica JJ.1982. Management of cancer pain. Acta Anaest Scand 74:75–82.
3. Ahles TA, Blanchard EB, Ruckdeschal JC. 1983. The multidimensional nature of cancer-related pain. Pain, 17:277–288.
4. Brown GK, Nicassio PM, Wallston KA. 1989. Pain coping strategies and depression in rheumatoid arthritis. J Consult Clin Psychol 57:652–657.
5. Davis M, Vasterling J, Bransfield D, Burish T. 1987. Behavioral interventions in coping with cancer-related pain. Br J Guid Couns 15:17–28.
6. Chapman CR. 1988. Effective pain management: Lessons learned from patient-controlled analgesia. Hosp Ther 19–20:26–28.
7. Redd WH. 1989. Behavioral interventions to reduce child distress. In JC Holland JH Rowland (eds), Handbook of Psychooncology. New York, Oxford University Press pp. 573–581.
8. Ross DM, Ross SA. 1982. A study of pain experience in children. Final report, Ref. no. 1 ROI HD 13672–01, Bethesda, MD, National Institute of Child Health and Human Development.
9. Ross DM, Ross SA. 1988. Childhood Pain: Current Issues, Research and Management. Baltimore, Urban and Schwartzenberg.
10. Gardner GG, Olness K. 1981. Hypnosis and hypnotherapy with children. New York: Grune & Stratton.
11. Hilgard JR, LeBaron S. 1982. Relief of anxiety and pain in children and adolescents with cancer: Quantitative measures and clinical observations. Int J Clin Exp Hyp 30:417–442.
12. Kellerman J, Zelter L, Ellenberg L, Dash J. 1983. Adolescents with cancer: Hypnosis for the reduction of the acute pain and anxiety associated with medical procedures. J Adol Health Care 4:85–90.
13. Zelter L, LeBaron S. 1982. Hypnosis and nonhypnotic techniques for reduction of pain and anxiety during painful medical procedures in children and adolescents with cancer. J Pediatr 101:1032–1035.
14. Kuttner L, Bowman M, Teasdale M. 1988. Psychological treatment of distress, pain, and anxiety for young children with cancer. Dev Behav Pediatr 9:374–381.
15. Jacobson PB, Maune SL, Gorfinkle K, Schorr O, McEvoy M, Rapkin B, Redd W. 1990. Analysis of child and parent behavior during painful medical procedures. Unpublished manuscript, Memorial Sloan-Kettering Cancer Center.
16. Jay SM, Ozolins M, Elliot CH, Caldwell S. 1983. Assessment of children's distress during painful medical procedures. Health Psychol 2:133–147.
17. McCaul KD, Malott JM. 1984. Distraction and coping with pain. Psychol Bull 95:516–533.
18. Jay SM, Elliott CH, Ozolins M, Olson R, Pruitt S. 1985. Behavioral management of children's distress during painful medical procedures. Beh Rsh Ther 23:513–520.
19. Jay SM, Katz E, Elliot CH, Seigel SE. 1987. Cognitive-behavioral and pharmacologic interventions for children's distress during painful medical procedures. J Consult Clin Psychol 55:860–865.
20. Miser AW, Dothage JA, Wesley RA, Miser JS. 1987. The prevalence of pain in a pediatric and

young adult cancer population. Pain 29:73–83.

21. Peterson L, Harbeck C. 1988. The Pediatric Psychologist. Champaign, IL, Research Press.
22. Spirito A, Hewett K, Stark LJ. 1988. The application of behavior therapy in oncology. Adv Psychosom Med 18:66–81.
23. Jay SM, Elliott CH. (1983). Psychological interventions for pain in pediatric cancer patients. Cancer Treat Res 17:123–154.
24. Wadden TA, Anderton CH. 1982. The clinical use of hypnosis. Psychol Bull 9:215–243.
25. Hendler CS, Redd WH. 1986. Fear of hypnosis: The role of labeling in patients' acceptance of behavioral interventions. Beh Ther 17:2–13.
26. Ament P. 1982. Concepts in the use of hypnosis for pain relief in cancer. J Med 13:233–240.
27. Caracappa JM. 1963. Hypnosis in terminal cancer. Am J Clin Hyp 5:205–206.
28. Finer B. 1979. Hypnotherapy in pain of advanced cancer. In JJ Bonica, V Ventafridda (eds), Advances in Pain Research and therapy, Vol. 2. New York, Raven Press.
29. Hilgard ER, Hilgard JR. 1975. Hypnosis in the Relief of Pain. Los Altos, CA, Kaufman.
30. Lea PA, Ware P, Monroe R. 1960. The hypnotic control of intractable pain. Am J Clin Hyp 3:3–8.
31. Margolis CG. 1983. Hypnotic imagery with cancer patients. Am J Clin Hyp 25:128–134.
32. Sacerdote P. 1970. Theory and practice of pain control in malignancy and other protracted or recurring painful illnesses. Int J Clin Exp Hyp 18:160–180.
33. Spiegel D, Bloom JR. 1983. Group therapy and hypnosis reduce metastatic breast carcinoma pain. Psychosom Med 45:333–339.
34. Olton DS, Noonberg AR. 1980. Biofeedback: Clinical Applications in Behavioral Medicine. Englewood Cliffs, NJ, Prentice-Hall.
35. Fotopoulos S, Cook M, Graham C, Cohen H, Gerkovich M, Bond S, Knapp T. 1983. Cancer pain: Evaluation of electromyographic and electrodermal feedback. Prog Clin Biol Res 1320:33–53.
36. Jacobson E. 1938. Progressive Relaxation. Chicago, University of Chicago Press.
37. Bernstein DA, Borkovec TD. 1973. Progressive Relaxation Training: A Manual for the Helping Professions. Champaign, IL, Research Press.
38. Bayuk L. 1985. Relaxation techniques: An adjunct therapy for cancer patients. Semin Oncol Nur 1:147–150.
39. Levenson BS. 1981. A multidimensional approach to the treatment of pain in the oncology patient. Front Radiat Ther Oncol 15:130–141.
40. Payne R, Foley KM. 1984. Advances in the management of cancer pain. Cancer Treat Rep 68:173–183.
41. Graffam S, Johnson A. 1987. A comparison of two relaxation strategies for the relief of pain and its distress. J Pain Sympt Manag 2:229–231.
42. Tan SY. 1982. Cognitive and cognitive-behavioral methods for pain control: A selective review. Pain 12:201–228.
43. Turk DC, Meichenbaum D, Genest, M. 1983. Pain and Behavioral Medicine: A Cognitive-Behavioral Perspective. New York, Guilford Press.
44. Fishman B, Loscalzo M. 1987. Cognitive-behavioral interventions in management of cancer pain: Principles and applications. Med Clin North Am 71:271–287.
45. Breitbart W. 1989. Psychiatric management of cancer pain. Cancer 63:2336–2342.
46. Moos R, Tsu VD. 1977. The crisis of physical illness: An overview. In R Moss (ed), Coping with Physical Illness. New York, Plenum.
47. Fordyce WE. 1976. Behavioral Methods for Chronic Pain and Illness. St. Louis, C.V. Mosb.
48. Redd WH. 1982. Treatment of excessive crying in a terminal cancer patient: A time-series analysis. Beh Med 5:225–236.
49. Carey MP, Burish TG. 1988. Etiology and treatment of the psychological side effects associated with cancer chemotherapy: A critical review and discussion. Psychol Bull 104:307–325.
50. Kahneman D. 1973. Attention and Effort. Englewood Cliffs, NJ, Prentice-Hall.
51. Schneider W, Schiffrin R. 1977. Controlled and automatic human information processing: I. Defection, search, and attention. Psychol Rev 84:1–66.
52. Dolce JJ, Raczynski JM. 1985. Neuromuscular activity and electromyography in painful backs: Psychological biomechanical models in assessment and treatment. Psychol Bull 97:502–520.

53. Linton SJ. 1982. A critical review of behavioral treatments for chronic benign pain other than headache. Br J Clin Psychol 21:321–337.
54. Dolgin MJ, Katz ER, McGinty K, Siegel SE. 1985. Anticipatory nausea and vomiting in pediatric cancer patients. Pediatrics 75:547–552.
55. Bush JP. 1987. Pain in children. A review of the literature from a developmental perspective. Psychol Health 1:215–236.
56. Chapman CR, Syrjala K, Sargur M. 1985. Pain as a manifestation of cancer treatment. Semin Oncol Nurs 1:100–108.
57. Portenoy RK, Foley KM. 1989. Management of cancer pain. In JC Holland JH Rowland (eds), Handbook of Psychooncology. New York, Oxford University Press, pp. 369–382.

18. LOW-LEVEL LASER BIOMODULATION FOR CHRONIC PAIN MANAGEMENT

HANS CHRISTIAN COLOV

The sun has always been associated with vitality. Many ancient cultures, such as the Egyptians and Greeks, worshipped the sun, and in Central America the Mayas, and later the Aztecs, even made an annual human sacrifice to appease the sun god. Heliotherapy, which is treatment based upon the use of sunlight, has been popular in the cure and palliation of many different diseases, such as rickets, skin disorders, and tuberculosis. At the end of the last century, the first artificial light source for therapeutic purposes, the ultraviolet lamp, was invented by the Nobel Prize winner, Niels Finsen. Several decades afterward, the interest in light therapy seemed to diminish, but with the invention of the laser, this modality has now begun a renaissance.

Laser (*light amplification by stimulated emission of radiation*) is a relatively new invention. The first laser was built by T.H. Maiman in 1960, but its subsequent development has been rapid. Lasers are now being used for many purposes including, technical, military, and medical applications.

The basis for the action of the lasers is the "stimulated emission" as described by Albert Einstein in 1917. According to this theory, an atom in its excited state can lose its extra energy by sending out electromagnetic waves (light). This transmission may be either a spontaneous (if there is no external influence) or a stimulated emission. In order for a stimulated emission to occur, the atom has to be influenced by an irradiation quantum with the exact frequency or energy of the emittable quantum. The emitted quantum gains, therefore, not only the same frequency, but also the same direction and phase as the quantum that stimulated the process. If within a limited space, there are many atoms excited to the same energy level, a single quantum will at first be able to simulate emission from one atom, and the two resulting quanta may then stimulate other atoms. A cascade of light quanta is thereby created. Collectively, these constitute a wave of monochromatic coherent light.

The presence of a number of excited atoms is not the sole determinant in the effective function of the laser. It is a general physical principle that if a process can run in one direction, it can also run in the opposite direction. If, for example, an excited atom releases its energy, this can be absorbed by another atom in its resting state. The process of amplifying the light signal by stimulated emission, therefore, involves having so many more atoms in the higher energy level than in the lower, that emission will be more dominant than absorption. This phenomenon produces a "population inversion," and is accomplished by constantly exciting new atoms. The process is called pumping, and it can be accomplished by electrical, chemical, or optical means.

In order to construct a laser beam, the emitted quanta must travel a certain distance in a laser-active substance. This can be achieved in two different ways. A laser may be constructed as a very long stick or tube, which may be several kilometers long. An easier way to achieve the same result is to place the laser-active substance between two parallel mirrors. In order to get the light out of the laser, one mirror is usually partly transparent. When a laser beam is constructed, the beam will self-destruct if the population inversion is destroyed. By constant pumping, however, new atoms will be excited and the process will be repeated periodically, resulting in a pulsed laser. The power in the pulses can be very high. In some lasers the population inversion is not destroyed but an equilibrium is established between atoms excited by pumping and atoms excited by stimulated emission. This gives a continuous wave laser (CW).

Different materials can be used as the laser-active medium. Maiman used a ruby crystal, for example, pumped by a powerful flash lamp. Numerous different liquids, solids, and gases have been used (even the fumes from Scotch whisky). It is the lasing medium that determines the wavelength and therefore the degree of tissue penetration.

A mixture of helium and neon gases was the first laser-active medium used for biomodulation. This laser gives a visible red light of 632 nm and is normally used for superficial treatments, such as wound healing. For deeper penetration, which is necessary in muscular and articular pain disorders, semiconductors such as gallium (Ga), aluminum (Al), and arsenide (As) are used. These are called diode lasers and were all, until 1988, emitting in the infrared spectrum. Currently, visible diode lasers are also manufactured.

The unit for power of the laser is, as for other light sources, the watt. The biomodulating lasers give average powers less than 100 milliwatts (mW.) Lasers are classified according to the degree of retinal damage they can impose as type 1, 2, 3a, 3b, and 4. Class 3b are the biomodulating lasers and class 4 are the strongest surgical lasers. Class indication 3b lasers are often called MID laser, soft laser, or biolaser. Although they all have the same therapeutic application, they have been introduced by different manufacturers, possibly to attract attention to their particular product.

Lasers do not differ from ordinary light with respect to their capacity to reflect from different surfaces. However, the absorption of the light is different, and this concept is the key to understanding the low-level laser action. In the tissues of the body, there are several compounds that absorb light at very specific wavelengths. These include melanin, bilirubin, hemoglobin, water, and beta-carotene. These compounds are called *chromophores*. Only lasers with wavelengths between 530 and 1000 nm can be used for biomodulation. The wavelengths that fall outside this range will be absorbed by some of these chromophores and will never reach their intended target, which may be a synovial membrane or a myofascial triggerpoint.

Laboratory investigations have shown that within this rather limited part of the electromagnetic spectrum, some wavelengths are more therapeutically effective than others. T. Karu, using cell culture studies, found that the synthesis of DNA and RNA was specifically stimulated at 400, 614, 680, 780, and 820 nm [1]. Lund et al. [2] demonstrated similar results after irradiation of the retina of rhesus monkeys. In their study, the total energy necessary to produce retinal damage at a specific wavelength was registered. The highest energy dose was found at 820 nm, but peaks at 660–680, 720, and 900 nm were also seen. These results make it possible to speculate that there are within our cells various compounds of indeterminate molecular structure (possibly chromophores) that may absorb light at specific wavelengths. Recently, it has been shown that enzymes such as NADH-dehydrogenase and cytochrome-c oxidase are activated by laser irradiation at the specific wavelengths and that these probably act as chromophores. These enzymes play an important role in the production of ATP in the mitochondria. Increased ATP production and associated morphological changes in this organelle have been shown after laser therapy [3,4]. This might be one of the explanations of the mechanisms of action by which a low-level laser can inactivate an ATP-depleted myofascial trigger point.

But why are some wavelengths laser active while others are not? The "particles" of light, the photons, all carry a specific amount of energy, which is calculated as the product of Planck's constant (6.62×10^{-34} J × sec) and the frequency characteristic for each wavelength. For example, light with a wavelength of 1200 nm and a frequency of 2.5×10^{14} Hz has a photonenergy of 1.655×10^{-19} J. Normally these very small energy amounts are given in electron volts (eV). For biomodulating lasers, the photonenergy or quantum energy is 1–2 eV, with highest values attained by the visible, shorter wavelengths.

The transfer of energy from the laser to the chromophore is accomplished by a collision between single photons and electrons. The electrons circling around the nucleus in various "energy shells" are hit and "pushed" or excited into a higher and more energy-holding shell. The photons then cease to exist. For the energy transfer to take place, the quantum energy of the incoming photon has to be exactly identical to the resonant energy of the electron, i.e., the difference in energy between the shell it is leaving and the one toward which it is excited. However, the excited state is very labile, and the electron quickly relapses to the original state, thereby releasing energy in the cell [5–7].

Recent studies [8] have indicated that, in addition to the wavelength, the repetition rates of the laser light are also important if the laser is being electrically pulsed. The division rate of E. coli has been increased or inhibited depending upon the pulsing frequency.

There are two main indications for low-level laser therapy: pain control and wound healing. The late Professor E. Mester of Hungary was the first to use low-level laser in the treatment of nonhealing ulcers. He and his colleagues have described the beneficial effect of the laser in a large series of patients [9]. Unfortunately, these early reports and many subsequent studies were not randomized and were improperly controlled. His work, however, has inspired several scientists, not only in Eastern Europe, but also in the West, to further investigate the therapeutic efficacy of the laser [10,11]. Both animal and human studies have subsequently been performed. Cell counts of embryonic foreskin and adult skin fibroblasts showed a significant increase in the number of cells in the laser-treated group compared to a nonirradiated control group [12]. Increased collagen production has also been shown [13]. Flap survival in rats increased significantly in laser-treated groups as compared to controls, and proliferation of new blood vessels has also been observed [14]. In the instance of bilateral full-thickness skin wounds made dorsally on New Zealand white rabbits, a significant increase in the tensile strength of the wounds was observed. It is interesting that the increase was seen not only in the treated side, but also on the nonirradiated lesion [15], implying that some release of tissue factors had taken place. In a double-blind placebo-controlled study, patients with reopened, infected abdominal wounds were treated with either an infrared (invisible) or a "placebo dummy laser diode." The time for 50% reduction of the wound area was registered. The laser group reached this reduction significantly faster (6.8 days) compared to the placebo group (14 days) [16].

Five years after the first reports on lasers for wound healing was published, the idea of using this new modality for pain management was introduced. As with the wound-healing reports, there have been a huge number of anecdotal reports and uncontrolled studies in this area. A beneficial effect has been claimed in both acute and chronic pain conditions, varying from acute inflammatory diseases — such as tendinitis, bursitis, and different kinds of muscular disorders — to more chronic conditions, such as rheumatoid arthritis. The literature is very controversial on this subject, some claiming good results while others seeing only a possible placebo effect.

Until recently, low-level laser utilization has been hampered by one major problem: the lack of standardization of the technical parameters. It is not sufficient to indicate the type and wavelength of the laser (He-Ne, Ga-As), the power, and perhaps the energy density (J/cm^2; 1 joule = 1 watt × 1 second). Two apparently identical study designs differ in parameters, such as emission mode (single or multiple mode), pulsing versus continuous wave, frequency modulation and power density (angle of divergence), or purity of the light source (spectral width). Since too little is known about the importance of each of these parameters with respect to the mode of action of the lasers, it is mandatory that these be indicated in all papers. It is interesting to note that there is one factor, namely, the coherence or the "definition" of laser, that seem to be of relatively little importance [11].

It is the author's opinion, however, that there is now sufficient support to conclude that low-level laser or noncoherent monochromatic intense light has an effect beyond placebo in a number of pain conditions. Sports injuries, for example, have been shown to improve faster with low-level laser treatment as compared to placebo [17,18]. However, other studies have failed to show this beneficial effect of low-level laser treatment [19–21]. Laser analgesia in experimentally induced ischemic pain was shown to be significantly greater compared to a control group [22]. Another study showed a significant rise in the pain threshold and the pain tolerance in the laser group compared to placebo in experimentally induced pain [23].

Thirty-six patients suffering from chronic pain (lasting more than 6 months) were divided into two groups receiving either low-level laser or a "placebo laser." The chronic pain syndromes treated were trigeminal neuralgia, postherpetic neuralgia, osteoarthritis, and sciatic pain. By use of a visual analog scale, it was concluded that the active laser group experienced significantly less pain than the placebo. Further, it was demonstrated that there was a statistically significant rise in the urinary excretions of 5-hydroxy-indole acetic acid (5-HIAA) in the patients who were treated with low-level laser compared to the patients treated with placebo laser [24]. In this study, only peripheral areas, as over the median, ulnar, radian, and saphenous nerves, were treated. 5-HIAA is a breakdown product from serotonin. These findings might indicate that a local reaction is involved and that a specific action is present in the nervous tissue, giving rise to an afferent impulse. It is well established that different biostimulation techniques (TENS, acupuncture) activating A-beta fibers can cause pain reduction, both through segmental (gate theory) [25] and central pain modulating systems, i.e., the serotonergic descending pathways [26].

In another study, the sciatic nerve in rats was exposed surgically, with the animals divided into different groups. In one group the sciatic nerve was crushed before it had received low-level laser treatment, and in another group the laser treatment was performed after crushing. In all groups, the electrical activity in the nerve was monitored throughout the whole study. In the group in which the laser treatment was given before crushing, there was a rise in the compound action potentials (AP) to 150% of the normal value. After the nerve crushing, there was an immediate decrease in the activity to 90%, but subsequently another rise and stabilization around 110%. In a third group, in which crushing resulted in a decrease to 40% of the precrush value, the following laser treatment gave a restoration AP value up to 70%. No such rise was seen in the control group. This study indicates that there might not only be a therapeutic action, but perhaps also a preventive action, of the laser in connection with surgery in which larger nerves are being traumatized [27]. Earlier published data in a similar study showed not only electrical recovery, but also morphological normalization in a group of animals in which the crushed sciatic nerves were laser treated as compared to the nonirradiated group [28].

Several studies have also been performed on the effect of low-level laser therapy on patients with rheumatoid arthritis. The rationale for this choice is probably due to the rather well-defined classification criteria and the existence of more objective parameters, such as swelling, grip strength, range of movement, and laboratory tests. The lack of such objective measures always constitutes a problem in interpreting the effect of different therapeutic modalities in pain conditions. With respect to the patients with rheumatoid arthritis, various beneficial effects have been shown. In a placebo-controlled double-blind study, a statistically significant reduction of the size of the finger joints, improved grip strength, and improved joint mobility were found in the laser-treated group compared to the placebo group. Furthermore, the morning stiffness and the pain measured on a VAS scale was reduced in the active group. It is surprising that a variety of immunological alterations have also been shown, for example, in c-reactive protein and in platelet aggregation. In the above-mentioned study, a significant falling trend was seen in the leukocyte count and in the sedimentation rate in the laser-treated group [29–31].

Human cultured lymphocytes were irradiated with low-level laser, and the proliferation of the cells assessed by radioactive labelling was monitored. A strong inhibition of the proliferation of the cells was seen in the treated group compared to a control group. Similarly, lymphocyte reaction to antigen stimulation as a functional response was reduced as a result of the laser treatment [32]. Bilateral tuberculin reactions were tested on sensitized guinea pigs. One group of animals received laser irradiation of low energy densities at one of the two injection sites. Both the irradiated side and also the contralateral nonirradiated side showed a suppression of the immune response. This may indicate that the laser has an inhibitory effect on delayed hypersensivity reactions [33].

In current research, the importance of free oxygen radicals in the inflammatory reaction is being strongly suggested. When phagocytes are activated, very reactive oxygen-derived free radicals are subsequently formed.

This is part of the normal defense mechanism, and cytokines, interleukin 1, and tumor necrosis factor, which are released from the phagocytes, do in fact enhance the production of these radicals. The oxygen radicals seem to play a very important etiologic role in chronic inflammatory conditions, such as arthritis, and in the development of ischemia, cancer, and radiation injuries. Being nonselective in their mode, the radicals can cause cell damage in the host, and therefore natural defense systems to counteract the production of the radicals must be activated. Enzymes, such as superoxide dismutase, catalase, and glutathione peroxidase, and compounds known as radical scavengers, such as vitamin C and E and betacarotene, belong to the complex of protective controlling systems [34]. The concentrations of superoxide dismutase and catalase are enhanced after low-level laser irradiation [11]. Unfortunately, these protective enzymes are not very resistant. The same radicals that they are supposed to neutralize can damage them [35]. Even acidification of the medium seen during ischemia and inflammation can deactivate the enzymes. In one study, incubation of bovine erythrocytes in an acid medium was found to show this deactivation, but following irradiation with low-level laser reactivated the enzymes [36].

The current literature suggests that the low-level laser acts through different functional systems, i.e., nervous tissue, connective tissue, and the immune system. Renewed studies will probably produce more knowledge about the biological importance of the diverse physical parameters of lasers.

Extensive testing and both experimental and clinical research remains to be done to determine if low-level laser therapy could become an acceptable and effective modality of chronic pain management.

REFERENCES

1. Karu TI. 1985. Biological action of low-intensity visible monochromatic light and some of its medical applications. Presented at International Congress on Laser in Medicine and Surgery, Bologna.
2. Lund D, Sliney D. Letterman Army Institute of Research, San Francisco. 1986. Absorbtions maxima between 500 and 950 nanometers. Personal communication.
3. Bolognani L, et al. 1985. Effects of GaAs pulsed laser on ATP concentration and ATPase activity in vitro and in vivo. Presented at International Congress on Laser in Medicine and Surgery, Bologna.
4. Passarella S. 1988. Recent discoveries on mitochondria bioenergetic mechanism after low power laser irradiation. Abstracts from the Second International Biotherapy Laser Association Congress on Laser Biomodulation, November.
5. Anderson RR, Parrish JA. 1982. Optical properties of human skin. In Regan, Parrish, et al. (eds), Science of Photomedicine. New York, Plenum.
6. Sliney D. Wolbasht M. 1982. Safety with Lasers and other Optical Sources. A Comprehensive Handbook.
7. Kubasova T, et al. 1984. Biological effect of He-Ne laser investigations of functional and micromorphological alterations of cell membranes in vitro. Laser in Surgery and Medicine, Vol. 4. New York, Alan R. Liss.
8. Karu T, Tiphlova O, Sanokhina M, Diamantopoulos C. 1989. Effects of near infrared laser and superluminous diode irradiation on E. coli division rate. The effects of different pulse repetition rates and pulse durations at 950 nanometers. Abstracts from the Third International Biotherapy Laser Association Congress On Laser Biomodulation, September.

9. Mester A, et al. 1985. Basic experiments and clinical praxis of laser biostimulation. Presented at International Congress on Laser in Medicine and Surgery, Bologna.

10. Trelles MA. 1981. The biostimulatory effect of the He-Ne laser beams for osseous regeneration. In W. Waidelich (ed), Optoelectronics in medicine. Proceedings of the 5th International Congress in Laser 81. 153–163, Springer-Verlag.

11. Karu TI. 1987. Photobiologial fundamentals of low-power laser therapy. IEEE J Quant Electron QE-23(10):1703–1716.

12. Boulton M. 1986. He-Ne laser stimulation of human fibro-blast proliferation and attachment in vitro. Lasers Life Sci 1(2):125–134.

13. Lam TS, Abergel RP, Meeker CA, Castel JC, Dwyer RM, Uitto J. 1986. Laser stimulation of collagen synthesis in human skin fibroblast cultures. Lasers Life Sci 1(1):61–77.

14. Kami T, Yoshimura Y, Nakajima T, Ohshiro T, Fujino T. 1985. Effects of low-power diode lasers on flap survival. Ann Plast Surg 14(3):278–283.

15. Braverman B, McCarthy RJ, Ivankovich AD, Forde DE, Overfield M, Bapna MS. 1989. Effect of helium-neon and infrared laser irradiation on wound healing in rabbits. Lasers Surg Med 9:50–58.

16. Palmgren N, Dahlin J, Beck H, Colov HC. 1988. Low energy laser treatment of infected abdominal wounds. Poster at the International Surgery Congress, Copenhagen, September.

17. Emmanouilidis O, Diamantopoulos C. 1986. CW I.R. low power laser application significantly accelerates chronic pain relief rehabilitation of professional athletes (abstr). A double blind study. Lasers Surg Med 6:173.

18. Minden D. 1989. A double blind crossover study on chronic achilles tendonitis with a 820 nanometers laser diode. Abstracts from the Third International Biotherapy Laser Association Congress On Laser Biomodulation, September.

19. Mcauley R, Ysla R. 1985. A treatment for osteoarthritis of the knee. Arch Phys Med Rehabil 66:553.

20. Basford JR, Sheffield CG, Mair SD, Ilstrup DM. 1987. Low energy helium neon laser treatment of thumb osteoarthritis. Arch Phys Med Rehabil 68:794.

21. Bliddal H, Hellesen C, Ditlevsen P et al. 1987. Soft-laser therapy of rheumatoid arthritis. Scand J Rheumatol 16:225.

22. Baxter GD, Bell AJ, Ravey R. 1989. A single blind cross-over study of laser analgesia in experimentally induced ischaemic pain. Abstracts from the Third International Biotherapy Laser Association Congress On Laser Biomodulation, September.

23. Martin D, Baxter GD, McCoy P, Ravey R. 1989. The effect of laser acupuncture on pain tolerance and pain thresholds in a single blind crossover study. Abstracts from the Third International Biotherapy Laser Association Congress On Laser Biomodulation, September.

24. Walker J. 1983. Relief from chronic pain by low power laser irradiation. Neurosci Lett 43:339–344.

25. Melzack R, Wall P. 1965. Pain mechanisms: A new theory. Science 150:971–978.

26. Han JS, Terenius L. 1982. Neurochemical basis of acupuncture analgesia. Ann Rev Pharmacol Taxicol 22:193–220.

27. Rochkind S, Nissan M, Lubart R, et al. 1988. The in-vivo-nerve response to direct low-energy-laser irradiation. Acta Neurochir 94:74–77.

28. Rochkind S, Barrnea L, Razon N, et al. 1987. Stimulatory effect of the He-Ne low dose laser on injured sciatic nerves of rats. Neurosurgery 20:843–847.

29. Goldman JA, Chiapell J, Casey H et al. 1980. Laser therapy in rheumatoid arthritis. Lasers Surg Med 1:93.

30. Walker J, Akhanjee LK, Cooney MM, et al. 1987. Laser therapy for pain of rheumatoid arthritis. Clin J Pain 3:54–59.

31. Palmgren N, Jensen GF, Kaae K, Windelin M, Colov HC. 1989. Low power laser therapy in rheumatoid arthritis. Lasers Med Sci 4(3), in press.

32. Ohta A, Abergel R, Uitto J. 1987. Laser modulation of human immune system Inhibition of lymphocyte proliferation by a gallium-arsenide laser at low energy. Lasers Surg Med 7:199–201.

33. Inoue K, Nishioka J, Hukuda S. 1989. Suppressed tuberculin reaction in guinea pigs following laser irradiation. Lasers Surg Med 9:271–275.

34. Ward P, Warren J, Johnson K. 1988. Oxygen radicals, inflammation, and tissue injury. Free Rad Biol Med 5:403–408.

35. Yoshikawa T, Tanaka H, Kondo M. 1984. The increase of lipid peroxidation in rat adjuvant arthritis and its inhibition by superoxide dismutase. Biochem Med 33:320–326.
36. Vladimirov Y, Gorbatenkova E, Paramonov N, et al. 1988. Photoreactivation of superoxide dismutase by intensive red laser light. Free Rad Biol Med 5:281–286.

19. NEUROSURGICAL APPROACHES TO CHRONIC PAIN MANAGEMENT

BENNETT BLUMENKOPF

For probably more than any other reason, people seek medical attention because of some painful affliction. Whether it be headache from a brain tumor, angina from coronary artery disease, or right upper quadrant abdominal pain from cholecystitis, a common denominator throughout is pain. This experience of pain generally subserves a "protective usefulness" to the organism. However, at times, this usefulness is lost and pain then becomes a debilitating effect.

Neurosurgeons are intimately involved with the management of painful disorders. Their involvement may attempt to resolve the underlying mechanism of the pain, for example, through discectomy, as in the case of a radicular syndrome due to a ruptured lumbar disc. Additionally, the neurosurgical approach may seek palliation of the pain, as in hypophysectomy for the diffuse bone pain associated with metastatic cancer. The following discussion reviews some aspects of pain management from a neurosurgical standpoint. First, a review of the basic anatomy and physiology involved in pain transmission is presented. Second, with this basic understanding, a number of the neurosurgical procedures performed to alleviate pain are presented. Finally, an interesting subclass of pain — deafferentation pain — will be discussed. This type of pain is less understood scientifically and is certainly more difficult to manage clinically. A new neurosurgical approach to this problem will also be presented.

297

NEUROANATOMY AND NEUROPHYSIOLOGY OF PAIN

A basic appreciation of the anatomy and physiology of pain transmission is required to understand not only the many causes of pain, but also the available procedures employed to alleviate the pain [1–3]. The nervous system involves the peripheral nerves, which convey the important sensory information about the organism to the central centers, i.e., the spinal cord, brain stem, and the brain itself. Additionally, the skin, mucous membranes, and periosteum may be considered the most peripheral expanse of the nervous system, for these structures contain the sensory receptors. These receptors, of which there are probably billions, are quite varied. Some receptors are very specific for a single modality, while others are polymodal.

With respect to considering the perception of pain, free nerve endings in the integument, viscera, and periosteum are generally believed to represent the receptor. The impulses generated by these free nerve endings thus serve to inform the organism of potentially noxious, damaging influences. These impulses are then conveyed to the central centers by the peripheral nerves. Among the various subtypes of peripheral nerve fibers, two appear to be especially concerned with nociceptive transmission — the nonmyelinated C-fibers and the thinly myelinated A-delta fibers. These two types of nociceptive afferents seem to subserve different types of pain experience. The A-delta fibers are faster conducting and reflect a sharp, localized pain. The unmyelinated C-fibers, being slower conducting fibers, convey a poorly localized dull, burning, or aching sensation.

The cell bodies or neurons of all the nociceptive afferent fibers are located within the dorsal root ganglia of each spinal root or the Gasserian ganglia of the trigeminal roots. Two subpopulations of neurons, one large and one small, are related to each fiber type, the A-delta and C-fibers, respectively. These neurons are bipolar, with their central connections in the spinal cord or brain stem. The spinal cord is topographically divided into the dorsal and ventral horns, and furthermore, into laminae (of Rexed) related to the cell types present. The central fibers of the primary nociceptive afferents — the A-delta and C-fibers — terminate in the superficial regions of the dorsal aspect of the spinal cord, specifically laminae I, II, III. In this region — the dorsal root entry zone (DREZ) — the first integration of pain information occurs.

The neurons in laminae I and II, along with other cells more deeply situated in laminae IV and V, project their fibers — the secondary nociceptive afferents — to the thalamus. These fibers constitute the spinothalamic tract. The spinothalamic tract decussates within a segment or two of its segmental level and traverses the anterolateral column of the spinal cord. An additional pathway of secondary afferents projects to the brain stem reticular formation. Both the direct spinothalamic tract and the indirect spinoreticulothalamic tract terminate mainly in the ventrobasal complex of the thalamus. From the thalamus, tertiary projections go to the cerebral cortex, specifically the primary and secondary somatosensory areas. The actual role of the thalamus and cortex in pain is more complex and certainly is not very clear.

Additional neural systems exist and they may play a part in pain modulation. In the peripheral nerves, the large myelinated A-alpha and A-beta fibers have an inhibitory effect on the spinothalamic neurons. This effect is probably mediated by inhibitory interneurons locally at each level of the dorsal horn laminae II and III. Also, the dorsal column nuclei and other brain stem locations project caudally to lamina I or IV, and V. With direct stimulation, these nuclei inhibit the activity in the nociceptive thalamic projecting cells.

A discussion of the neurochemistry of the DREZ must, therefore, include at least three interacting neural systems: 1) the descending projections of the supraspinal (primarily bulbospinal) pathways that terminate in the dorsal horn region, 2) the segmental interneuronal circuits operating solely within the dorsal horn region, and 3) the primary sensory afferents to the dorsal horn whose cell bodies reside in the dorsal root ganglia [4]. A vast variety of compounds appear to be involved in the processing of nociceptive information at the DREZ level. Among these are the "classical neurotransmitters," such as the excitatory and inhibitory amino acids and the catecholamines. In addition, the recent discovery of a number of previously described gastrointestinal tract peptides in the central nervous system has significantly advanced the understanding of neural transmission, especially of pain signals. When considering the latter, the concept of a neuromodulator has been advanced — a compound that modifies the responses of neurons to other transmitters and, thereby, modulates synaptic transmission. Neuropeptides have been identified in those small ganglia cells mentioned above, in the axons of the dorsal roots, and in axon terminals in the superficial dorsal horn laminae, especially I and II. These neuropeptides include substance P, somatostatin, cholecystokinin (CCK-8), calcitonin gene-related product (CGRP), vasoactive intestinal polypeptide (VIP), neurotensin, and the endogenous opiates or endorphins. Substance P, somatostatin, CCK-8, CGRP, and VIP are important products of the primary sensory neurons. The endorphins reduce the responsiveness of dorsal horn neurons to noxious stimulation both through interneurons at a segmental level and through a descending inhibitory system. Intracisternal neurotensin produces a potent antinociceptive response that is naloxone insensitive.

NEUROSURGICAL PAIN PROCEDURES (TABLE 19-1)

Peripheral procedures

Based upon this knowledge of the anatomy and physiology of neural tissues involved in pain, a variety of neurosurgical procedures can attempt to alleviate pain (Figure 19-1). The role of the peripheral nerve in carrying the pain fibers from the periphery can be addressed in this respect. One may suppose that cutting a nerve — *peripheral neurectomy* — would abolish future pain impulses conveyed from the periphery and, thereby, abolish pain. However, a number of problems with this approach limit its applicability. There is a significant overlap (both dermatomal and sclerotomal) in the distribution of innervation among the peripheral nerves. Thus, rarely is a pain limited to the zone of a

Table 19-1. Neurosurgical pain procedures

PERIPHERAL
Peripheral neurectomy [2,3]
Rhizotomy [7,8,9]
Selective posterior rhizotomy [10]
Ganglionectomy [11]

CENTRAL — SPINAL CORD
Cordotomy [12]
Midline myelotomy [13]
Spinal stimulator [14]
Intrathecal narcotic analgesia [15,16]
Dorsal root entry zone (DREZ) lesion [23,24]

CENTRAL — BRAIN
Mesencephalotomy [17]
Brain stimulator [18,19]
Hypophysectomy [20]

single peripheral nerve. Furthermore, most peripheral nerves are mixed motor and sensory. A peripheral neurectomy procedure could, therefore, incur an unacceptable neurological deficit. Finally, the development of a deafferentation pain (as discussed below) is a major complication of peripheral nerve section. Accordingly, this procedure is rarely done for pain. A possible exception would be neurectomy performed for pain following injury to the superficial radial nerve. [5,6]. In contrast, compression of peripheral nerves is often painful, and a variety of decompression procedures are routinely done, including carpal tunnel release and ulnar nerve transposition. Stimulation of the peripheral nerve has also been utilized in the management of chronic pain, particularly that following nerve injury. This approach attempts to stimulate selectively the large myelinated fibers that inhibit the nociceptive pathway at

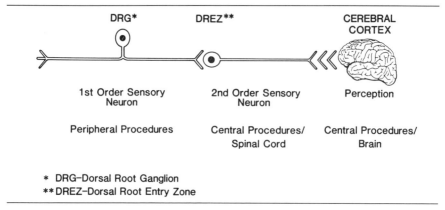

Figure 19-1. Schematic representation of the anatomy of pain transmission, and the loci of the variety of neurosurgical procedures performed to alleviate pain.

the level of the dorsal horn. This may be performed with either a transcutaneous or implanted stimulation device.

The next most proximal approach involves sectioning the sensory fibers that make up the peripheral nerves. This procedure — *rhizotomy* — may be performed extradurally or intradurally [7–9]. In the former, the entire dorsal root is sectioned, while in the latter the multiple rootlets that make up the dorsal root are cut. *Selective posterior rhizotomy* has also been described; this procedure limits the involvement to the ventrolateral aspect of the rootlet, where the small fibers (small-myelinated and unmyelinated) are organized [10]. In these procedures, a segmental region of analgesia is usually created, corresponding to the dermatomal levels included. Rhizotomy has proven useful in the management of pain due to malignant involvement of the brachial plexus (Pancoast syndrome), the chest wall, and occasionally the pelvis; its usefulness is limited in benign processes due to the frequent development of a deafferentation syndrome — postrhizotomy dysesthesia. The nerve roots are also sensitive to compression, such as occurs with intervertebral disc herniation or foraminal stenosis. Here again, decompression of the root through discectomy or foraminotomy may result in pain relief.

Excision of the sensory ganglia — *ganglionectomy* — has also been proposed for segmentally restricted pain [11]. This procedure removes the dorsal root ganglia at multiple levels. There is a suggestion that this procedure is an advantage over sensory rhizotomy, because a percentage (up to 20%) of the nociceptive afferents traverse the *ventral* root.

Central procedures — Spinal cord

A number of procedures are performed on the spinal cord itself in an attempt to palliate pain; both ablation and stimulation have been done. Included among these are procedures designed to destroy the spinothalamic tract — *cordotomy* [12]. An anterolateral cordotomy may be accomplished either through a formal hemilaminectomy with sectioning of the ventral spinothalamic tract, or more recently, through a percutaneous approach using a radiofrequency electrode. This results in contralateral analgesia below the level of the procedure. An anterolateral cordotomy is remarkably effective in the situation of malignant pain that is predominately one sided, e.g., a metastasis in the femur. Unfortunately, bilateral cordotomies are generally not performed due to respiratory complications. Furthermore, the deafferentation syndrome — postcordotomy dysesthesia — severely limits its usefulness in benign pain syndromes.

A procedure that simultaneously divides the decussating nociceptive fibers from both sides of the body at the level of the anterior commissure — *midline commissurotomy* or *myelotomy* — has been utilized in cases of midline perineal, pelvic, and rectal pain of malignant etiologies [13]. Through a single cord incision, bilateral effects are thereby produced, providing the site of the pain is limited. This procedure does, however, have a significant morbidity risk and is not generally popular.

Stimulation of the spinal cord, particularly the dorsal columns — *dorsal column stimulator (DCS)* or *spinal cord stimulator (SCS)* — has been applied to cases of chronic benign pain, particularly the failed back syndrome following a ruptured intervertebral disc [14]. The stimulation current presumably activates the bulbospinal inhibitory pathways to provide pain relief. Paresthesiae are perceived with the stimulation; these paresthesiae should be perceived throughout the distribution of the pain.

Finally, an approach to pain relief at the spinal level that takes advantage of the basic neurochemistry of pain — *intrathecal narcotic analgesia (ITNA)* — has gained popularity [15,16]. Small doses of morphine, when instilled directly into the cerebrospinal fluid or into the epidural space, provide profound and prolonged analgesia in a number of circumstances. ITNA has been employed mostly for cases of metastatic malignancy, but more recently in cases of benign pain. A variety of pump devices have been designed for chronic therapy. Tolerance to the opiate remains a problem and a long-term concern. Other potential complications of ITNA include unpredictable respiratory depression, nausea, vomiting, pruritis, and urinary retention.

Central procedures — Brain

As is the case at the spinal cord level, both stimulation and ablation procedures for pain have been described. Regions in the mesencephalon and diencephalon may be approached surgically using stereotaxic techniques. *Stereotaxic mesencephalotomy* is indicated for cephalo-brachial pain due to carcinoma and thalamic syndrome pain [17]. It is interesting that not only the pain itself, but also the suffering component of the pain experience, is relieved by this procedure. Stimulation of areas in the midbrain and thalamus — *deep brain stimulation (DBS)* — has been utilized in cases of chronic benign pain and malignant pain [18,19]. The analgesia following midbrain stimulation appears to be opiate mediated, while that following thalamic stimulation is not. Currently, DBS is investigational and performed in only a limited number of neurosurgical centers for specific indications.

A central procedure that is particularly effective in palliating the pain of metastatic (especially osseous metastases) cancer is *hypophysectomy* [20]. The pituitary gland may be surgically excised by the trans-sphenoidal route, or chemically ablated using absolute ethanol injections (Figure 19-2). In cases of hormonally responsive malignancies, such as breast or prostate, a remarkable, long-lasting pain relief is often achieved. The mechanisms responsible for this effect of hypophysectomy are not understood.

DEAFFERENTATION PAIN

A pain problem conceptually different from most pain, and probably less familiar to most physicians, is *deafferentation pain* [21]. In fact, deafferentation

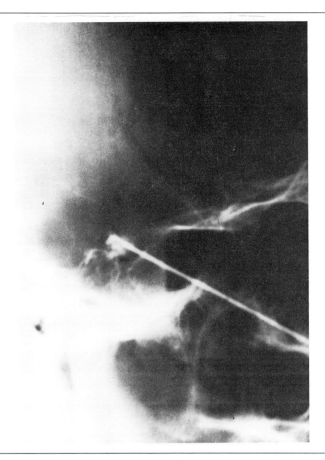

Figure 19-2. Lateral skull radiograph showing placement of a spinal needle within the sella tur-cica for the injection of absolute alcohol — chemical hypophysectomy for pain.

pain is quite common in clinical medicine and is very difficult to manage effectively. Deafferentation pain, or central pain as some refer to it, involves the perception of painful sensations, such as burning, tearing, throbbing, etc., in a region of the body that is partially or totally sensorially deprived. Thus, all or some of the peripheral nociceptors are physically disconnected from the central centers. Among the deafferentation pain syndromes are amputation phantom pain, root avulsion pain, peripheral nerve injury pain, quadriplegic and paraplegic pain, and postherpetic neuralgia. The prevalence of deafferentation pain in these conditions is surprisingly high, and each of these situation is quite common. Fifty to 90% of amputees, 80–90% of brachial plexus avulsions, and 10–20% of paraplegics suffer some sort of deafferentation pain.

In cases of deafferentation pain, the pain does not result from an ongoing, peripheral noxious stimulus. Rather, this phenomenon results from changes at the central nervous system level. The mechanisms to explain this unusual phenomenon involve again anatomy and physiology. The nervous system and the pain pathways, in particular, are arranged as a circuitry with positive or excitatory and negative or inhitory influences. These actions are mediated by the neurotransmitters or neuromodulators, e.g., substance P, somatostatin, and the endorphins. Each transmitter acts upon its particular receptor to create its influence. An analogous situation exists for hormonal actions on their target tissues.

Recent discoveries on the receptors in the nervous system have revealed a finding that may explain the phenomenon of deafferentation pain. This finding suggests that when the influence upon a receptor is removed (i.e., the loss of transmitter substance due to the sensory disconnection), the neuron attempts to compensate by increasing its number of receptor sites to ensure a response to even the most trivial amount of transmitter substance present. Thus, a situation of supersensitivity or hypersensitivity develops. An example relates to the ineffectiveness of cutting nerve roots to relieve pain. By so doing, the primary afferent fibers are lost and, consequently, the afferent excitatory transmitters diminish. Those cells in the dorsal horn laminae responsive to these substances increase their receptor sites and become hypersensitive [22]. These central neurons become hyperirritable, as demonstrated by single-cell recordings in the dorsal horn of the spinal cord following dorsal root section. This hyperirritability would then be transmitted throughout the nervous system circuitry to higher brain regions. Clinically this may present as deafferentation pain. The same may hold true if an attempt at cutting a central pathway is done, e.g., the cordotomy. Hypersensitivity in the brain stem or thalamus may create a deafferentation pain. Interestingly, the onset of deafferentation pain may be delayed, thus the usefulness of rhizotomy or cordotomy for the malignant pain situation in a patient with limited life expectancy — generally less than 1 year.

The pain syndromes that develop after brachial plexus avulsion, amputation, quadriplegia, and paraplegia, etc. may involve similar mechanisms. These forms of pain are often quite disabling. Previous treatments for these syndromes have included rhizotomy, cordotomy, dorsal column stimulation, and stereotactic mesencephalotomy, all of which were generally unsuccessful. Recently, a new procedure has been developed to attempt to deal with these pains. Based upon the hypothesis that the pain is due to hypersensitivity of neurons in the dorsal horn laminae, an attempt is made to diminish or silence the hyperirritability, and thereby, to relieve the pain. The procedure — *dorsal root entry zone (DREZ) lesion* [23,24] — involves the placement, under microscopic guidance, of a very small needle electrode into the spinal-cord dorsal horn. Then, using a radiofrequency lesion generator, serially placed lesions are created, with the destruction of those hyperactive, hyperirritable neurons.

The DREZ procedure was initially performed in a group of patients with

Table 19-2. Dorsal root
entry zone (DREZ) procedure

Brachial plexus avulsion pain
Paraplegic/quadriplegic pain
Amputation phantom pain
Postherpetic neuralgia

---

brachial plexus avulsion pain [24]. Long-term relief (5 years) has now been described in 66% of those cases [23]. Additional groups who have undergone the procedure now include paraplegic/quadriplegic pain, with 55% obtaining pain relief; amputation phantom pain, with 62% pain relief; and postherpetic neuralgia, with 57% relief. These indications are listed in Table 19-2. In addition, a *trigeminal nucleus caudalis DREZ* procedure has been developed for patients with pain after herpes zoster ophthalmicus and carcinoma of the orbit. These results are only preliminary [23].

One question may be, why does the DREZ operation not create a deafferentation situation more distally in the circuitry? Perhaps this is due to limiting the damage to nerve cells and not fiber tracts. However, deafferentation is a concern and continued follow-up is required. For the moment, an encouraging new procedure exists for these difficult pain problems.

REFERENCES

1. Albe-Fessard D, Berkley KJ, Kruger L, Ralston HJ III, Willis WD Jr. 1985. Diencephalic mechanisms of pain sensation. Brain Res Rev 9:217–296.
2. Basbaum AI, Fields HL. 1984. Endogenous pain control systems: Brainstem spinal pathways and endorphin circuitry. Ann Rev Neurosci 7:309–338.
3. Fields HL, Heinricher MM. 1985. Anatomy and physiology of a nociceptive modulatory system. Phil Trans R Soc Lond B308:361–374.
4. Blumenkopf B. 1988. Neurochemistry of the dorsal horn. Appl Neurophysiol 51:89–103.
5. Dellon AL, Mackinnon SE. 1984. Susceptibility of the superficial sensory branch of the radial nerve to form painful neuromas. J Hand Surg 9B:42–45.
6. Dellon AL, Mackinnon SE. 1986. Treatment of the painful neuroma by neuroma resection and muscle implantation. Plast Reconstr Surg 77:427–435.
7. Esposito S, Bruni P, Delitala A, Canova A, Hernandez R, Callovini GM. 1985. Therapeutic approach to the Pancoast pain syndrome. Appl Neurophysiol 48:262–266.
8. Loeser JD. 1972. Dorsal rhizotomy for the relief of chronic pain. J Neurosurg 36:745–750.
9. Onofrio BM, Campa HK. 1972. Evaluation of rhizotomy. J Neurosurg 36:751–755.
10. Sindou M, Goutelle A. 1983. Surgical posterior rhizotomies for the treatment of pain. In H Krayenbuhl (ed), Advances and Technical Standards in Neurosurgery, Vol. 10. Wien, Springer-Verlag, pp. 147–185.
11. Smith FP. 1970. Trans-spinal ganglionectomy for relief of intercostal pain. J Neurosurg 32:574–577.
12. Spiller WG, Martin E. 1912. The treatment of persistent pain of organic origin in the lower part of the body by division of the anterolateral column of the spinal cord. JAMA 58:1489–1490.
13. Sindou M, Daher A. 1988. Spinal cord ablation procedures for pain. In R Dubner, GF Gebhart, MR Bond (eds), Proceedings of the Vth World Congress on Pain. Amsterdam, Elsevier Science, pp. 477–495.
14. De La Porte C, Siegfried J. 1983. Lumbosacral spinal fibrosis (spinal arachnoiditis). Its diagnosis and treatment by spinal cord stimulation. Spine 8:593–603.

15. Auld AW, Maki-Jokela A, Murdoch DM. 1985. Intraspinal narcotic analgesia in the treatment of chronic pain. Spine 10:777–781.
16. Penn RD, Paice JA, Gottschalk W, Ivankovich AD. 1984. Cancer pain relief using chronic morphine infusion. J Neurosurg 61:302–306.
17. Nashold BS Jr. 1982. Brainstem stereotaxic procedures. In G Schaltenbrand, AE Walker (eds), Stereotaxy of the Human Brain. New York, George Thieme Verlag, pp. 475–483.
18. Adams JE, Hosobuchi Y, Fields HL. 1974. Stimulation of internal capsule for relief of chronic pain. J Neurosurg 41:740–744.
19. Hosobuchi Y. 1986. Subcortical electrical stimulation for control of intractable pain in humans. J Neurosurg 64:543–553.
20. Levin AB, Katz J, Benson RC, Jones AG. 1980. Treatment of pain of diffuse metastatic cancer by stereotactic chemical hypophysectomy: Long term results and observations on mechanism of action. Neurosurgery 6:258–262.
21. Nashold BS Jr. 1988. Deafferentation pain in man and animals as it relates to the DREZ operation. Can J Neurosci 15:5–9.
22. Ovelmen-Levitt J, Johnson B, Bedenbaugh P, Nashold BS Jr. 1984. Dorsal root rhizotomy and avulsion in the cat: A comparison of long term effects on dorsal horn neuronal activity. Neurosurgery 15:921–927.
23. Nashold BS Jr. Higgins AC, Blumenkopf B. 1985. Dorsal root entry zone lesions for pain relief. In RH Wilkins, SS Rengachary (eds), Neurosurgery. New York, McGraw-Hill, pp. 2433–2437.
24. Nashold BS Jr. Ostdahl RH. 1979. Dorsal root entry zone lesions for pain relief. J Neurosurg 51:59–69.

INDEX